T. T. Liang's Tai Chi Ch'uan

The Tai Chi Solo Form with Rhythm

Jonathan Russell

with photographs of T.T. Liang

Ride Books

Berkeley, CA

Published by RIDE Books

ISBN: 978-0-9828471-0-7

Library of Congress Control Number: 2015948062

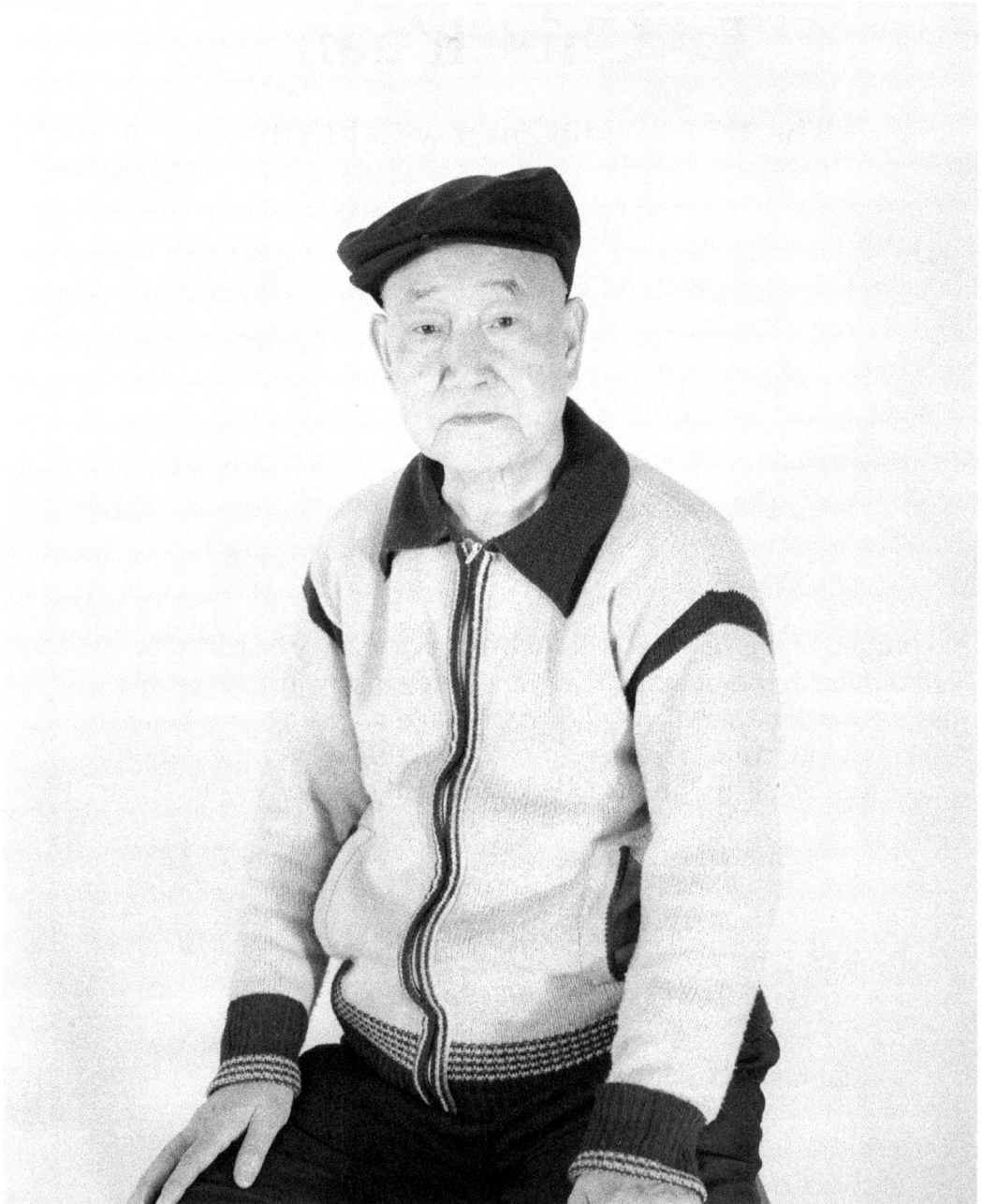

Liang Tung Tsai, 1900 – 2002

Acknowledgements

First and foremost I want to express my gratitude for having had the benefit of T.T. Liang's patience and kind understanding and, in the end, his confidence and trust that someday this book would be written and published. I think I speak for all of his students in expressing my thanks to him for providing such a fertile ground from which to grow and learn the art of Tai Chi Ch'uan.

To my wife Saori. It was through her critiques and persistent questioning that what started out as a three-page article eventually became the entire manuscript for this book.

To my students for their encouragement and support. They are the ones who forced me to develop a vocabulary to express the ideas in this book.

To Jael and Vicki Weisman, for their tireless examination and questioning of the Tai Chi movements and principles. All of us have had to stay sharp to keep up with them.

And last, to my friends in the publishing business whose attentionto detail, in both expression and presentation, has been an inspiration for me.

Table of Contents

Dedication

For my two sons, keep up the good work guys!

"I have opened the door. It's up to you to go in and steal my art"

T. T. Liang

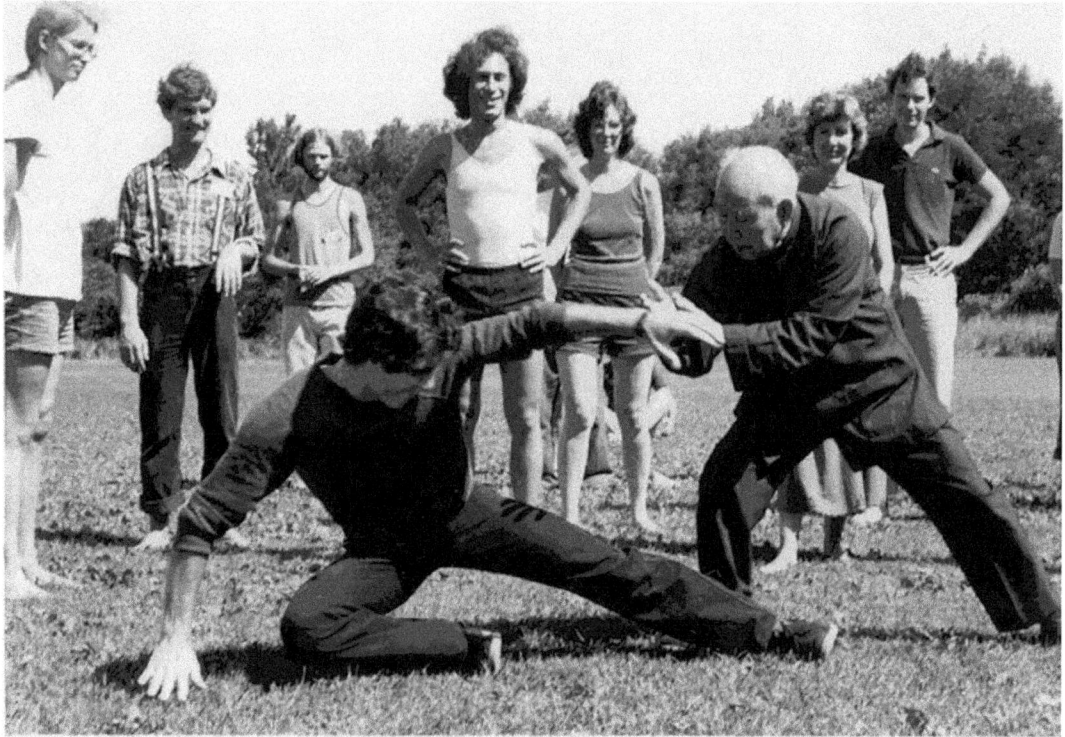

Liang demonstrating the posture *Press* on the Author, 1980

"Tai Chi Ch'uan is an ancient form of calisthenics created by a Taoist priest named Chan San Feng about 700 years ago. Tai Chi means "round form" as pictured in the Yin Yang symbol (Tai Chi Shu) so when you practice you must simulate that form, everything a round shape. You must practice it slowly, effortlessly and continuously, then it will be good for your health. Tai Chi is first for Health, second for Self-defense, third for mental accomplishment and last to become an Immortal."   *T.T. Liang*

Preface

When I first started studying Tai Chi with T. T. Liang over 45 years ago, a great deal of our time together was spent reviewing the manuscript he was working on with his editor (and student) Paul Gallagher. The result being his now classic book, Tai Chi for Health and Self-Defense.* This book was the first English-language translation and explanation of the ancient Chinese texts on Tai Chi commonly referred to as "the Tai Chi Classics." It also included Mr. Liang's personal anecdotes and interpretations of the theory and practice of Tai Chi. The book is still in print and I recommend it to any serious student. For me, working with him on these papers was a great way to be introduced to Tai Chi. They are a treasure trove of information regarding the foundations of how to understand this exercise.

One thing troubled me though: he barely mentioned anything about his use of rhythm as an integral part of his classes. Not

published in 1977 by Vintage, a division of Random House - revised edition April 6, 2011

included in his book were any details of how to perform the postures of his Yang style form or, more importantly to me, any description of his unique use of beats in the practice of Tai Chi. Why was this, especially when this was at the core of how he taught? I asked Liang and his reply was that he wanted his book to address the underlying principles of Tai Chi so that it would be accessible to students of all the different styles and teachers, not just his own. He went onto say "but as far as my own style of teaching is concerned, I leave that for you to do."

Liang had many students before, during and after my time with him who are now spread around the world. Many have gone onto become accomplished practitioners. While some like to label their relationship with him in some kind of hierarchical order, all of our associations with Liang were unique. I had the good fortune to set up and run with him the Tai Chi Dance Association in Boston, Massachusetts, where we taught together in the '70s and '80s. I taught the beginner students and he taught the advanced. It was during these years that he and I started to work on this book; I would photograph him performing all the postures as well as review with him the techniques and underlying principles related to them. To write this book I have drawn upon my notes from our endless conversations as well as the interviews I recorded with him over our 15 years together.

T.T. Liang's Yang Style Tai Chi Ch'uan is intended to serve as a companion book to Mr. Liang's classic. My intention is to provide an introduction to the art, including an overview of Liang's methodology and goals. This will be particularly useful to potential students who wish to have some understanding of Tai Chi before they begin to take classes. Reading it will provide a good foundation and referring to it periodically will, I hope, help students avoid mistakes. But no one can learn Tai Chi from books alone. Indeed, and I emphasize this, without a teacher, aspects of this practice can be detrimental. Liang often said to me regarding the advanced techniques that they can be dangerous and should not be attempted without proper supervision.

I will detail how each posture is performed as well as give an overview of how he used rhythm to facilitate the training and understanding of the fundamental principles he describes in his book – both physical and mental. My aim is to make clear what Liang was doing while practicing Tai Chi with music and to fulfill a long overdue obligation.

Without using obscure Chinese terminology I have attempted to explain the intricacies of Liang's Tai Chi and create a practical, hands-on approach to day-to-day learning – one that shows how the theories and principles of his use of rhythm can be used and applied. The chapters that follow are T.T. Liang's Tai Chi as seen, experienced and understood by me, and I take full responsibility for any mistakes, misrepresentations or omissions.

Since Liang introduced his use of rhythm in practicing Tai Chi in the late '60s, it has met with mixed reactions from the international community of Tai Chi practitioners. Some have embraced it as a useful tool while others find it too difficult to learn. There are still others who feel it is offensive to the traditions of Tai Chi. When I asked Liang about the latter reaction, his reply was, "This is common when anything new is introduced … but, no matter, for some it will always be like playing the violin before a cow." Whatever the case, Liang's use of rhythm as a teaching tool is his unique contribution to the legacy of Tai Chi Ch'uan.

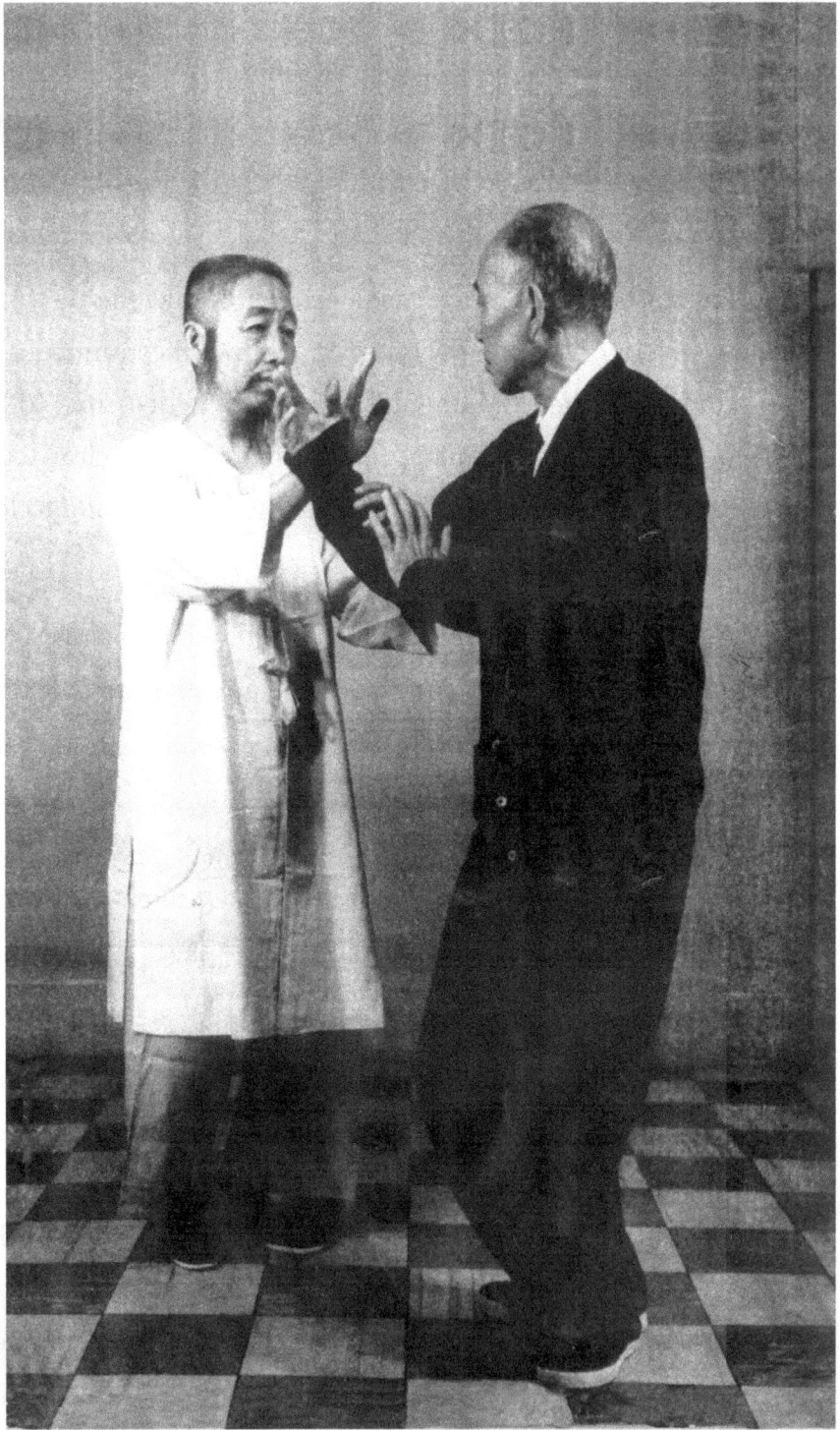

Cheng Man Ching and T. T. Liang demonstrating Pushing Hands, 1972

1 A Little History

Liang Tung Tsai, or T.T. Liang as he was known, lived in the United States for the latter part of his life. He was 70 years old when I first met him living in Boston in 1969. He had perfected his Tai Chi skills under the tutelage of Cheng Man Ching in Taiwan, and while there he developed the use of music and rhythm for the purpose of learning and practicing the Tai Chi forms. He felt that music most efficiently helps the student learn the mechanics of the Tai Chi postures and effectively joins the mind and body in movement.

Liang's Tai Chi can best be understood in the context of an art of refining one's nature; something he embraced fully. He was fond of saying, "to move a mountain is easy, but to change a man's nature … now that is really difficult." He must have had some personal success in the latter: I recall many visitors to our studio who knew him from his past years in China who would comment that his current gentle and humorous nature was not at all the same as the hot-tempered man they once knew.

When I asked Liang how Tai Chi had affected him personally he answered,

"Of course, Tai Chi has affected me personally a great deal. When I was young I did a lot of notorious things. My temper was very, very hot and I gave my parents a lot of trouble. I was always ready to fight with the other boys and did a lot of bad things as I grew up. Later I joined the Maritime Customs Service where I received a good salary and life became a little easier. I was able to help provide for my parents and siblings. But I still didn't know how to curry favor with my boss and as a result my boss sometimes blamed me saying, 'you should not do this … you should not do that'. So I still got into trouble. Two times at least I was 'dis-rated' (this means your pay is not increased). I still don't care at that time. I served in customs 20 years and afterward retired. In the beginning I had to work hard, then gradually after 12 years I was promoted from Tide-waiter to the highest rank, called Chief Tide-Surveyor." [He became

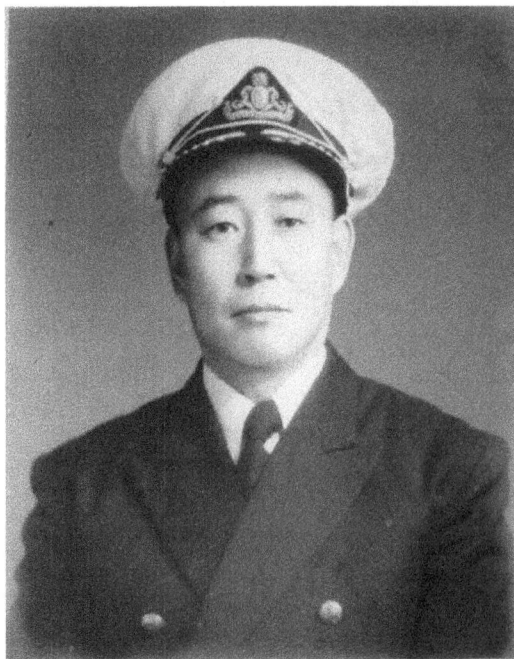

the senior customs officer overseeing boarding of ships to check goods in the port and outlying waters of Shanghai.] "At this time I had many body guards, subordinates and junior officers. I deemed myself to be just like a commander or an Admiral. As soon as I gave orders everyone has to obey. This made me feel very proud and I thought of myself as the top authority. I didn't depend on anybody else. I had many bad habits though and I dissipated too much (gambling, alcohol, and women) and became very ill. At 45 years old I went into the hospital for 60 days. Before this I had learned Kung Fu, Shaolin, Baseball, Basketball, football (soccer), all the 'hard' styles of exercise. Now I was so weak I could do none of them. The only thing I could do was Tai Chi."*

Due to his illness Liang was transferred to Taiwan in 1948. It was here that he sought out the Tai Chi teacher Cheng Man Ching. Cheng, who was also skilled in Chinese medicine, informed Liang that although he would take him on as a student, he was really too sick to learn and there was little prospect of recovery. It was from this point on that Liang took up the study of Tai Chi in earnest. According to him it took ten years to regain his health fully. He attributed his recovery and subsequent robust health to his consistent practice of Tai Chi. Liang died in 2002 at the age of 103 years old.

The teacher he regarded as the most influential in his understanding of Tai Chi was Cheng Man Ching. Liang eventually came to be his "chief disciple," though in later years, as Liang's skill improved and he sought out other teachers, this relationship soured.

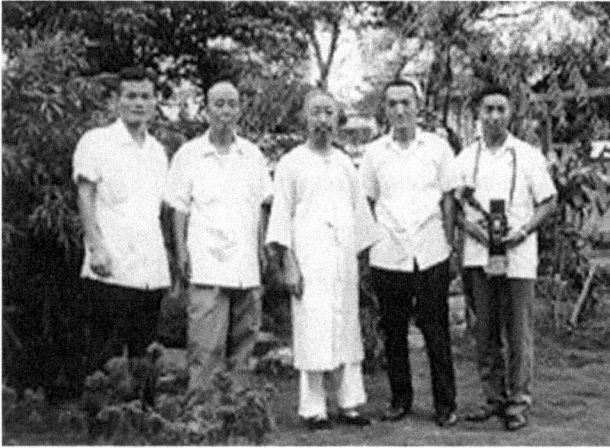

Ben Lo, T.T.Liang, Cheng Man Ching, Yi Ching Bo, Hsu Fun Yuen

Taiwan was a refuge for a number of highly skilled Tai Chi teachers fleeing Mao's new regime in mainland China in the late 1940's. Liang took advantage of this and sought out teachers who specialized in different aspects of Tai Chi study. The following are a few of the notable teachers that Liang had contact with and what they taught:

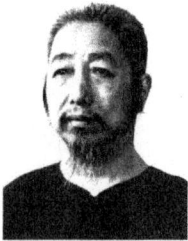

Cheng Man Ching

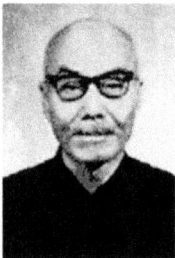

Hsiung Yang Ho

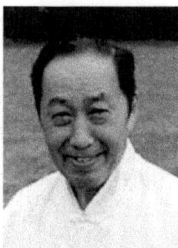

Wan Yen Nien

• Prof. Cheng Man Ching: (studied under Yang Cheng Fu): Tai Chi solo form and pushing-hands (basic two-person sparring set).

• Hsiung Yang Ho (studied under Yang Shao Hou): pushing-hands, *san-shou* (advanced two-person sparring set), sword and sword fencing.

• Wang Yen Nien (studied under Chang Ching Ling): pushing-hands.

• Li Jin Fei: Tamo sword and the practical use of the tassel.

It was this quest to improve his skill and understanding of Tai Chi that eventually brought him to the use of music. There was one event in particular that he related as impressing him greatly. He happened upon a Judo master in Taiwan giving a demonstration in which he used music to accompany his forms. Liang thought this was a brilliant idea and foresaw how it could be utilized in the practice of Tai Chi. While employed as senior customs officer, Liang had frequented the dance halls of Shanghai and had learned the dances of the time, such as the fox trot, tango, and waltz. He drew on this experience now to create the timing of the postures. "As I got better and had further experience with Tai Chi," he said, "I gradually became more and more interested in trying to make the art both more scientific and more aesthetic. In order to do this I introduced rhythm so that the postures can be practiced slowly, effortlessly, evenly and continuously in order to make the body and mind in co-ordination."

In 1964 Cheng Man Ching was invited to teach Tai Chi at the United Nations in New York City and he asked Liang to come with him as his assistant and interpreter. From there they were invited to teach at numerous universities and colleges on the east coast. According to Liang, a minor dispute regarding a payment became the catalyst for the two to split, and Liang moved to Boston in '69 while Cheng stayed in New York City. Neither had contact again.

It was in Boston in 1969, in a tiny apartment (with the Murphy bed up) that doubled as a studio, I first started classes with Liang. After fours years of studying with him, much to my dismay, Liang decided to return to Taiwan. He asked me to continue teaching his beginner students while he was gone but gave no indication as to when he would return. During his time in Taiwan, he sought out the Tai Chi teacher Li Jin Fei. Liang learned from him the practical use of the tassel for the Tai Chi double-edged sword as well as continued studies in the *Wu Tang* two-person sword fencing sets.

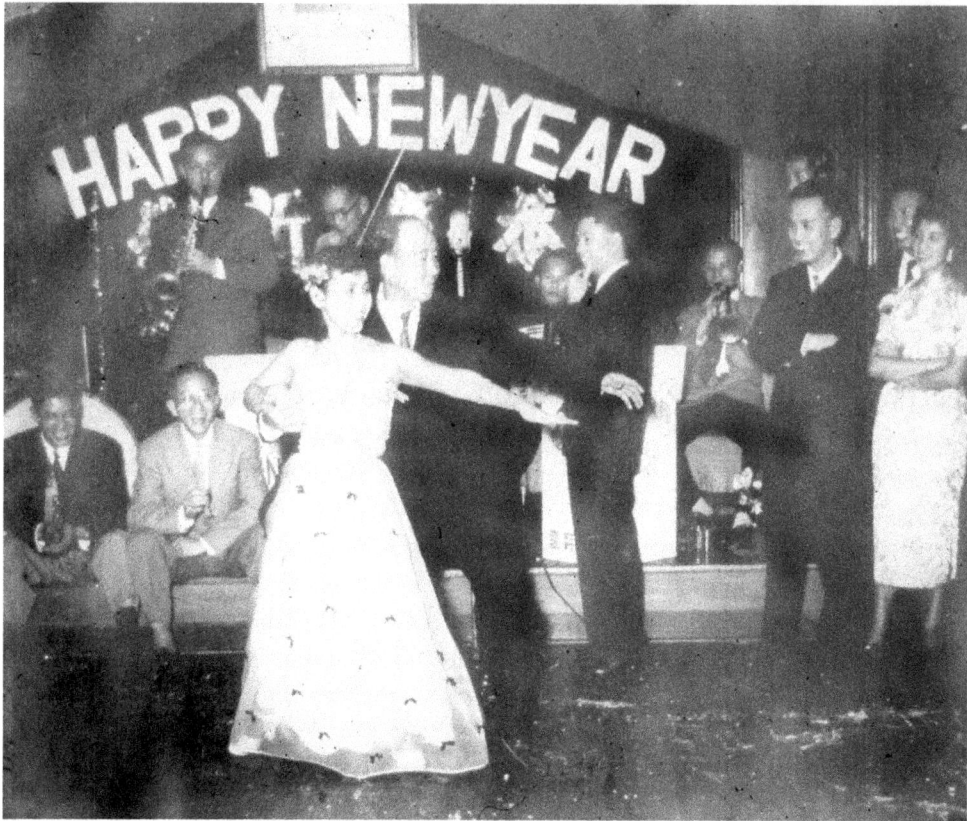

Liang demonstrating his moves, Shanghai, 1942

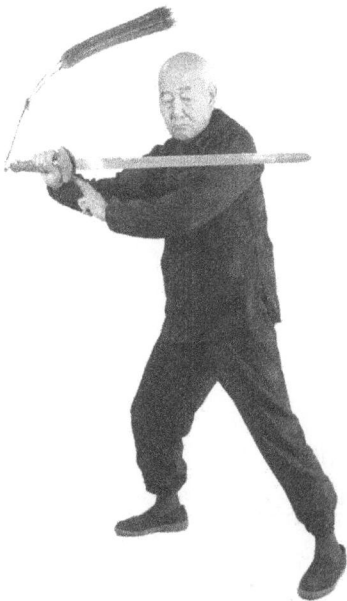

Liang demonstrating the Tai Chi double-edged sword form with tassel

I kept in touch with him by phone during this time and tried in vain to convince him to come back. I even set up a Tai Chi studio in Boston's Chinatown and let him know it was waiting for his return. Finally, I remembered a story he had told to me how he "curried favor" in order to meet a renowned, yet reclusive Tai Chi practitioner who was refusing to see him. Liang very much wanted to meet this man but had no way of contacting him. He knew, though, that this teacher's wife lived in Taipei, so he arranged to have gifts delivered to her in the hopes that she could arrange an introduction. Liang finally did get his meeting.

I decided to try this same indirect technique on Liang. He had told me that his wife was a devout Buddhist. At the time I was studying art so I sculpted a seated Buddha figure and a Chinese incense burner, cast them both in bronze and sent them as gifts to her in Taipei. It worked, or at least I like to think it did. He kept these two sculptures with him until the day he died.

Liang returned to Boston in late 1974. Together we founded the "Tai Chi Dance Association" and for the next eight years we taught together. Again, I worked with the beginner students while he taught private and advanced classes. It was during this time with him that I inherited a lifelong interest in this art. As he described it, "the more I learn, the less I feel I know. The theory and practice of Tai Chi is so profound and abstruse! I must

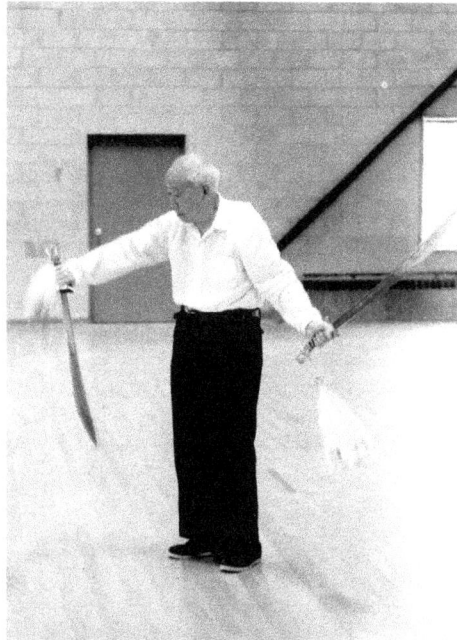

Liang demonstrating the Double Saber form

Poster for Boston Chinatown studio, 1974

continue to study forever and ever … it is the only way to better myself."

In 1983 he informed me that his time in Boston was ending and our partnership in The Tai Chi Dance Association would come to an end as well. His daughter, who lived in St. Cloud, Minnesota had bought him and his wife a house and they were moving there to retire. This "retirement" became a new chapter in Liang's teaching Tai Chi in America and one in which he met and taught many new and talented students.

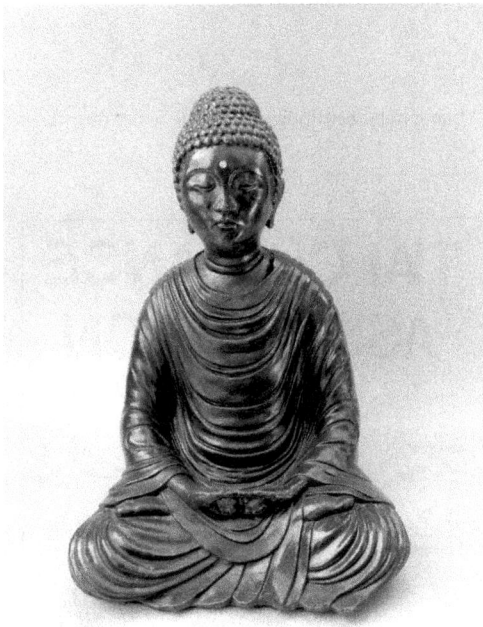

Bronze Buddha by the Author

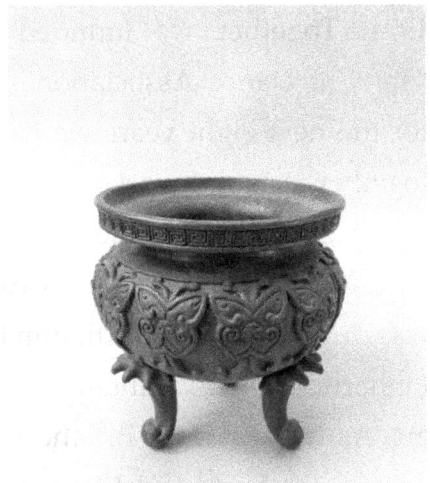

Bronze incense burner by the Author

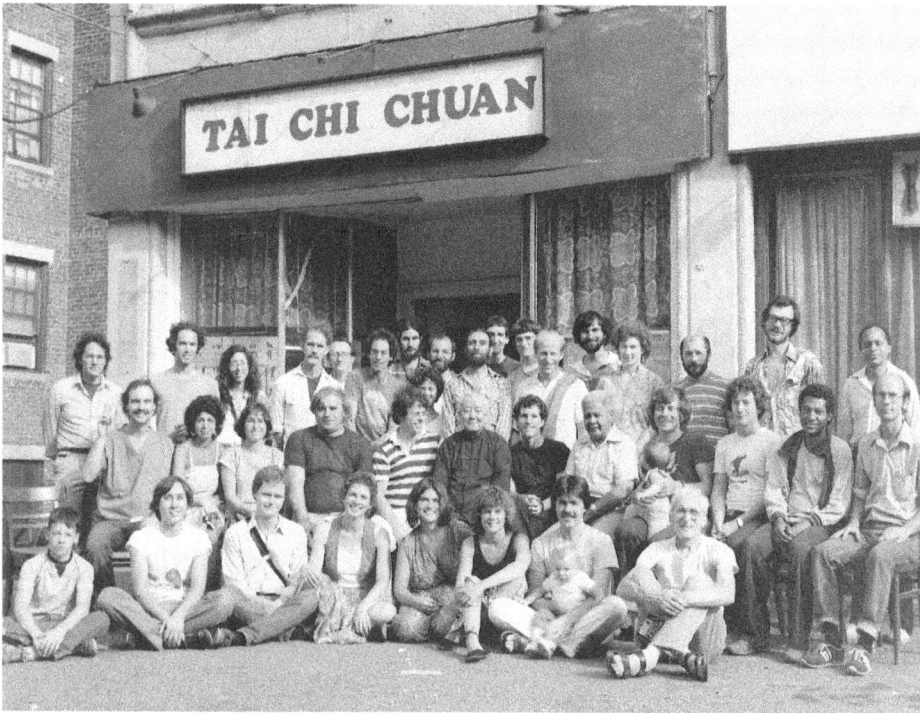

The Author and T.T. Liang with students in front of their Peterborough Street studio, Boston, 1983

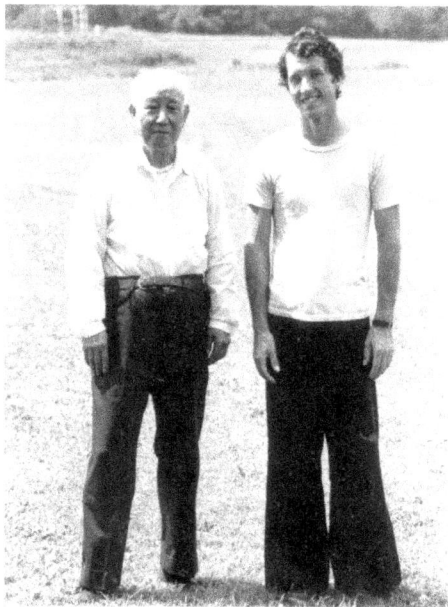

T.T. Liang and the Author, 1980

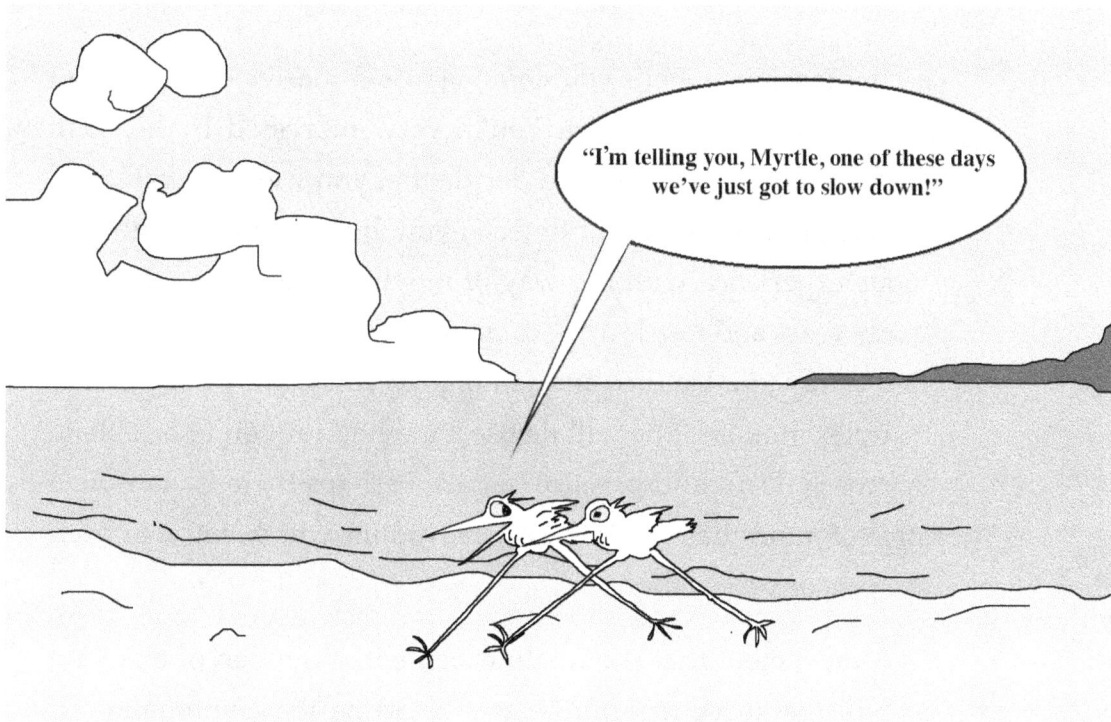

2 Why Tai Chi is Practiced Slowly

Almost everyone has seen people practicing the slow motion exercises of Tai Chi. You can find in almost any city in the world people silently moving through the postures of the solo exercise routines. What are they doing? … Why are they moving so slowly?

I think the best way to answer these questions is to describe Tai Chi as the product of a particular way of teaching. Imagine a circumstance where you come across a master of some kind of physical movement art. You're very impressed by her skill and economy of gesture and decide that you want to learn from her. She might be willing to teach you, but as you have no previous experience with her way of moving, and it has taken her many years and much work to perfect her skills, she will need to find a way to introduce and familiarize you with her subtle and complex motions. She will devise a method for you to be able to approach, learn and practice her art. Perhaps there is, as well, a state of mind that needs to be achieved for which you will need the proper preparation.

A movement that she might execute in a fraction of a second and in the space of a millimeter could be the combination of many subtle turns of her body and shifts of her weight. In order for her to make this explicit, she will have to slow it down and give you the movement broken up into many separate increments that take up much more time and space. She will then take care to guide you through these practice movements in exactly the right sequence of shifting and turning and then leave you to practice this prescribed sequence repeatedly until it becomes familiar. Over time, with observation and practice, you will begin to understand the subtleties of her way of moving, become familiar with the nuances of balance involved and incorporate them as your own. She will now be able to begin to teach you about her art.

This is the situation that every Tai Chi student finds himself or herself in. They're performing a series of movements that have been slowed down and stretched out in order to clearly delineate movements that in actual use are very small and very fast. Most people practice Tai Chi as a slow-moving exercise for health that focuses on relaxation, balance, unifying the movements of the limbs and focusing the mind. They are in fact gaining benefit from the first stage of study of a very effective martial art, which in itself is an integral aspect of a progressive system of developmental study.

The slow-moving solo exercise that most people are familiar with is the first step in a long process of studying the art of Tai Chi. The student will progress from solo exercises to working with a partner, from empty hand to learning the use of hand-held weapons. All are based on the underlying principles one learns in the solo form: the foundation upon which everything else in Tai Chi is built.

Each movement of the solo form comprises a complex series of shifts and turns that are not random. To learn it requires an experienced teacher who has a firm understanding of the nuances within the movements and knows their end purposes in order to guide the student correctly. Without this, it becomes just another movement exercise where the gestures of the limbs and turns of the body, however beautiful they might be, will have lost their context and meaning as pertaining to the art of Tai Chi Ch'uan.

The nuances of the Tai Chi movements are easily lost as the exercise gets passed on from instructor to instructor. Like the game of "Telephone" that I played in school where my classroom would sit in a circle and one student would be given a sentence to whisper into the ear of the person sitting next to them. Each student would repeat the sentence to the student next to him or her until it came around to the last student in the circle. This student would then say the sentence out loud to the rest of the class. Always, to the great amusement of the class, the result was nothing near to the original sentence. This same situation happens in the teaching of Tai Chi, among other things. Following and mimicking movements of a teacher can have great benefits, but often it is not precise enough to learn their intent and meaning fully. T.T. Liang created his system of counting as a way to standardize some of the basic movements and principles that are so easily lost.

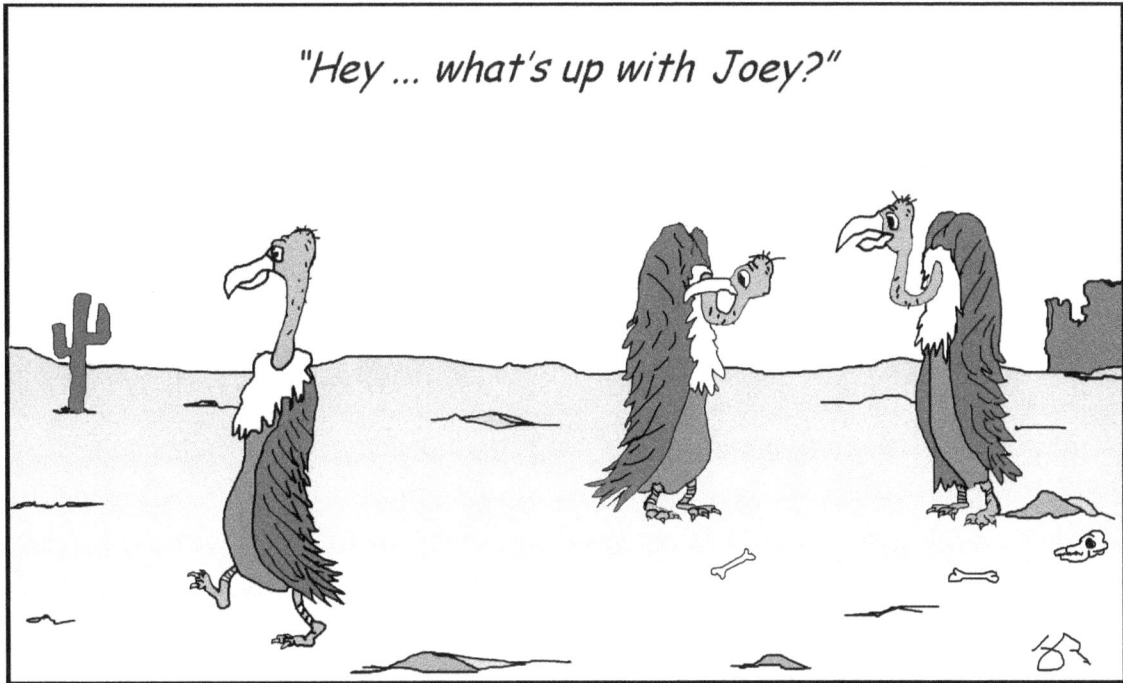

"Hey ... what's up with Joey?"

3 Fundamentals

If you have spent time in a cold climate then you have most likely experienced "sheet ice." This is when it rains and then immediately after freezes, leaving a thin sheet of ice over everything. When someone tries to walk on ice they have to be very careful or their feet will slip out from under them. In order to stay upright and move in this environment the most important thing is to completely relax. Next is to bend your knees and sink your weight downward. Then you carefully shift your weight directly over each foot while at the same time keeping your back straight and not leaning. Not moving your limbs independently of each other, but instead moving your body as a single unit, will help to achieve greater balance.

Walking on sheet ice like this exactly describes what is needed in the practice of Tai Chi. The following points elaborate on these fundamentals and are what Liang liked to call his "guiding principles."

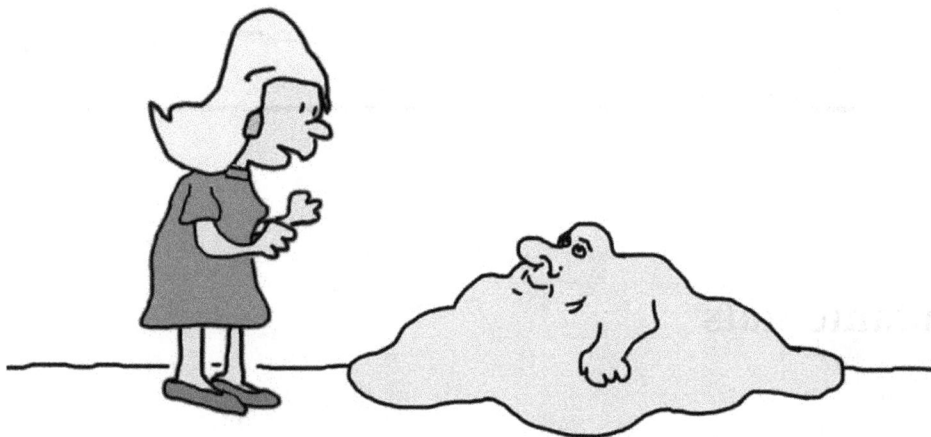

"Really Frank, - you're taking this relaxing thing an bit too far."

Relaxing

A lot of attention is paid to keeping your body relaxed while practicing Tai Chi. Becoming aware of where in your body you are holding tension and then trying to relax that area is an ongoing concern. Most of us are unaware of how much tension we hold, especially in our neck and shoulders. Breaking that habit is very difficult and is the first concern for beginning students.

Your goal is to use the least amount of muscular tension possible while still holding your body upright. As Liang would say, "relaxed, but not collapsed." This kind of relaxation can appear to the casual observer to be very simple and easily achieved. Completely relaxing while moving through the varied postures of the Tai Chi solo form requires much more work than you might think. Beginners will often comment on the fact that they are using muscles that they didn't know they had.

Relaxing your muscles while slowly moving can have the effect of making your limbs feel very heavy. This was made clear to me when I had to undergo surgery on my left hand. I was given a nerve block to anesthetize my entire left arm. The doctor, after having administered the nerve block, lifted my good hand and said, "here, please hold onto this. I'll be right back." I was surprised to see that he had placed my anesthetized left forearm into my right hand. But even more surprising was to feel how heavy it was! When you relax entirely, to the point where you are using just enough energy to remain upright, it feels like you have become very heavy, as gravity tries to pull you down. With the least amount of muscular tension possible, you try to resist that gravity. I've seen students sweating and shaking while attempting to maintain this state of "relaxation."

Stepping

Researchers have noted that Emperor penguins, who are not particularly well suited for walking on land, conserve energy while making the long trek inland to their breeding grounds by leaning from side to side to create locomotion. The action of leaning to the left lifts their right foot and leaning to the right lifts their left foot. With little effort they can travel great distances. Unlike Emperor penguins, we are well adapted for walking on land, yet a lot of us unknowingly resort to the same energy-saving technique that penguins use. We lean and throw our weight from foot to foot. This allows us to use less energy and involves using fewer muscles to move, but it also keeps us in a perpetual state of imbalance. The very simple act of shifting your weight from one foot to the other, when looked at closely, is much more difficult (and complex!) than you might imagine.

In addition to sometimes leaning side-to-side, we have a tendency to lean forward while walking. This way, as you lift your foot, the forward lean will propel you forward. For most people this is a natural way of walking and has no ill effect. If you are carefully observing your balance, though, you realize that this leaves you, for a brief moment, out of balance. I've heard this described as "controlled falling. " What would happen, as your weight is being propelled forward, if the ground under your forward-stepping foot, before it landed, suddenly shifted? You would most likely stumble and, at worst, crash to the floor. While we are young and active this tendency to throw our weight onto our stepping foot is hardly noticed. Where it becomes a problem is when we get older and cannot rely so much on our coordination and muscular agility. From a martial arts perspective it is a serious defect.

To overcome this tendency, Tai chi is asking us to clearly differentiate our weight on each foot as we move and walk. This means that before I take a step (in any direction) I will need first to shift 100% of my weight onto my stationary foot while I pick up the stepping foot. I will then place that foot down on the floor without shifting any weight onto it. My other foot is still bearing 100 percent of my weight. Then, like pouring water from one glass to another, I will shift my weight onto my other foot.

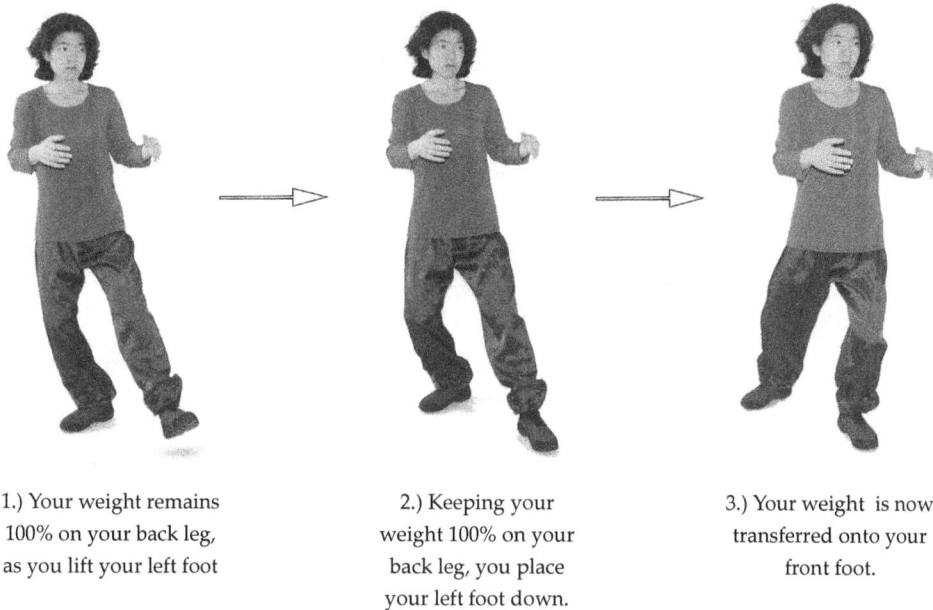

1.) Your weight remains 100% on your back leg, as you lift your left foot

2.) Keeping your weight 100% on your back leg, you place your left foot down.

3.) Your weight is now transferred onto your front foot.

Beginning students will often lean with their upper body as a counterweight, similar to the Emperor penguin, to make it easier to lift their legs. Tai Chi corrects this tendency by requiring you to keep your head up and your spine plum erect. This upright position will make you bring your weight, as you are stepping, in a vertical line directly over your weighted (stationary) leg. This keeps your body in perfect balance while walking.

Knees

When practicing Tai Chi, you try to stay flexible and pliable at all times, the joints are never fully extended or "locked." Locking the knee joint can be observed in another energy-saving device that most of us use to support our weight. A perfect example of this can be observed in Michelangelo's sculpture of David. This classic pose (contrapposto) shows David with his weight shifted over onto one leg so that his locked knee and torqued hip support his weight. In this position, David's leg muscles can relax as his weight is mostly supported by the "locked" bones in his leg. Tai Chi asks you not to use this technique when shifting your weight from foot to foot but instead to bend your knees and move from a lowered position in order to increase mobility. Because this low stance is difficult to maintain as one moves through the Tai Chi postures, beginners will often rise up and straighten out their legs while transitioning their weight from foot to foot in order to give their tired muscles a brief respite.

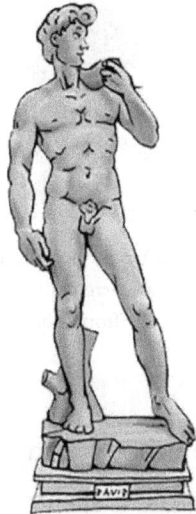

Feet

Keeping your feet relaxed allows your weight, in a sense, to sink into the floor. The importance of this for maintaining your balance can be observed with a beach ball. If you blow it up completely, it will roll along the floor at the slightest push. If you take one-third of the air out of it, you will see that it doesn't want to roll at all. It is hugging the floor instead. The same idea applies to your feet. If you tense them up with your toes trying to grip the floor, you create a hard object that can be uprooted or separated from the floor easily. If your feet are soft and relaxed, however, they can, like the deflated beach ball, "hug" the floor.

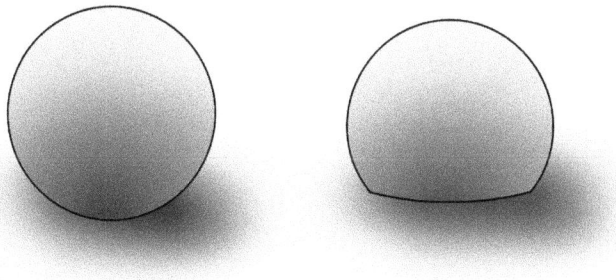

It may seem counterintuitive, from a martial arts perspective at least, that if someone is pushing you, you should relax your arms, knees and feet as well as the rest of your body. A good way to understand this is in the comparison of a chain and a solid pipe. If you were asked to pick up a solid steel pipe, you would most likely grab it from anywhere along the shaft and simply pick it up. If on the other hand that same pipe was melted down and forged into a linked chain and then piled on the floor, you would find it much more difficult to pick up. Unlike the solid pipe, the chain has no static center of gravity, so simply grabbing a handful would not help you lift it. In this sense, the chain becomes heavier and more connected to the floor. The same principle applies to our feet and body. If we can keep them relaxed and not rigid and tense, then like the deflated beach ball and the linked chain, our weight stays "rooted" to the floor.

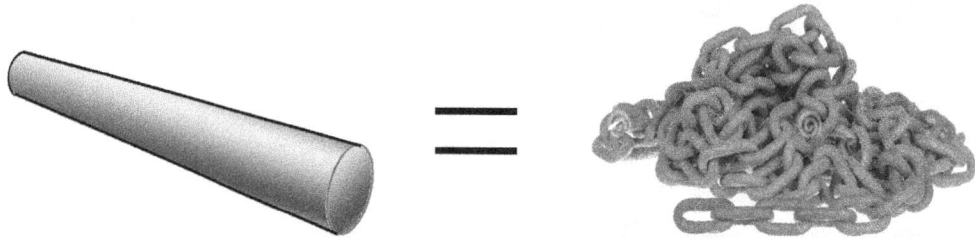

Hands

In Tai Chi you are asked to move the whole body as a single unit. This specifically applies to the hands where you are asked not to move them independently. They instead become mere extensions of your forearm. The practitioner tries to release any tension in his/her fingers and prevents the thumbs from sticking out. The hands remain relaxed but contained.

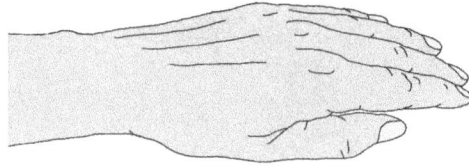

Tai chi hand position

Not using one's hands may seem a simple idea, but for anyone who has tried, it is actually quite difficult to do. I've noticed that if you ask someone not to touch something, try as he might, he will often reach out for it with his hands. For example, as an artist, I have for years worked with assembling very small parts for casting. When I have visitors come to see what I am doing, I will always say to them, "please don't touch." Invariably my guests, in a moment of enthusiasm, will reach out with their hands first as they say, "oh, look at this!" This is understandable; when we are infants of barely six days old, we are already reaching out to the world around us with our hands. People can be observed thinking and speaking with their hands.

When responding to any situation, most people will move their hands before any other part of their body, including their mouth. The Tai Chi exercise, on the other hand (as it were), is asking you not to react with your hands but instead to respond with your whole body. For the Tai chi practitioner this means not using your hands to react to every block, parry and punch, but instead to relax and not focus on specific actions of your partner/opponent and attempt to perceive a larger picture, a view of the whole situation.

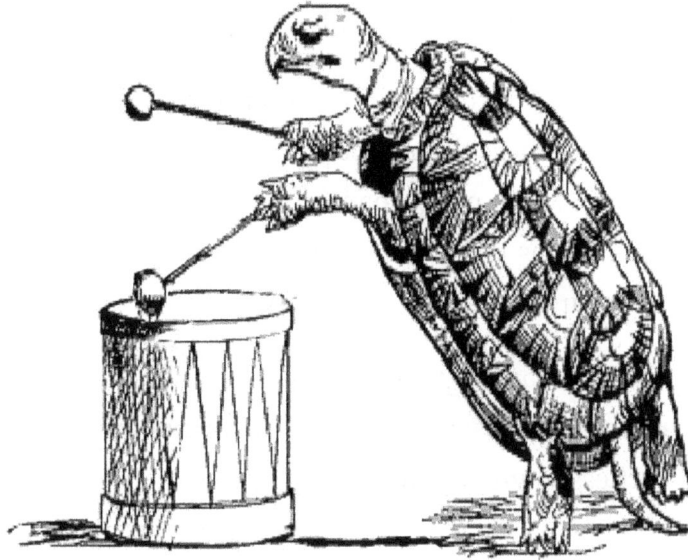

4 Liang's Counting System with Beats

Many people, and I include myself as having been among them, are put off by the idea of practicing Tai Chi to music or with a metronome. I think this is because there is a common misconception that in practicing this way you're going to give up active control of your movements and instead are mindlessly moving to the flow of the rhythm as one feels it. Actually, depending on what "flowing with the music" means, this might be a good idea ... but not until the student has gained a thorough understanding of the mechanics of each of the individual postures that comprise the whole of the Tai Chi solo exercise.

When practicing Tai Chi with music, T.T. Liang was not listening so much to the melody. He was instead paying attentionto the beat. More often than not, he would practice with a metronome. It was the evenly timed beats that were important to him and around which he structured his method of practice.

A useful analogy of how Liang employed the use of rhythm in Tai Chi is in observing how a great jazz musician seems to flow effortlessly with the music he is playing. In order to gain that fluidity, the musician must have prepared himself by studying how to hit a note accurately and then have practiced those notes using scales, arpeggios, and chords. The seemingly effortless interaction with these notes would come, no doubt, much later. Liang uses beats to facilitate this same progression of study as it applies to Tai Chi.

A musician working with a set tempo has to learn when to hold a note, when to give it emphasis with volume and when to differentiate the speed of which the notes are played. Similarly, the Tai Chi practitioner will learn within the beats which parts of his/her body needs to speed up or slow down in relationto each other and where emphasis needs to be placed.

Connecting the Dots

When a child is first learning to draw, he or she has very little idea how to begin. How can the child think of creating, for instance, a face? One way to help her/him is to lay out sequentially numbered dots to lead the child's pencil over the paper. In this way, the child can conceive of how this is accomplished and, although the results will be a little rough in terms of detail, he or she can visualize the process of creating a facsimile of a face.

In this same way, following the beats can be likened to connecting the numbered dots of a child's drawing book. The beginning Tai Chi practitioner uses beats as points of reference to move with. On certain beats the foot or hand is to arrive at exactly the right moment or the waist turned before a step is taken. On another beat there will be a specific and separate expression of mental intent or a slight movement made for issuing force. This requires of the student an exacting participation with the rhythm.

When you adhere to and move within the beats in this manner, it can, in the beginning, feel somewhat awkward. Your moves will tend to be a little staccato while you try to be at a particular point at a precise time and the turns of your waist may sometimes feel like they are moving at right angles. All this can seem counterproductive when one of the expressed goals of Tai Chi is to move in a circular and flowing fashion. The purpose, though, is to comprehend fully the individual components that make up a posture. When this is accomplished and you have mastered the

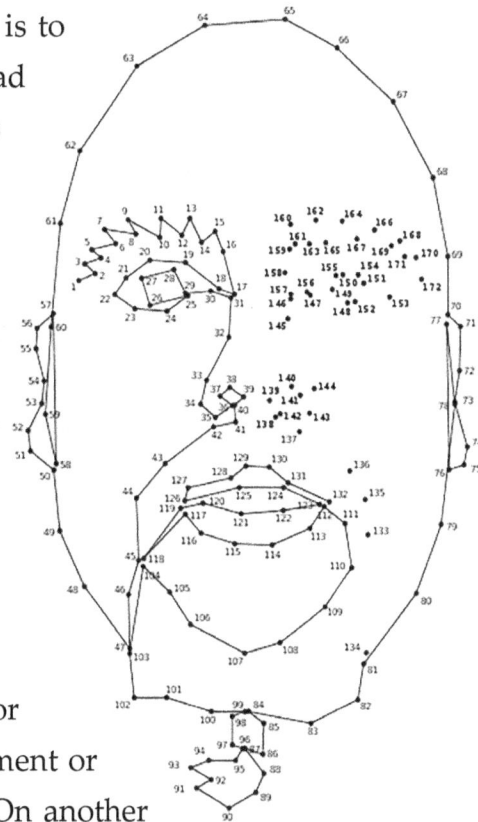

use of rhythm, you will no longer need to stop at any given beat, but instead will flow through it at exactly the correct moment. In fact, while practicing with the beats, you eventually will not consciously think about them at all. Proceeding from angular movements, the student will progress to using open circular gestures in their practice. The attentionto where specific body parts are, at any given beat, is no longer necessary. What remains in your mind, and is expressed by your body, is the intent and idea inherent within each posture.

This learning progression is sometimes referred to as "finding the circle within the square." When a specific posture is first studied, the individual aspects of the movements are clearly defined and delineated – as in the sharp corners of a square. After the student has thoroughly understood the mechanics and can express them through movement, she then should round off these "sharp" angular edges so that the form becomes circular and fluid. Retained within their rounded movements, though, is the knowledge and memory of the "square," i.e., the use and intent of the posture. From this point on, as the advanced practitioner begins to employ the movements for practical use, the circular gestures will become smaller and less pronounced.

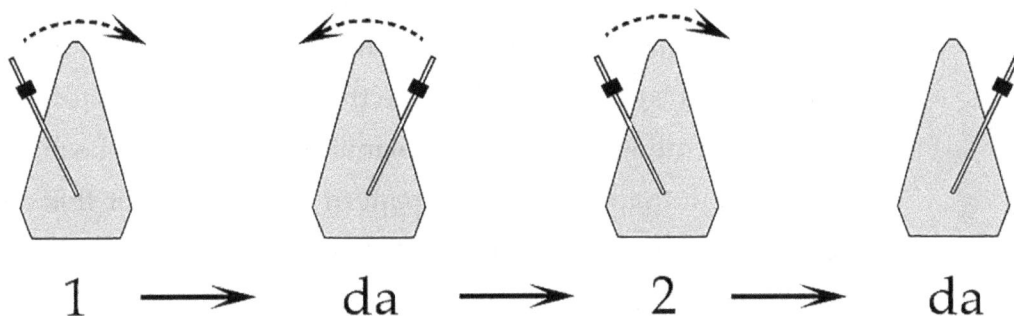

1 → da → 2 → da

5 Anatomy of a Single Posture with Beats

In the Tai Chi solo exercise as Liang taught it, there are 150 postures, each with a specific sequence of movements. Liang broke down every one of these postures so that each gesture, and shifting of the weight within it, is represented by a count. Each count he then divided in two, creating a specific timing counted as "one-and-two-and" - or in his case – "one-da-two-da," etc. The practitioner uses these beats as points of reference during the execution and performance of the postures.

How to apply Liang's system of counting to the postures of the Tai Chi solo form can be learned with the close examination of just a single posture. This was demonstrated to me when I was first studying with Liang. I was averse to the idea of learning and practicing with beats, so I managed to learn the whole of the 150 postures solo form without them. Liang never mentioned anything to me about this during all our lessons until one day he placed a metronome in front of me and said, "OK, now do it with the beats." Of course I couldn't. He then proceeded to show me a single posture with detailed explanations of how the beats are used. I found that knowing the pattern of the beats for this one posture was enough to apply to the rest of the postures in the solo form (with a few exceptions).

As I started to practice using the beats, I came to understand my practice in a different way. The movements were a lot more complex than I had realized. There were many things I had not noticed previously about the sequence and relationship of my gestures. I was unaware of the compound movements within movements. It was from this point on that Liang and I would endlessly review and examine the nuances of the Tai Chi postures using the beats as our reference.

General Guidelines on Counting

The 1st count is almost always for shifting your weight off the weighted front foot in preparation for stepping or adjusting it if necessary. Oftentimes, though, this [weighted?] foot does not need to be adjusted, so instead the weight will gradually shift fully onto it (without first taking the weight off of it).

In Liang's Tai Chi, he pays close attention to the Tai Chi "Clas-

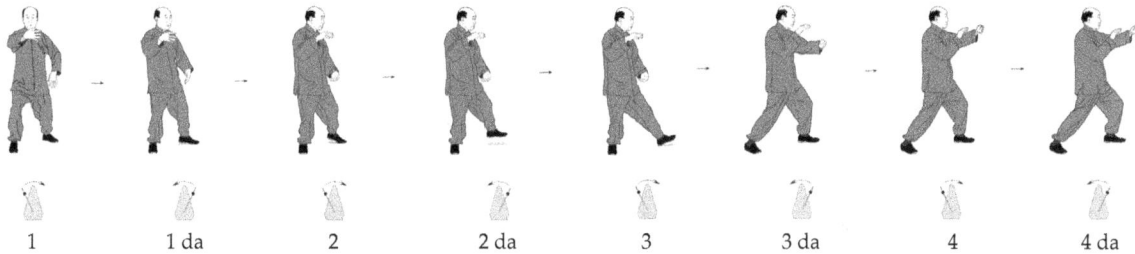

1	1 da	2	2 da	3	3 da	4	4 da

sics" where it is said: "The substantial and the insubstantial must be clearly discriminated." In regards to moving your feet this means that you must completely take the weight off of one foot first before moving it. Liang manifests this in the solo form by making sure that you never turn on a weighted foot. Instead, when it is necessary to adjust your foot's position, you will shift your weight off of it first. This principle is clearly emphasized by Liang throughout all the postures of the solo form.

The 2nd count in a four-count posture is used for fully shifting your weight onto the now adjusted or positioned foot and preparing to step with your unweighted foot. After your weight is fully shifted onto the stationary or "rooted" foot, your other foot simultaneously pivots on your toes as your waist turns 45 degrees in preparation to step forward.

The 3rd count: The final forward stepping foot lands on the 3rd count in a 4-count posture (the 5th count in a 6-count posture). **On the second beat of this count** you shift your weight onto it [the "stepping foot"] as you turn your waist forward and turn in your back foot, pivoting 45 degrees on the heel.

You are now fully turned to face your imagined opponent. The hands on this count turn with the waist to come into a position ready to execute the intent of the posture. Your weight will shift 60% onto the forward foot.

On the last count your weight shifts directly forward (and into the ground) 10% and the imagined issuing force is directed forward in a focused direction.

On the last beat of the last count of every posture the movement comes to a complete stop. This last beat is always reserved for the last final focused expression of completing the posture's intent. Liang sometimes described a posture as: "you stick the key in the lock, slowly turn it … and then, at the last moment …. CLICK." The click represents this final beat.

As can be seen from the above brief description, there is a specific progression of movements that Liang is delineating with his use of beats. He is always insuring that one never steps without being in perfect balance and takes care to position the practitioner so that he/she is facing the imagined partner before expressing the intent of the posture.

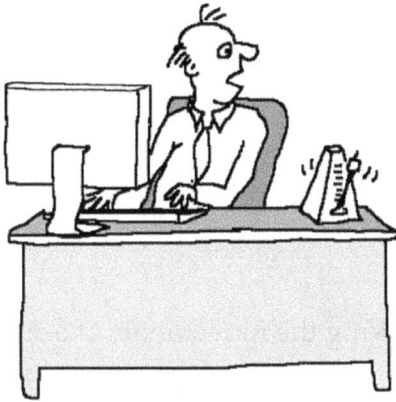

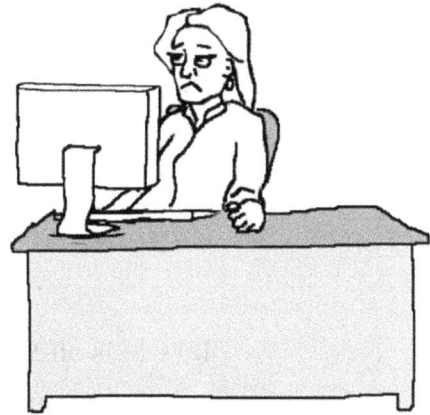

"I hope you don't mind ... it helps me focus"

6 Tai Chi Principles Within the Beats

When students have achieved an understanding of how to perform the postures using rhythm, they can now go onto use the beats as a tool for exploring the fundamental principles that are the basis of Tai Chi. The beats create a structure for understanding how to approach and employ Tai Chi concepts such as adhering to an opponent, moving from a center point, the use of focused imagination, issuing force as well as building momentum in the moment or space between postures. While some of these concepts are observed in the overall use of the beats, some individual beats will often delineate a specific use.

Benefits of Following a Beat

Tai Chi is often described as mimicking the movements of a river: continuous and flowing. It's no wonder then that some people will feel that following a beat while practicing is too restrictive and against the principles of Tai Chi. In the beginning it probably is restrictive, but if you can persevere with this practice there is an important skill to be gained. This is the ability to follow.

With Liang's use of rhythm while practicing the form, you match the movements within the postures exactly to the pre-scribed beat. By precisely following an externally generated cadence when you are stepping and moving, you develop the ability to give up your own self-motivated movements. This capacity to let go of one's own initiative in order to be able to follow something else (in this case the rhythm or beat) in turn prepares the practitioner for the development of an advanced skill that is known in Tai Chi as "listening." This is the ability to interpret ("hear") your partner's or opponent's movements. You achieve this by not initiating your own actions but, instead, following and adhering to your partner's every move. Similarly, follow-ing the beats accurately within the form requires you to take the same attentive attitude.

This "listening" skill can aptly be described in terms of a conversation. If two people are going to be able to communicate effectively, they have to be able to hear what the other is saying. This means that each, in turn, has to stop talking (or thinking extraneous thoughts) in order to follow what the other is saying; and this requires a momentary giving up of one's own preoccupations in order to listen attentively and comprehend the other person's intentions. In this same way, if you can give up your own initiative and instead follow and adhere to the beats of each posture, at whatever speed, you are laying a foundation for developing the skills needed to follow and interpret your partner's intent as expressed through movement or otherwise.

"Find the center of the circle within you and

you can respond to any situation"

Attributed to Cheng Man Ching

Finding the Center of the Circle within You

In order to give up your own initiative so that you can follow an external beat, you have to know where in yourself your movements originate. In Tai Chi this careful self-observation is part of what is called an "internal art" – it is inward seeing.

A common response for most people is to lead their actions and reactions with their hands, head or shoulders. The goal in Tai Chi is instead to initiate your movements from a central point within your body - not from your limbs externally. This central point is called the Tan-Tien in Chinese and is located in the center of your hips about four inches below your belly button (I will refer to this point from now on as your "center core").

The advantage of responding and moving from a central point is that it economizes your movements by eliminating extraneous actions. The movement of a bicycle wheel is a good way to describe the correct connection between your hands and your waist. The hub of the wheel represents your waist and the rim your hands. The outside perimeter of the wheel only moves if the center hub initiates the movement; and the hub only has to

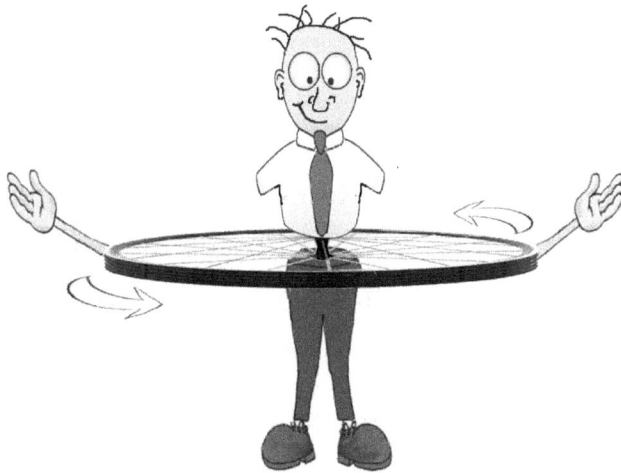

turn a small amount for the outside of the wheel to turn a much greater distance.

Even with more complex actions, the movements are always connected to and derived from the action of the center core (or center of the circle within you). This can be likened to a drive-shaft moving force through multiple gears. Although the gears are possibly moving at different speeds, all are deriving their force from the movement of the central driveshaft. In this same way, the Tai Chi practitioner will not use her limbs to initiate her movements but will instead derive the movements from the center core of the body.

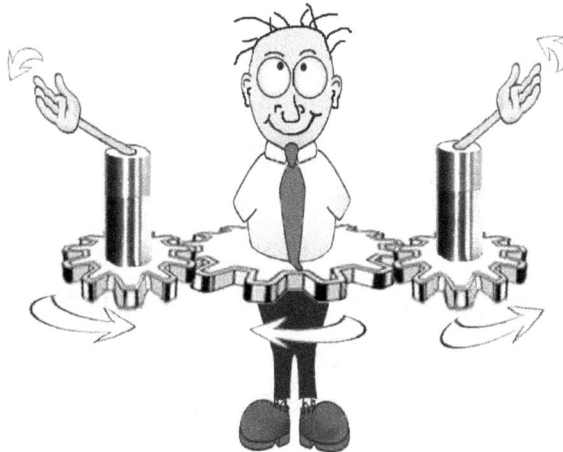

Liang made reference to this on numerous occasions by pointing it out in an indirect way. We would often have visitors come and demonstrate their Tai Chi forms for us. After what I thought to be excellent performances, Liang would invariably exclaim to our guest, "beautiful, beautiful! You are number one!" Then he would lean over to me and quietly say, "nothing to do with Tai Chi, but beautiful!"

You have hands all over your body, but it has nothing to do with hands"

Tai Chi saying

I eventually came to understand that what he meant by this was that although our performers were long-time and accomplished practitioners, and their gestures were well coordinated and often beautifully complex and powerful, they lacked the one necessary ingredient to qualify, according to Liang, as "Tai Chi." The defect was that they did not initiate their movements from their center core. Technically they looked perfect except for this almost imperceptible subtlety. At any given moment, our performer's hands, head or shoulders would initiate a movement independently of, or without a connection to, the center point in their torso. This is where the idea in Tai Chi that "the hands don't move" comes from. They move, but only in conjunction with the entire body, motivated by the center core, not separately.

Liang would add to the above quote by Cheng Man Ching that after you find and become familiar with the center of the circle within you, *you must then learn to respond and move from within it.* This is what he is asking the practitioner to do while following the beats. Again, on each beat you initiate your movement from within the center of the circle within you (the center core). If the student can practice in this way and incorporate this as a natural action, then, as Cheng says, "you can respond to any situation."

This ability to respond is a direct result of moving from your center core point and can be experienced while working with a metronome. For example, try to practice with the metronome turned up to the fastest speed possible. You'll notice that if you are trying to keep track of and animate all the separate parts of your body, you'll never be able to keep up with the beats. On the other hand if you only move from your center core and let everything else follow, you'll find that it is actually quite easy to keep time with the metronome's fast pace. I sometimes describe this as "slowing down time" because with so much less effort you can accomplish so much more that is extremely useful in a martial context.

Mirroring (Squaring up)

When dance couples are performing their routines, they will often try to face each other. This is known as mirroring and Li-ang paid a great deal of attentionto this. He contended that in order for one to stay in balance effectively while executing the intent of a posture, he must be directly facing the opponent. Li-ang stressed this positioning because, according to him, a Tai Chi posture rarely ends when you're turning your waist forward. This would indicate that you were executing the active intent of the posture while you were turning.

In doing this there's a potential problem: there will be a brief moment as you're turning and shifting your weight forward when your weight will be evenly distributed on both feet; a defect known as "double weighting." This presents a brief moment of vulnerability. Your opponent, if he or she is sensitive to it, can push across your evenly weighted feet, causing you to lose your balance (in Tai Chi terminology this is called being "uprooted"). But there is a solution!

The correct placement of your feet for optimum balance when executing the intent of most Tai Chi postures follows what is referred to as a "square stance." This is where the heels of your feet are positioned on diagonally opposite corners of a square, the sides of which are approximately your shoulders' width. Your forward heel is placed on a front corner with the toes facing forward and your back heel is placed on the diagonally opposite corner positioned at a 45-degree angle outward. Your waist and torso face directly forward in the direction of the forward foot. This stance gives you the maximum amount of standing stability (see diagram).

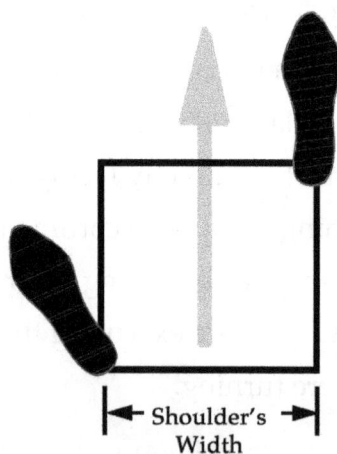

Shoulder's Width

In Liang's counting system this forward-facing stance is achieved on the second-to-last count of every forward-stepping posture. On this count you step with your forward leading foot, landing heel first. Then you shift a little more than 50% of your weight onto it before you turn your waist forward to face your imagined opponent directly. As you turn your waist forward, you use this movement to turn in your rear foot, pivoting on the heel, to the angled 45-degree position. Your weight distribution now should be 60% on the forward foot and 40% on the back. With your waist and torso now facing your opponent directly, you are now ready to execute the intent of the movement.

Many readers who are advanced in their study of Tai Chi and are familiar with working with a partner/opponent will have difficulty with the above concept. I also questioned Liang in detail about it, since I'd worked with many other teachers who did not adhere to this method. The common understanding was if someone pushes you on your left side you would respond by yielding on that side while simultaneously responding with force on your right side (this had been explained to me as "Yin transitioning to Yang," or the soft and yielding becoming hard and forceful).

Liang's response was that this interpretation is a misunderstanding of the commonly used Tai Chi saying: "to neutralize means to attack." He explained that although it's true that as you yield on your left side, your right side immediately responds, that does not mean – and he stressed this - that your right side should blindly strike. You first should, in this order:

1. adhere to the opponent

2. interpret his lines of balance

3. create a superior position of your own

When these three conditions are met, then (and only then) would you push or issue force. To quote him, "otherwise it's nothing more than a blindman's bluff." What Liang is saying is that after you neutralize an incoming push, you need to re-gain a superior position in relationto your partner before you act. You do this by establishing your balance (equilibrium) in the above-mentioned "square stance," aligning your body correctly to face your partner directly.

This, he said, was an often overlooked and subtle aspect of mar-tial skill, and he emphasized this preparatory awareness-train-ing by explicitly teaching it within the beats as students executed each posture of the Tai Chi solo form.

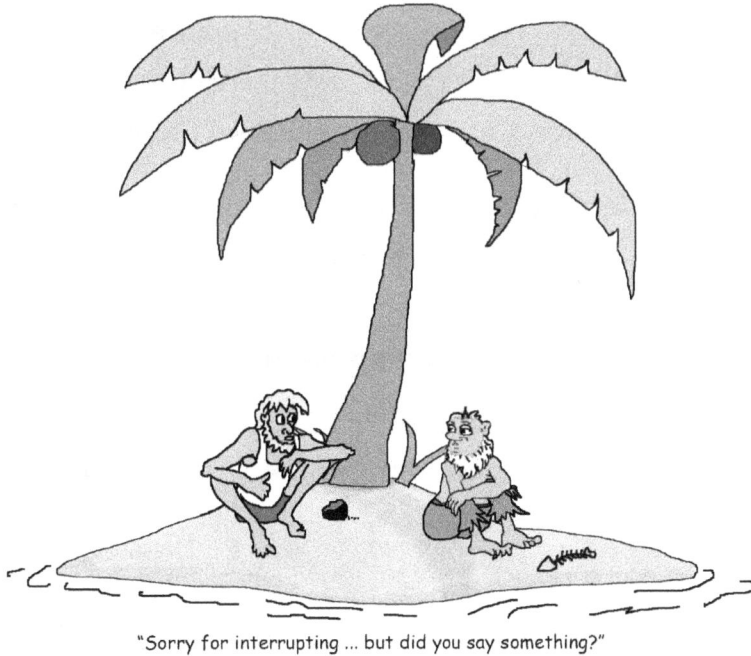

"Sorry for interrupting ... but did you say something?"

Listening and Interpreting

Now that your body is correctly aligned (with your imaginary opponent), the first beat of the last count is always reserved for feeling and interpreting your partner/opponent's movements and intentions. In Tai Chi this is described as "listening" to your opponent.

If the intent of the posture is being expressed through the hands, your hands will move with your body as you shift your weight. During this beat they remain completely relaxed as they try to "feel" the opponent. Like a blind person reading braille, you feel with your fingers for any nuances of resistance or imbalance. When this is detected, you are now in a position to issue energy or force during the beat that follows.

Relaxing and feeling first, ensures that your push is well informed. This prevents what Liang liked to refer to as the "blindman's buff" situation: one never blindly pushes someone; one feels, or "listens," and interprets first.

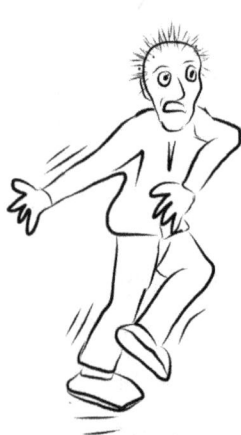

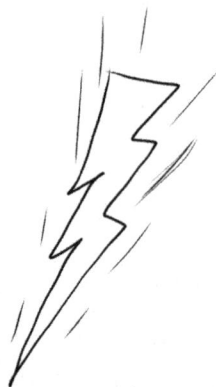

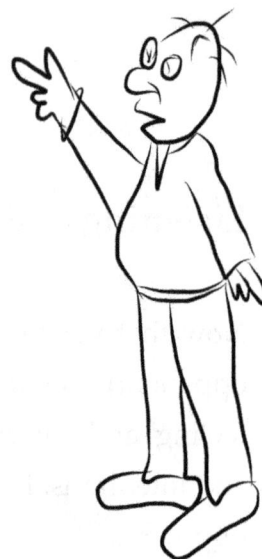

"Sorry George ... my aim is off today!"

"Strength is shot out of the legs like an arrow is from a bow... The waist is the bow that directs the arrow."

Tai Chi saying

Issuing

The very last beat of the last count of every posture in the solo form is always reserved for issuing force or energy.

When one strikes or pushes someone in Tai Chi it is unlike the kind of push that most of us are accustomed to. Usually, when you want to push something or someone, you extend your arms outward from your body with as much muscular force as you can gather. In Tai Chi a push is not like this at all. The pushing force does not entail the rigid use of one's muscles or bones but instead employs your body's more supple (elastic) sinews and tendons.

This kind of striking in Tai Chi is commonly referred to as "issuing." The use of this word is carefully chosen: it refers to force being generated from the feet and legs, gathering in the hips and waist and from there, directed outwards. If this is done properly, no rigid muscular tension is needed to generate the force. It's like a whip, which can generate a huge amount of force (as witnessed by the loud snapping "crack") but at no time is the whip itself ever rigid. The force travels through the whip in a wave like motion and "issues" out of its tip. In this same way, when issuing force, the Tai Chi practitioner's body is never rigid. It stays relaxed, like a whip, as the energy passes through it.

This force or energy can exit from anywhere on your body, it is not limited to just the use of your hands or limbs. This is sometimes described by the phrase, "you have hands all over your body, but it has nothing to do with your hands." In other words, any place on your body can be used as a hand, the point from which the energy is projected.

To understand how force or energy is used in Tai Chi, it is useful to look at the following example:

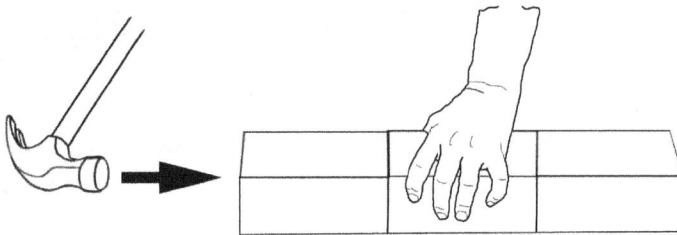

Place three blocks on a table, end-to-end. With one hand, hold the middle block stationery and with the other hand pick up a hammer.

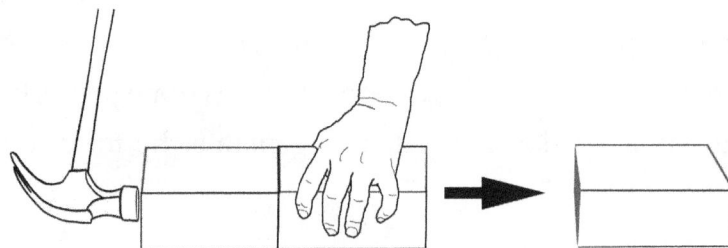

Hit the end of one of the outside blocks and observe what happens. The opposite block on the other side of the stationary middle block shoots away.

Why did it do this? The simple answer is that when you hit the block with the hammer it sent a wave or vibration (of energy) through the first block, which then traveled through the stationary block, resulting in the third block on the other side being propelled away. The block in the middle didn't move BUT the energy wave passed through it. In Tai Chi, the middle block represents the practitioner's whole body.

Like the middle, stationary block, the Tai Chi practitioner does not move while issuing force. Instead he or she develops the skill of allowing energy developed by the feet to go through the body. Alternatively, if you remember the analogy of a whip, then we could describe this as allowing the energy to roll through the body like a wave that goes through the length of the whip, resulting in the final "crack" of energy at the end (see image below). The difficulty for the practitioner here is that he needs to develop the ability to avoid any out of sequence or rigid movement within his body, because this would impede the directed wave-like flow of energy.

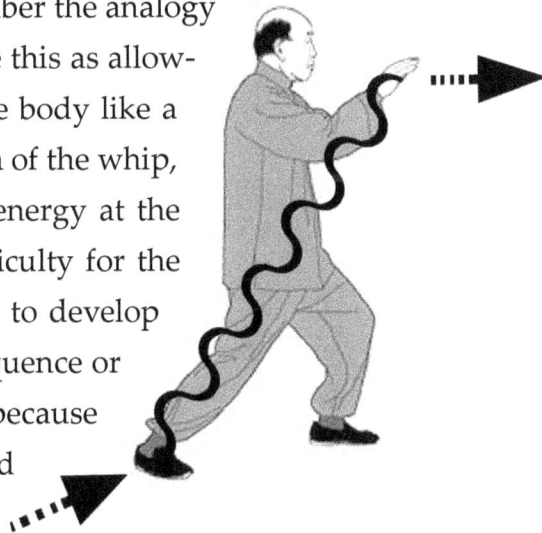

With both the "block" and "whip" analogies the energy is projected in an instant and then is gone. Similarly in Tai Chi, when the energy is issued it is instantaneous and leaves no residual tension in your body.

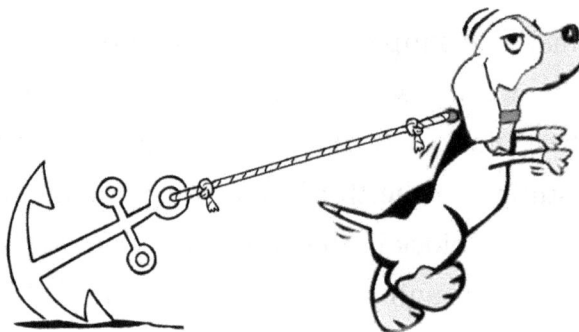

Sinking in

One cannot mention "issuing" in Tai Chi without also talking about "sinking." They come hand-in-hand. This means that along with learning the technique of issuing the student must also combine the knowledge of how to keep his balance when pushing. In other words, you do not throw your weight forward with the push but, instead, culminate the push with sinking your weight into the floor. This is often referred to as "anchoring" your weight.

A common defect when someone is pushing or striking is to throw his/her weight forward along with the push. If the person being pushed can get out of the way in time, the pusher will often lose his balance when he finds no resistance. When I would try to push Liang, he would sometimes ask me "why are you giving me your energy?" He explained that in Tai Chi, when you do issue force, you never "throw it" at your opponent. Instead, at the end of issuing, you will always anchor it by shifting your weight into the floor. Most times your weight goes into your forward foot. In Liang's counting system this sinking in always occurs at the end of the last beat of the last count of every posture.

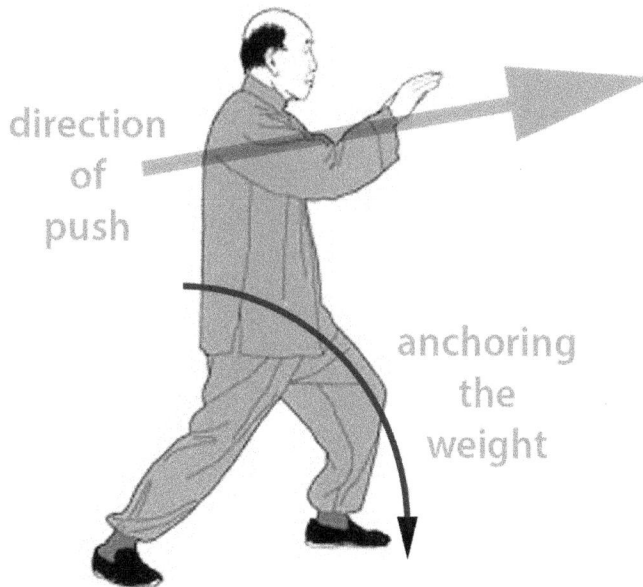

direction of push

anchoring the weight

"Hey man - why the hesitation?

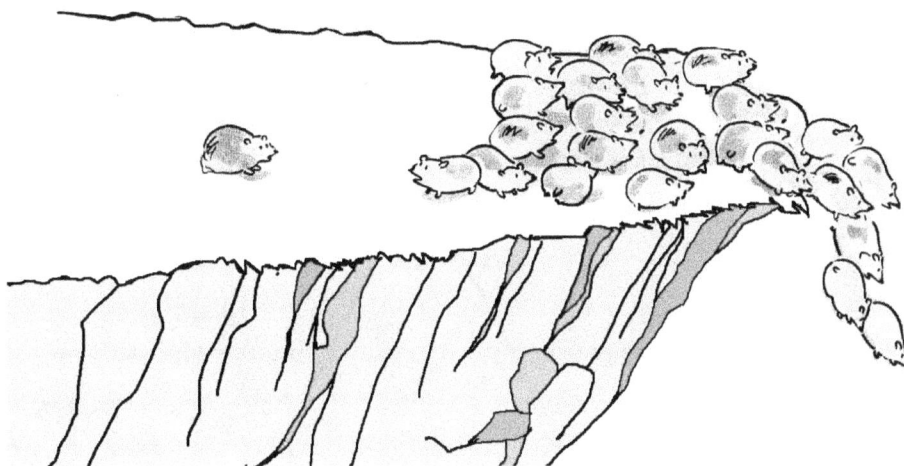

7 Pregnant Pause

I recently looked for a definition of the commonly used English phrase "pregnant pause" and found this answer: "a pause, which is expected to 'give birth' to something significant." Performers use this kind of a pause to build up tension and expectation in their audience; in interviews there's often a pause after a question, as the interviewee prepares and builds his answer. This idea of "building" and "expectancy" perfectly describes the momentary pause between every posture in the Tai Chi solo form.

The Space between the postures

To the outside observer there seems to be no separationto the flowing gestures, it looks as if the movements of Tai Chi continuously flow into each other for the duration of the exercise. But between every posture, there is a transitional pause where, according to Liang, a lot is happening

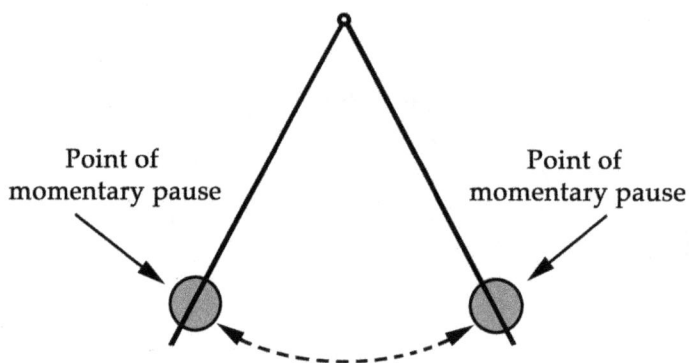

Point of momentary pause   Point of momentary pause

When you observe the movement of a pendulum, it also appears never to stop, but, in fact, as the pendulum reaches the end of each swing there's an infinitesimal pause as it gathers the momentum which enables it to swing in the opposite direction. In exactly this way, at the end of each posture of the Tai Chi form, there's a brief transitional moment where your momentum has been expended and you pause before heading into the next posture. This momentary charged stillness, or pregnant pause, is expressed internally by the practitioner and is barely, or not at all, visible to an outside observer.

To describe this, Liang would say, "The solo form is like a string of pearls." Each "pearl" is an individual posture with its myriad movements contained within it. The string is your imagination or mind's intent, which runs through each movement and connects one to the other. In Liang's counting system the space between the pearls or postures is represented by the transitional half-count. In other words, every posture ends on the last beat of the last count, and the next posture does not start until the first beat of the next count. That leaves a beat (or a half-count) where there is no movement (see chart below). It is in this slight pause that the expression or intent of the posture is brought to a focused, clearly defined conclusion.

Liang wrote, "Suppose one posture contains four beats – you must stop momentarily at the end of the fourth beat to complete the movement of the posture, then go onto the next posture. So during the transition of one posture to another, you must stop for just half a second. This momentary stoppage will be connected and joined to the next posture by the mind's intent. If one goes onto the next posture before the preceding one is fully completed, this is not the correct way of 'continuously moving.' It is confusion and one will not be able to determine clearly which of the postures is which."

Kinetic and Potential Energy

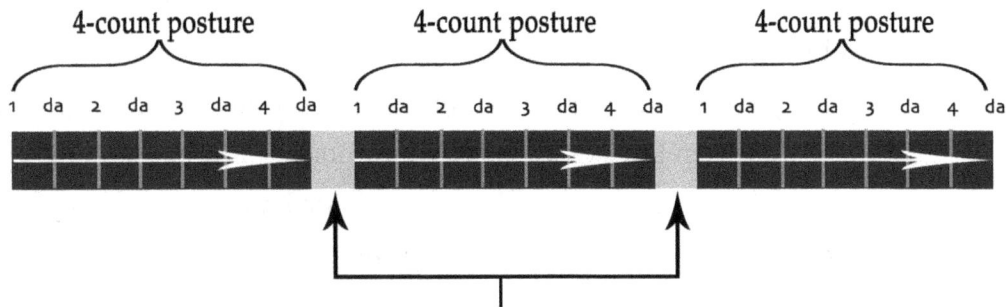

The above chart shows each individual count divided into 2 beats (or 1/2 counts).
Liang counted the second beat of each count with the sound or word "da".
The grey area here defines the beat or 1/2 count between each posture.

Another way to understand the kinetic and potential energy exchange that happens between each Tai Chi posture is to visualize a bouncing ball. The ball, falling through space, gains potential kinetic energy (the energy of motion), but when it hits the floor its shape compresses and the kinetic force is momentarily transformed into potential, or stored, energy until the ball, using this stored energy, moves back up and its shape is restored.

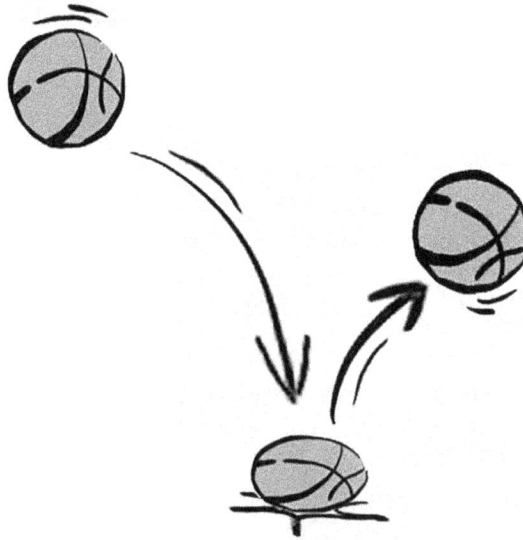

In this same way, on the last beat of each posture, as your weight sinks into the hard surface of the floor, the kinetic energy of the posture's movements transforms to potential energy. The space between the postures is this gathering of potential energy. The next posture begins, like the rubber ball, as your body, in a sense, recovers its shape and springs back into action (kinetic energy).

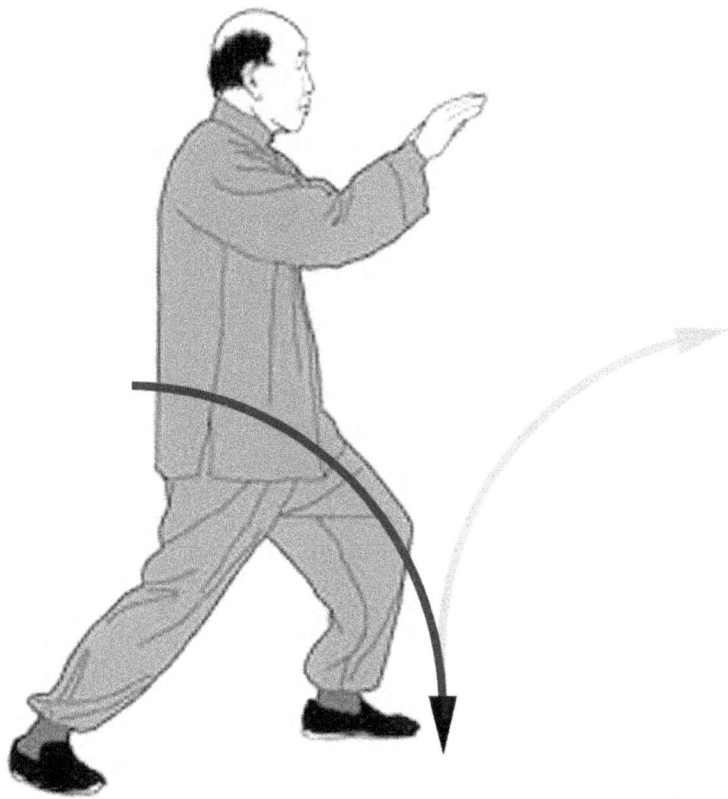

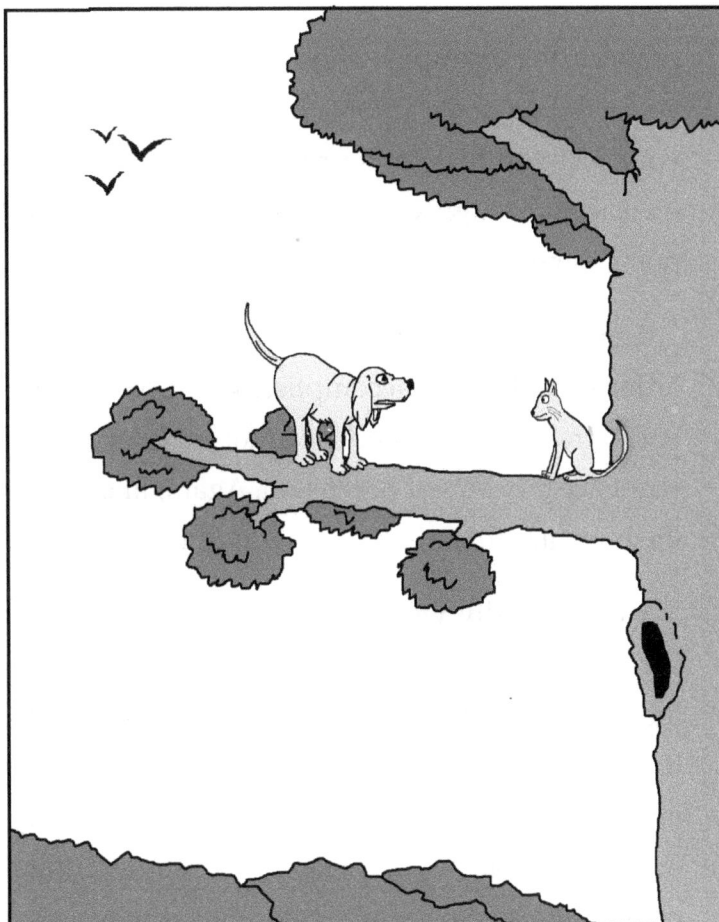

"I'm telling you, it's sheer will."

8 Imagination

The practice and development of Tai Chi is accomplished with the active use of visualization. "Imagination becomes reality" is a quote from the Tai Chi Classics that Liang often cited. He encouraged students to use imagination as an integral part of their practice. For example, when issuing energy through your hands, you will imagine the force coming from the ground up through your feet and legs to your waist where it gathers and emanates (projects) through your arm(s) and out the hand(s) to a focused point somewhere in the distance.

Correctly aligning the movement of your body in the right order is difficult to accomplish. The flow of energy through the body, from feet to hands, cannot be interrupted by any out-of-sequence movement or tension. Again, like the whip, the joints of the body are threaded together without gap.

By repeatedly visualizing this process, you gradually coordinate and train the complex muscular movements involved until they become automatic. This visualization helps students actualize what they are studying, and, at the same time, it trains their minds to lead their actions - not the other way around. Liang comments that, "When beginners practice, this kind of 'imagination' is indistinct and vague, but if they practice over a long period of time, they will be able to use this at will and the 'imagination' will become reality."

Modern-day athletes emphasize visualization techniques as part of their training. The following excerpt from an article on the use of these techniques by Steve J. Ayan (The Will to Win; April 2005; Scientific American Mind) is a good description of this:

> A high jumper must see in her mind exactly each step of her run up and takeoff and then watch her body glide over the bar. In most visualization training, this focus is achieved by learning to see and subsequently control each concrete component of a movement.

Visualization can benefit training too, by helping to transform complex motor procedures into automatic movements. The effects on the body of visualization were demonstrated more than a century ago. In the late 1800s English psychologist William Carpenter discovered that imagining movements could elicit reactions from muscles. When we see a soccer player strike the ball toward that goal, our own leg muscles may contract, imperceptibly if not noticeably. This "ideomotor" effect, with repeated visualization, can make the real motion easier to perform.

More recently, researchers have studied this phenomenon with imaging technologies. Stephen M. Kosslyn, a psychologist at Harvard University, discovered the imaging of movement activates the same motor regions of the cerebral cortex that light up during the actual movement. Most researchers theorize that repeatedly visualizing the movement strengthens or adds synaptic connections among relevant neurons. Some basketball players and coaches, for example, claim that repeatedly visualizing the ideal arm and hand motions for a free throw from the foul line improves players' success rates in actual games: bend the knees, flex the elbow, cock the wrist, then let the ball roll off the fingers.

Tai Chi involves active visualization by the practitioner. Like the basketball player imagining the movements of a free throw, the Tai Chi practitioner will imagine the "issuing" force moving through his limbs, as he directs it to a focused point outside his body. All of his intention then culminates at this single focused point. Liang reserved the last full count of every posture for the expression of this final projection of imagined energy or force. It is then that the posture's intent culminates in the focused action: when the action is funneled to a single point coinciding with that last beat. Your body and weight may shift slightly forward but most of the movement on this count takes place in your mind. This imagined intent will change and vary with each posture and, of course, this always means that the practitioner has to have an understanding of the posture's end use. As practitioners become more experienced, they will vary the intent and direction of their imagined issuing force within any given posture. According to Liang, "you must have a clearly formulated idea of the goal and a perfected technique of achieving it before giving it outward expression."

As the practitioner becomes more advanced, there is less need to focus on the external manifestation of the movements and the practice becomes more about the internal expression of them. Individual postures of the solo form become analogous to the brush strokes of Chinese calligraphy. At times when the calligrapher's brush doesn't completely finish a stroke it creates an empty space for the viewers' imaginationto fill in or complete. Similarly, each Tai Chi posture is not an exact reenactment of a complete martial movement. You will not physically delineate every minute aspect of a posture that you are performing, but will instead, like the Chinese calligrapher, complete it with your mind. By design, a posture is usually a close approximation because the emphasis is often more on the mental intent.

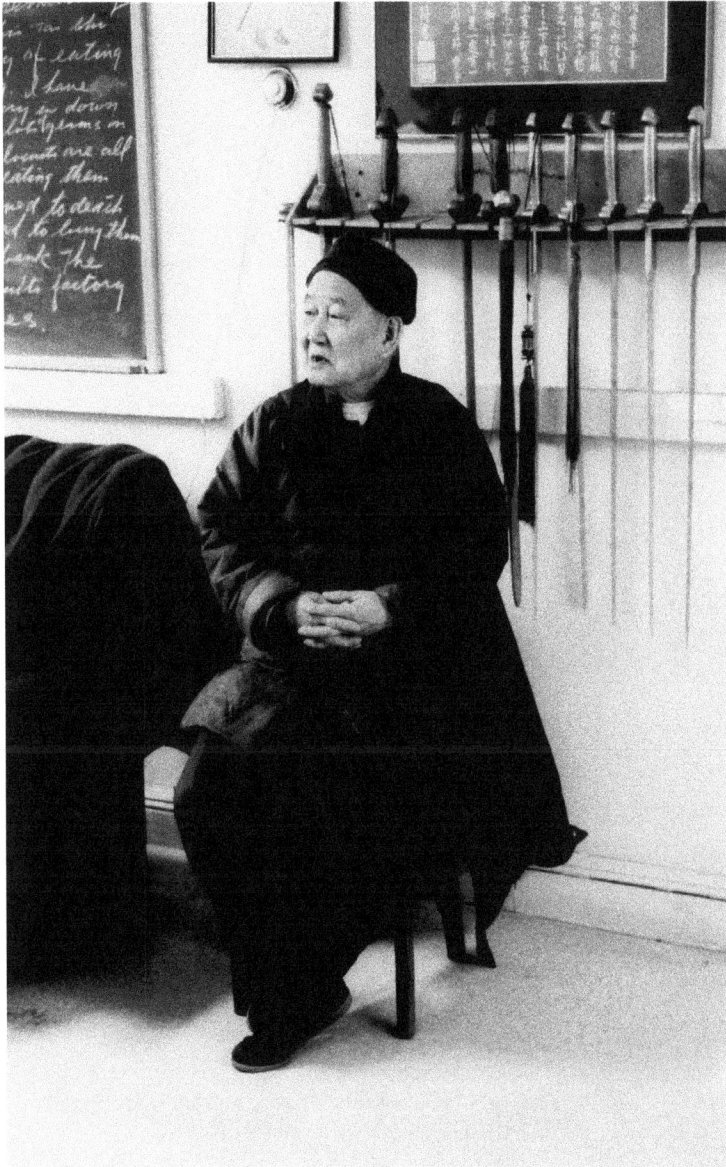

T.T. Liang at our Lincoln St. studio, Boston, MA 1981 (photo by R. Sturtevant)

9

T. T. Liang's
Tai Chi Ch'uan:
Solo Form

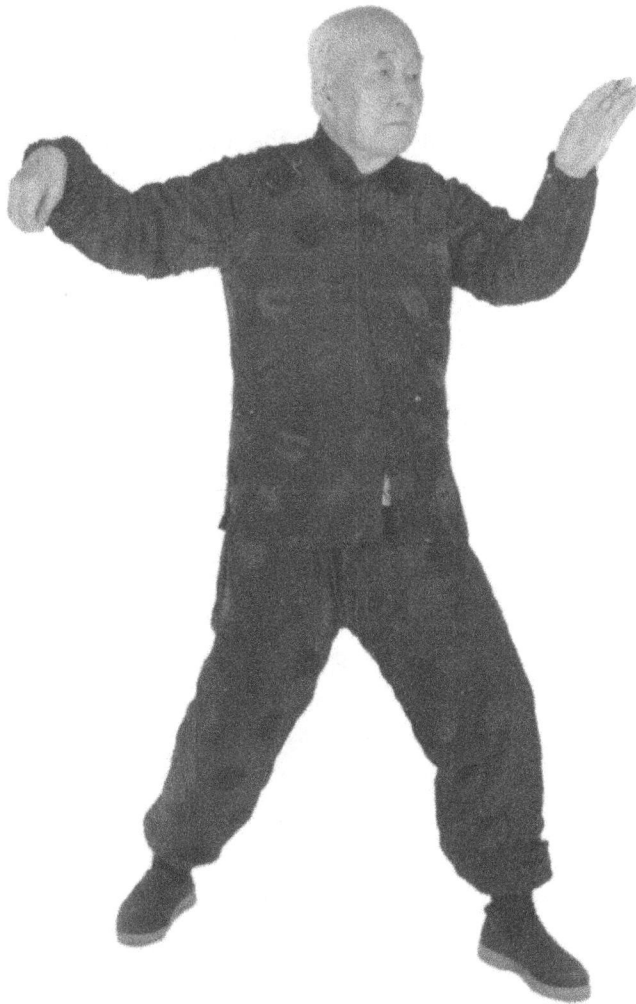

Solo Form - 150 Postures

How to make sense of the following posture descriptions:

Counts: Each posture is divided into 2, 4 or 6 counts depending on its complexity. The movements within each count are explained.

Photographs: For each posture there is a picture at the top of the page of the Tai Chi teacher T.T. Liang demonstrating the completed posture. Running vertically down the right side of the page is a numbered sequence of pictures of a student demonstrating that posture. Each of these pictures corresponds with the same numbered count and its description. The positioning and relationship of the feet, moving downward from picture to picture, is indicated by the vertical lines running though all the images.

View: You should view the photographs as though you are in the photograph yourself. You are on the page looking out (north) and moving accordingly.

Direction: For ease of explanation only, the four cardinal directions of north, south, east and west are used so that you can orient yourself within the 360 degree circle in which you will be performing the Tai Chi postures. Where you are facing when you begin the exercises will become north (whether it actually is or not does not matter). Each movement will be described in relationship to your chosen "north."

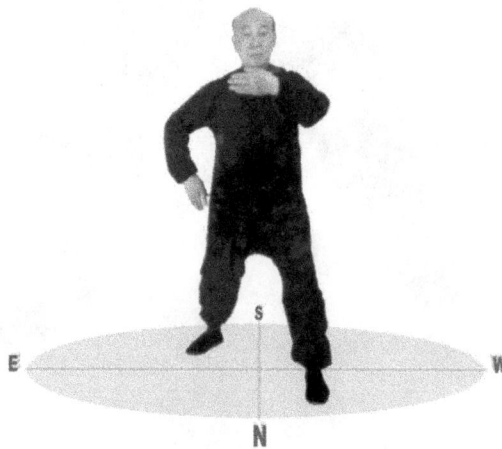

Preparing to begin ...

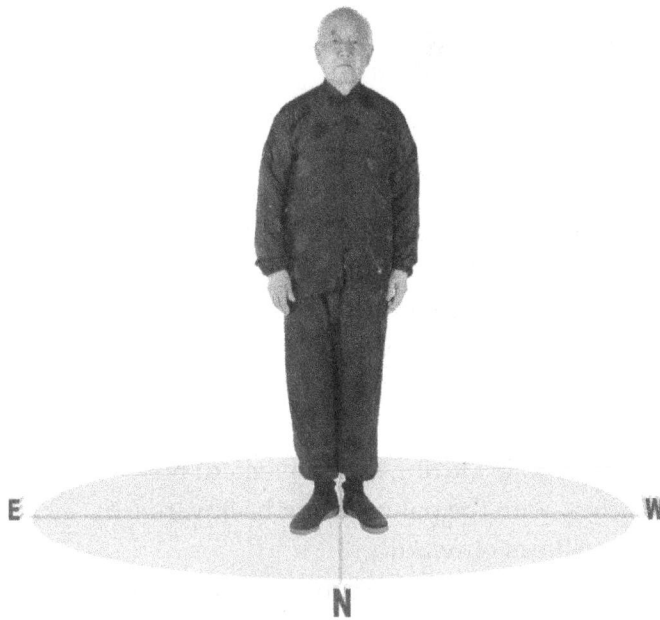

3.

Stand erect facing "north" with your heels touching and your toes apart forming a 90 degree "V." Your arms hang loosely down by your sides with the palms facing in.

1. Preparation

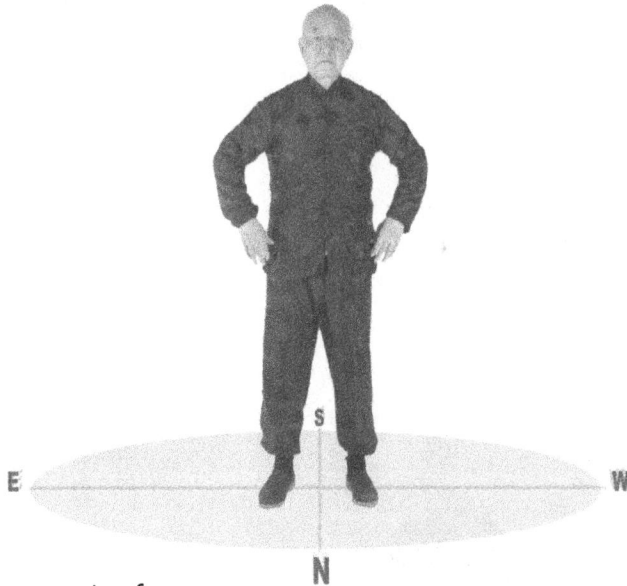

During the counts of:

1. Shift your weight, without leaning, completely onto your right foot. Raise your left foot off the floor and place it sideways to your left about 12 inches. Without shifting any weight onto it*, place your left foot down with the heel landing first and the toes pointing north.

2. Now shift your weight onto it. During this movement raise your hands a few inches, with the palms facing backwards, by slightly bending your elbows outward.
   Pivoting on your right heel, turn your toes inwards to point north. Now shift 50% of your weight back onto your right foot. Your feet are now parallel to each other and the toes are pointing north with approximately a shoulders' width between them. During the duration of this posture the hands rise up to about pocket level - at the hip bones.**

*All stepping movements in Tai Chi should be performed with this clarity of shifting your weight fully from foot to foot.

** This position of the hands next to the hips will be referred to in upcoming postures as the "position of attention."

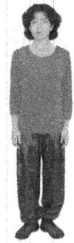

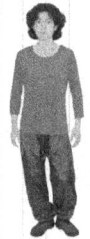

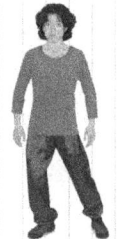

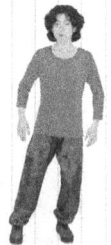

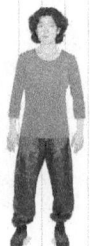

1.

2.

2. Beginning

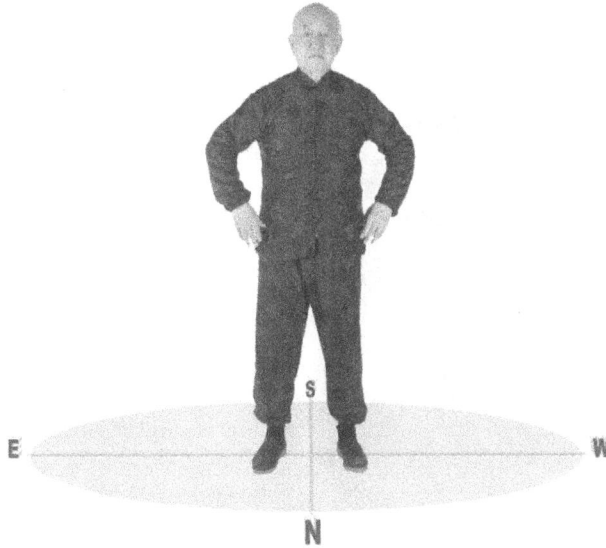

During the counts of:

1. Raise your arms, without bending your elbows or raising your shoulders, forward and upwards to the height of your shoulders. Keep your wrists bent and your fingers hanging down.

2. Straighten out the hands so that the fingers point forward to the north.

3. Draw your hands back towards your upper chest and let your elbows drop down.

4. Without lifting your elbows, raise your hands slightly upward (as though a puff of wind is lifting them upward).

5. Lower your hands straight down till the arms are by your sides with the hands opposite your thighs, palms facing backward.

6. Raise your hands back to the starting "position of attention" by bending the elbows slightly outward. Be careful not to raise your shoulders while raising the hands. Your back is straight, your head erect and your gaze is focused as though viewing a distant horizon.

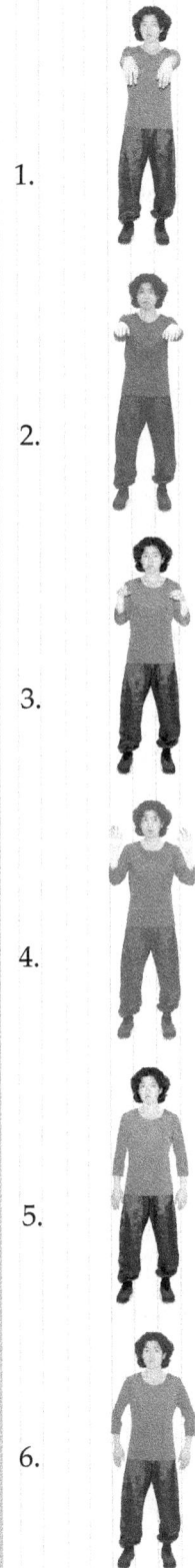

1.

2.

3.

4.

5.

6.

3. Ward Off Left

During the counts of:

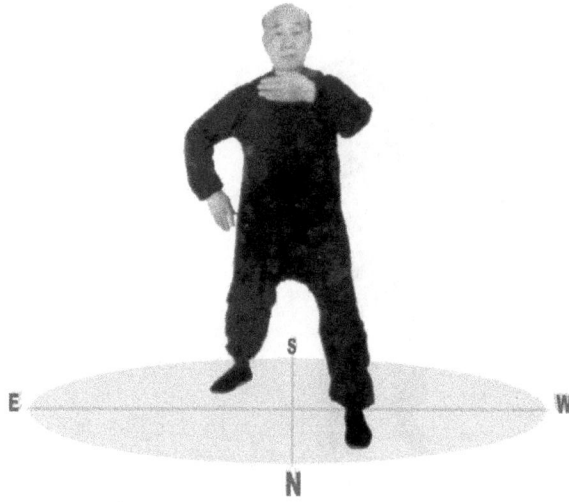

1. | Keeping your back straight, shift your weight to your left leg and turn your torso 45 degrees to your right.

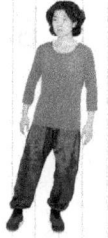

2. | Continue turning your torso to the right until it is facing east. Your right foot simultaneously turns, pivoting on the heel, to point east as well. The hands during these 2 counts come into a position of holding an imaginary beach ball in front of your torso. Your left hand is on the bottom with its palm facing up and your right hand is on the top with its palm facing down. Your arms and elbows are relaxed.

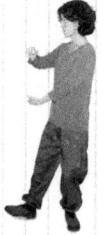

3. | Shift 75% of your weight towards the east onto your right foot.

4. | Shifting your weight 100% onto your right foot, turn your torso 45 degrees to the left to face northeast and simultaneously pivot on your left toes so that they point to the northwest.

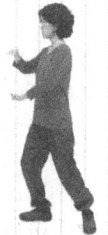

5. | Step forward to the north with your left foot, placing the heel down in front of where the toes were and point the toes to the north. Shifting your weight 60% onto the left leg, turn your torso to face north and bring your right hand down to the "position of attention" next to your right hip. Simultaneously bring your left hand up into a "ward off" position with your palm facing inward and opposite your neck. With the turning of your torso to face north, turn your right foot, pivoting on your heel, so the toes point to the northeast.

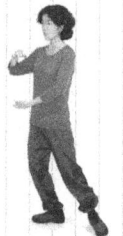

6. | Complete the positioning of your legs and feet (called a "bow and arrow" stance) by shifting an additional 10% of your weight (a total of 70%) onto your left foot. At the same time, using your whole body, ward off with the back of your left hand. Your left elbow remains relaxed and down.

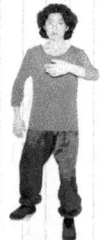

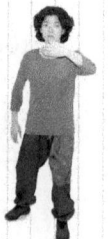

4. Ward Off Right

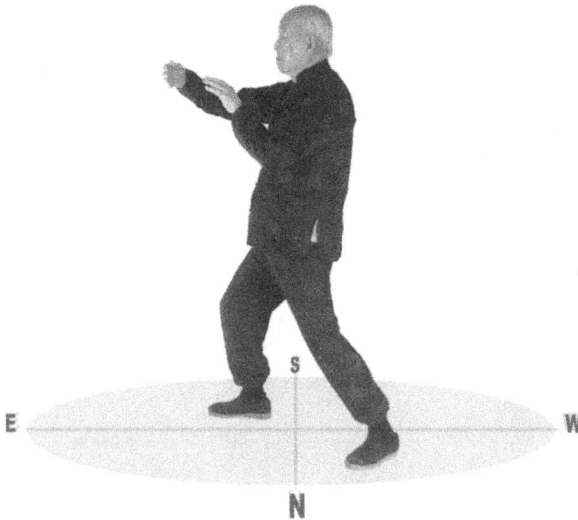

During the counts of:

1. | Shift all of your weight to your left leg while turning your torso to face northeast.

2. | Pivot on your right toes and turn your palms so that they face each other and ...

3. | ... step forward with your right foot to the east into a bow and arrow stance. Shift your weight 60% onto your right leg as you turn your torso to face east. Simultaneously pivot on your left heel, turning your left foot inward 45 degrees so the toes are pointing to the northeast. During this count, bring your right hand up in front of your neck with the palm facing in. Your left hand faces your right palm, as if holding an imaginary small ball. Your right arm remains rounded out and your left elbow is lowered.

4. | Complete the bow and arrow stance facing east by shifting an additional 10% of your weight onto your right foot. At the same time, using your whole body, push forward with the back of your right hand, both elbows remaining slightly bent.

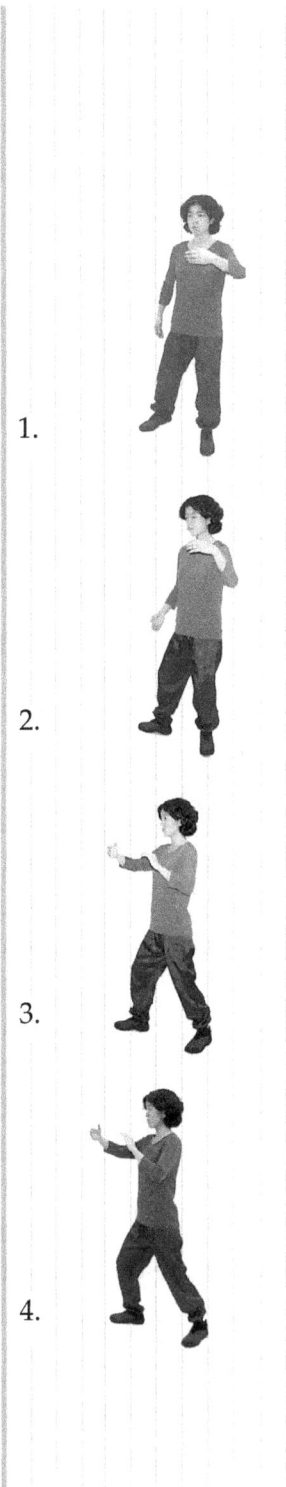

1.

2.

3.

4.

5. Roll Back

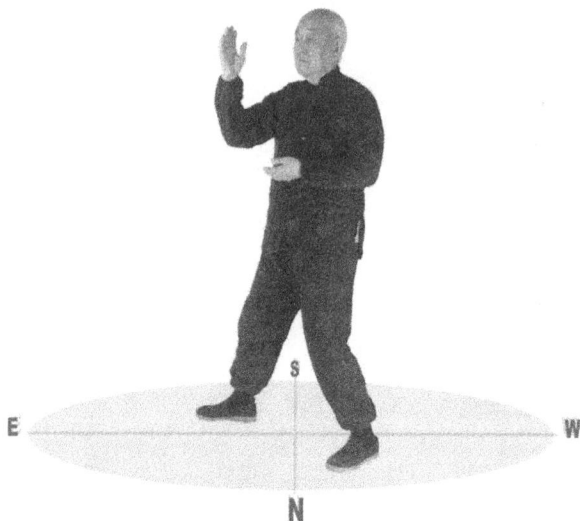

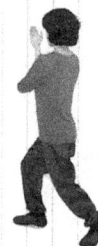

1.

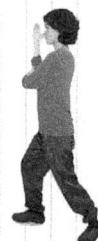

2.

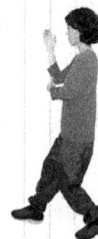

3.

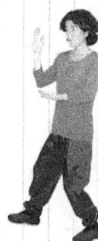

4.

During the counts of:

1. | Turn your torso to the right 45 degrees and bring your right forearm up into a 90 degree angle, perpendicular to your body. At the same time bring your left forearm across in front of the chest with your left palm facing in and the fingers almost touching your right elbow.

2. | Keeping your weight on the right foot, turn your upper torso back to the left 45 degrees to face east. Your waist, upper body, arms and hands move together as one unit.

3. | With your torso facing straight ahead to the east, withdraw your weight back onto your left foot.

4. | Turn your torso to the left 45 degrees to face northeast. At the same time turn your left palm upwards.

6. Press

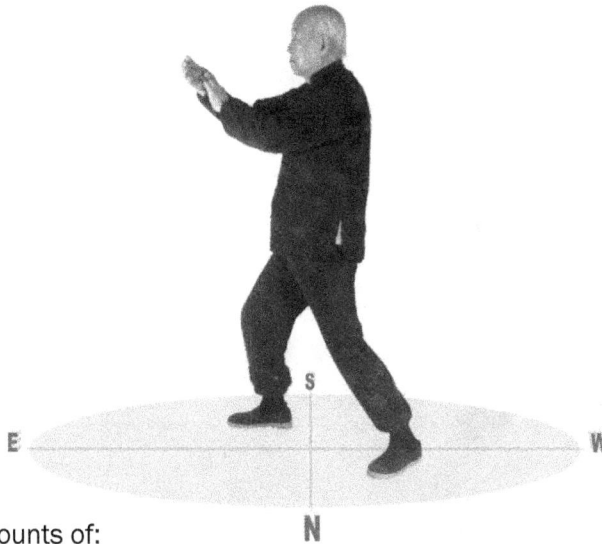

During the counts of:

1. Turn your torso 45 degrees to your left to face north. With the momentum of this turn let your left hand drop down and circle around (without lifting the elbow), heading up toward your left ear.

2. As your left hand is passing by your ear, turn your torso back 90 degrees to your right to face east and lightly attach your left fingers to the inside of your right wrist (as though you're feeling your pulse). Your right forearm drops slightly down into a diagonal position in front of your upper chest with the left elbow lowered.

3. Without letting your hands and arms move separately from your body, shift your weight onto the right leg and press forward with your right forearm. It's important here to move your whole body as one unit and not let your hands and arms move independently or initiate any movement.

4. Continue to press forward and slightly upwards until your right leg bears about 70% of your weight.

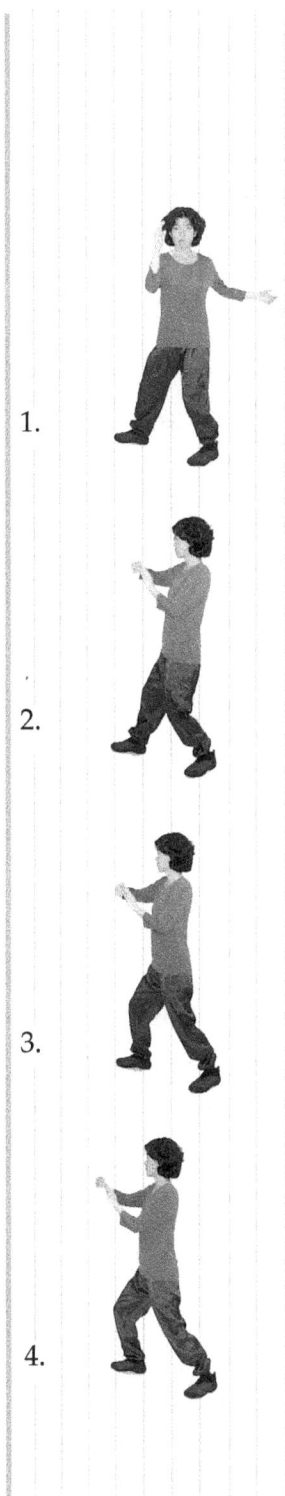

7. Push

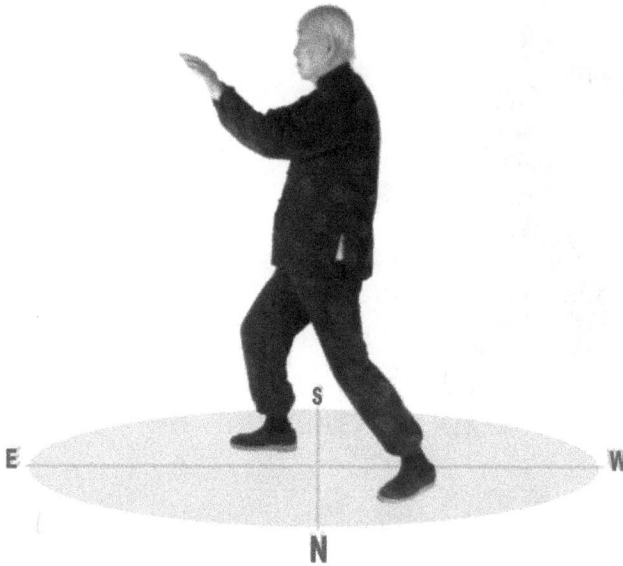

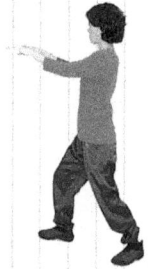

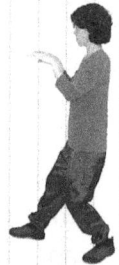

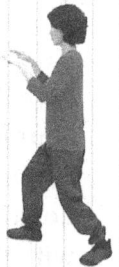

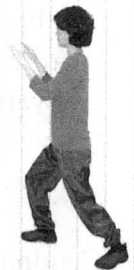

During the counts of:

1. | Separate your hands, palms down, at the level of your shoulders.

2. | Keeping your back straight, shift your weight back onto your left leg and simultaneously withdraw your hands slightly towards your upper chest. The fingers of both hands point forward and the elbows remain relaxed and bent downwards.

3 | Without moving your hands and arms separately from your body, shift 60% of your weight onto your right leg again. The push is coming from the forward movement of your whole body - not your arms.

4. | Complete the bow and arrow stance by shifting about 10% more of your weight into your right foot. At the same time slightly raise your fingertips so that the intention of the push is coming through your palms and directed to the east.

1.

2.

3.

4.

8. Single Whip

During the counts of:

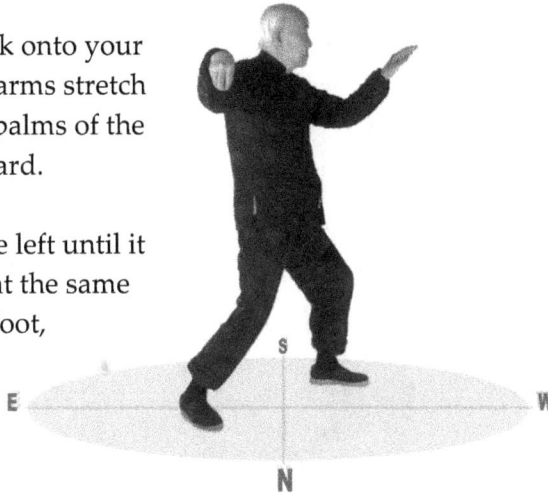

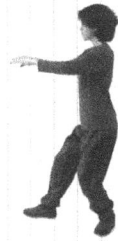

1. Shift your weight back onto your left foot and let your arms stretch out slightly with the palms of the hands facing downward.

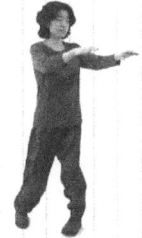

2. Turn your torso to the left until it faces northwest and at the same time turn your right foot, pivoting on the heel, so that the toes point north.

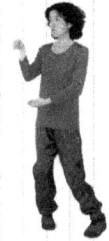

3. Shift your weight back to your right leg as you turn your torso to face northeast. Simultaneously withdraw both hands. The left hand comes down opposite the navel with its palm up and the right hand forms a "hook" (all 5 digits are touching at the tips and pointing downward) near your right armpit.

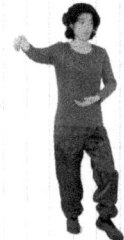

4. Turn your torso counterclockwise back to the northwest corner. With this movement strike to the northeast corner with your right hand "hook" and simultaneously pivot the left foot on the toes to point northwest.

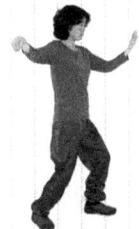

5. Continue to turn your torso to face west and step with your left foot, heel first, so as to form a shoulders' width stance facing west with 60% of your weight on your left foot. The movement of your torso brings your left hand, palm facing in, up in front of your body at face level. At the same time let this movement turn your right foot, pivoting on the heel, to point northwest. The right hand "hook" does not move.

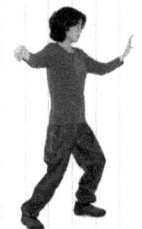

6. Complete the bow and arrow stance facing west by shifting 10% more of your weight onto your left foot. At the same time turn your left hand palm outward being careful to leave your arm slightly bent. Your eyes gaze over and past the fingertips.

9. Lifting Hands

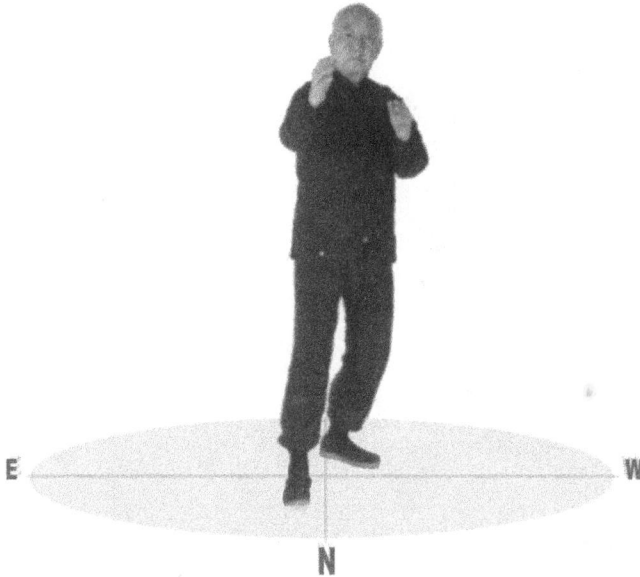

During the counts of:

1. Shift your weight all the way onto your left leg and turn
   your right foot, pivoting on the toes, to point northeast.
   Simultaneously turn your palms slightly inwards so that
   they face each other.

2. Bring your right foot to the north in front of your
   body and place it heel down, with the toes slightly off
   the ground, about 12 inches in front (to the north of)
   your left heel. Your right leg remains slightly bent. At
   the same time bring your arms together horizontally,
   without dropping them down, so that your right arm,
   with the elbow slightly bent, is aligned over your right
   leg. Your left hand comes over opposite the inside of
   your right elbow - leaving about 10" between them.

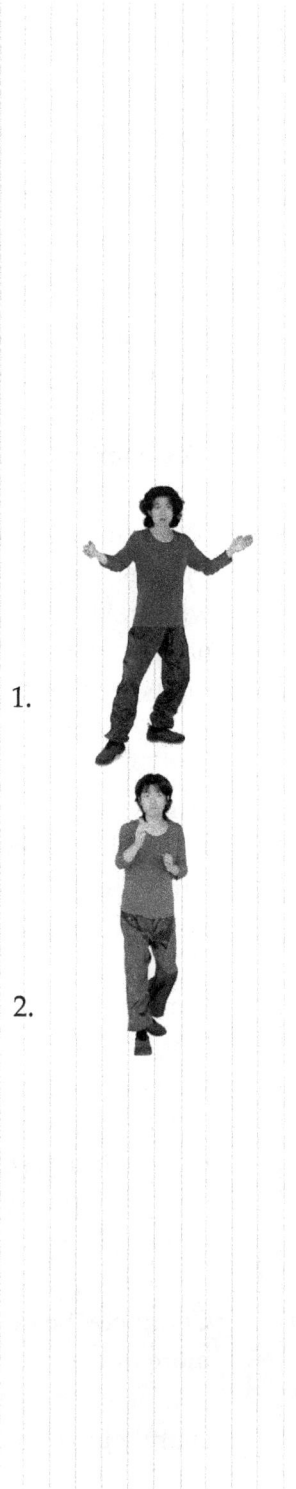

10. Shoulder Stroke

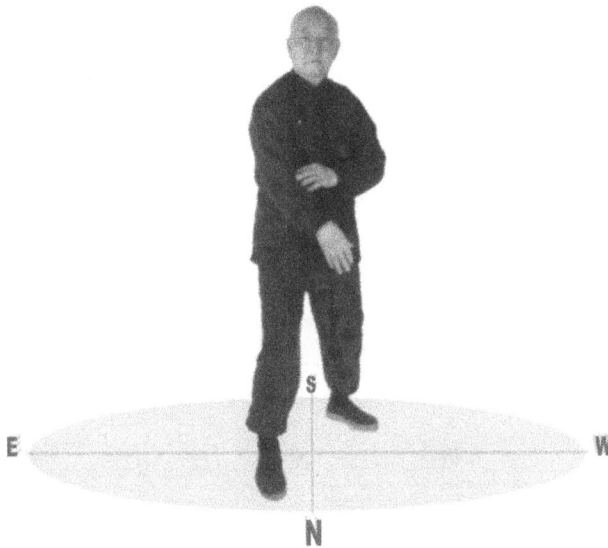

During the counts of:

1. Withdraw your right foot and place it down, heel up, toes touching the ground, directly in front of your left heel. At the same time, bring your arms down. Your right hand drops to the side of your right thigh with its palm facing backward toward the groin. Your left hand comes down with its palm facing the right palm. Your torso faces northwest.

2. Turn your torso to face north and step forward with your right foot (heel touching first and toes pointing very slightly to the northwest). Lightly adhere with your left fingers to the inside of your right forearm and simultaneously shift your weight about 70% forward onto your right foot, striking forward with your right shoulder and side.

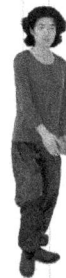

1.

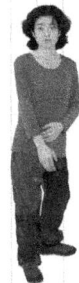

2.

11. White Crane Spreading Wings

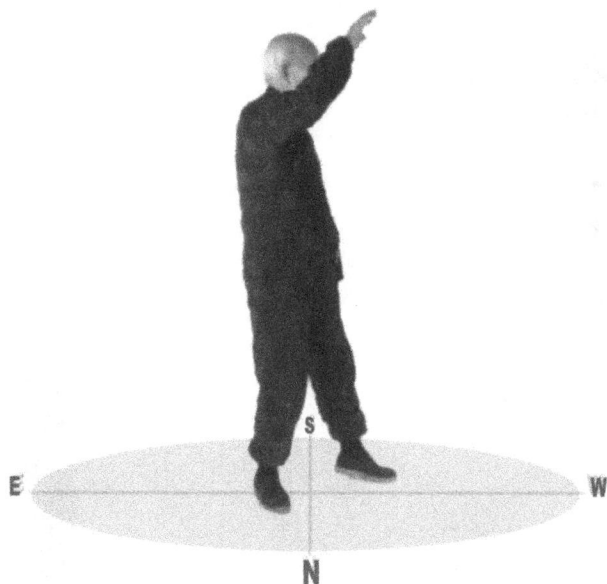

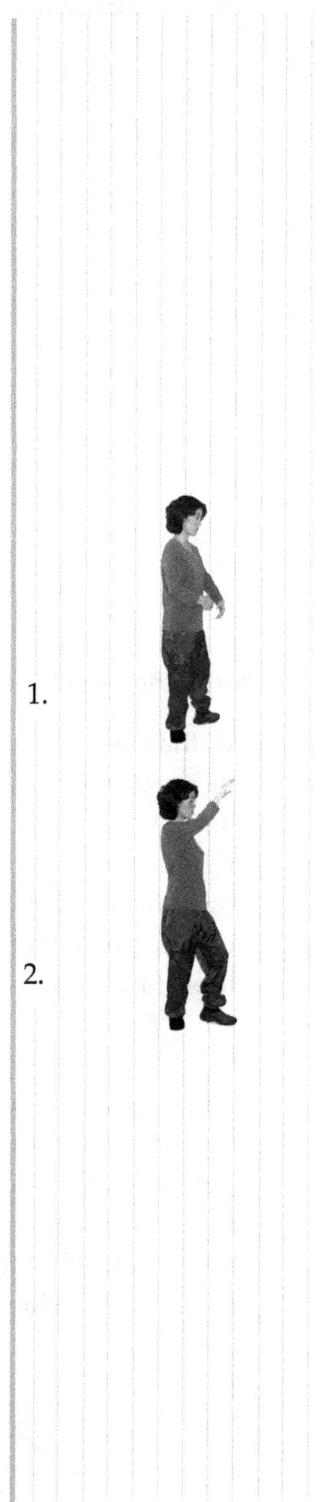

During the counts of:

1. | Shift your weight to your right foot as you turn your torso to face west, letting your left foot pivot on the toes to point southwest.

2. | Raise your body by straightening out your right leg. At the same time bring your left foot forward and place it toes down, heel up, in front of your right heel. Using this upward momentum, let your right arm come underneath your left and raise it up above your forehead, in a screw motion, to face angled diagonally outwards, elbow down. Your left hand simultaneously comes to the "position of attention" beside your left hip, palm facing backward.

12. Step Forward and Brush Knee (left)

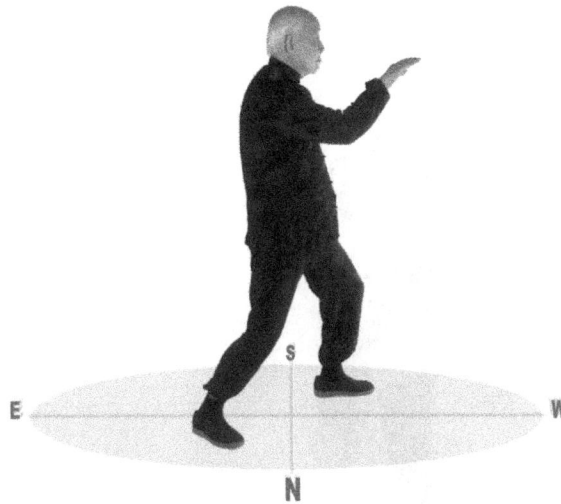

During the counts of:

1. Lower your body by bending your right knee and turn your torso slightly to the right. At the same time turn your right hand palm up to face you and let it begin to drop down in a counterclockwise motion.

2. Continue to turn your torso to the right until it is facing northwest (45 degrees) let your right hand continue its counter-clockwise motion until it comes full circle to your right ear with the fingers pointing towards the west and the elbow bent and hanging downwards. During this turning motion of your torso your left hand rises up into a "ward off" position opposite your chest with the fingers pointing north.

3. Step with your left foot, heel first to the southwest, so as to form a shoulders' width stance facing west. Turn your torso to face west. In conjunction with this turn brush your left knee with your left hand (fingertips) and let it come to rest in the "position of attention" by your left hip pocket. Your right foot, pivoting on the heel, turns in 45 degrees to point northwest and your weight is now 60% forward on your left foot.

4. Complete the bow and arrow stance facing west by shifting 10% more of your weight into your left foot. At the same, time using your whole body, push forward with your right hand, elbow slightly bent.

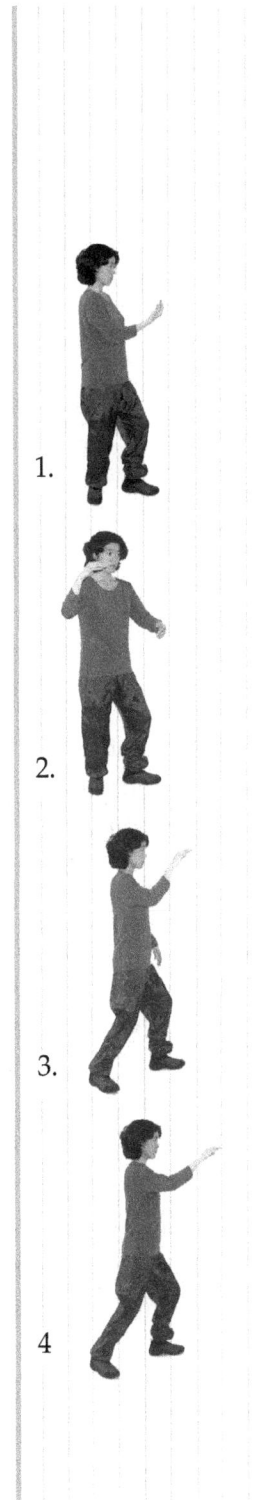

13. Play Guitar

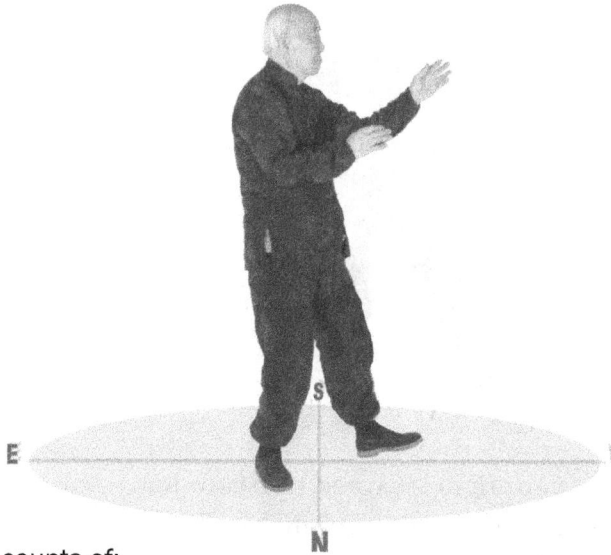

During the counts of:

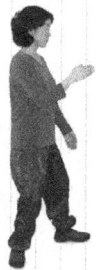

1. | Shift your weight all the way forward onto your left leg and pick up your right foot. Turn it out 45 degrees to the right so that the toes are pointing north and place it back down (approximately in the same place).

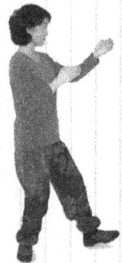

2. | Shift your entire weight onto your right foot and pick up your left foot, bringing it sideways to the right and place it down on the heel in line with your right heel. At the same time your arms create a scissors-like action with your left hand coming up and your right hand, palm facing south, coming down to a position opposite your left elbow. Your left palm faces north with the fingers pointing west in line with your mouth and the left elbow remains slightly bent. This position simulates playing a harp (or the Chinese intrument called the bipa).

14. Step Forward and Brush Knee (left)

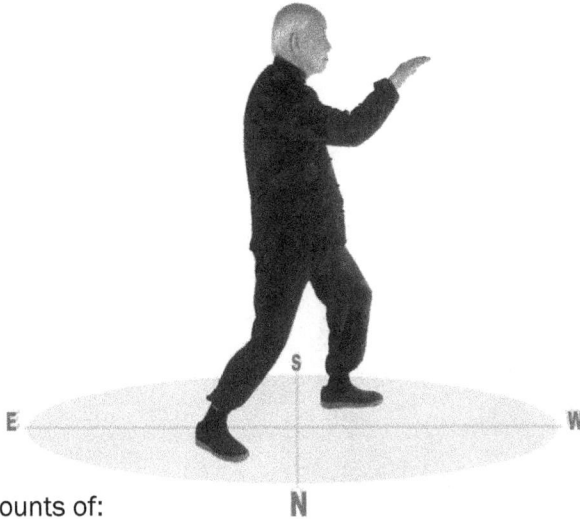

During the counts of:

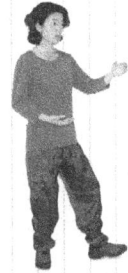

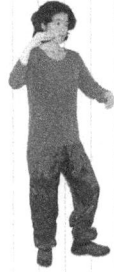

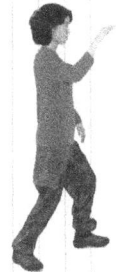

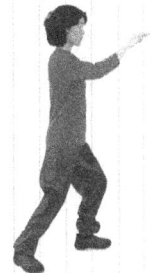

1. | Turn your torso slightly to the right and at the same time turn your right hand palm up, and let it begin to drop down in a counterclockwise motion.

2. | Continue to turn your torso to the right until it is facing northwest (45 degrees) with your right hand continuing its counterclockwise motion until it comes full circle to your right ear with the fingers pointing towards the west and the elbow bent and hanging downwards. During this turning motion of your torso your left hand lowers into a "ward off" position opposite your chest with the fingers pointing north.

3. | Step with your left foot, heel first to the west, so as to form a shoulders' width stance facing west. As you turn your torso to face west brush your left knee with your left hand and let it come to rest in the "position of attention" by your left hip pocket. Your right foot, pivoting on the heel, turns in 45 degrees to point northwest and your weight is now 60% forward on your left leg.

4. | Complete the bow and arrow stance facing west by shifting 10% more of your weight into your left foot. At the same time using your whole body, push forward with your right hand being careful to let your elbow remain relaxed and slightly bent.

15. Step Forward and Brush Knee (right)

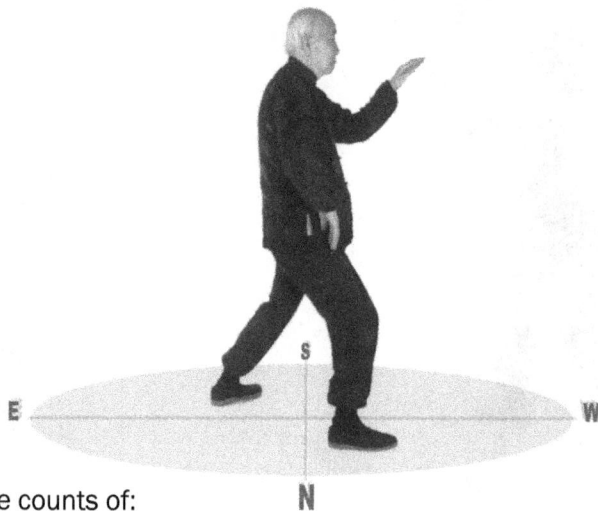

During the counts of:

1. Shifting your weight back onto your right leg, turn your torso slightly to the left and at the same time turn your left hand palm up, and let it begin to circle up in a counterclockwise motion.

2. Continue to turn your torso to the left until it is facing southwest (45 degrees) and turn the left foot, pivoting on your heel, to point almost to the south. Your left hand continues its counterclockwise motion until it comes full circle to your left ear with the fingers pointing towards the west and the elbow bent and hanging downwards. During this turning motion of your torso your right hand lowers into a "ward off" position opposite your chest with the fingers pointing south.

3. Step with your right foot, heel first to the west, so as to form a shoulders' width stance facing west. As you turn your torso to face west brush your right knee with your right hand and let it come to rest in the "position of attention" by your right hip pocket. Your left foot, pivoting on the heel, turns in 45 degrees to point southwest and your weight is now 60% forward on your right leg.

4. Complete the bow and arrow stance facing west by shifting 10% more of your weight into your left foot. At the same time using your whole body, push forward with your right hand being careful to let your elbow remain relaxed and slightly bent.

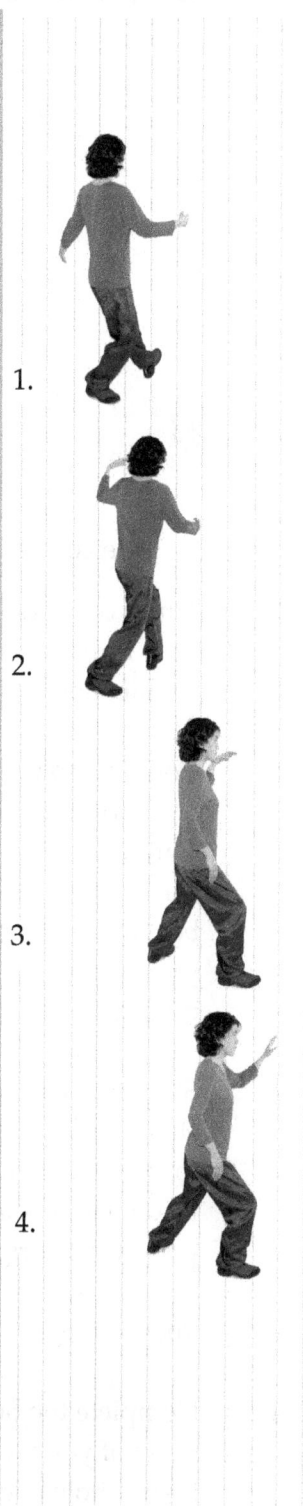

16. Step forward and Brush Knee (left)

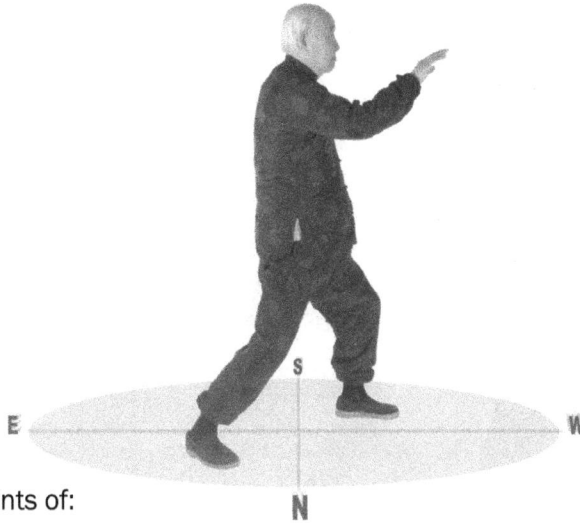

During the counts of:

1. Shifting your weight back onto your left leg, turn your torso slightly to the right and raise the toes of your right foot slightly. At the same time turn your right hand palm up, and let it begin to circle up in a counterclockwise motion.

2. Continue to turn your torso to the right until it is facing northwest (45 degrees) and turn the right foot, pivoting on your heel, to point almost to the north. Your right hand continues its counterclockwise motion until it comes full circle to your right ear with the fingers pointing towards the west and the elbow bent and hanging downwards. During this turning motion of your torso your left hand lowers into a "ward off" position opposite your chest with the fingers pointing north.

3. Step with your left foot, heel first to the west, so as to form a shoulders' width stance facing west. As you turn your torso to face west brush your left knee with your left hand and let it come to rest in the "position of attention" by your left hip pocket. Your right foot, pivoting on the heel, turns in 45 degrees to point northwest and your weight is now 60% forward on your left leg.

4. Complete the bow and arrow stance facing west by shifting 10% more of your weight into your left foot. At the same time using your whole body, push forward with your right hand, elbow slightly bent.

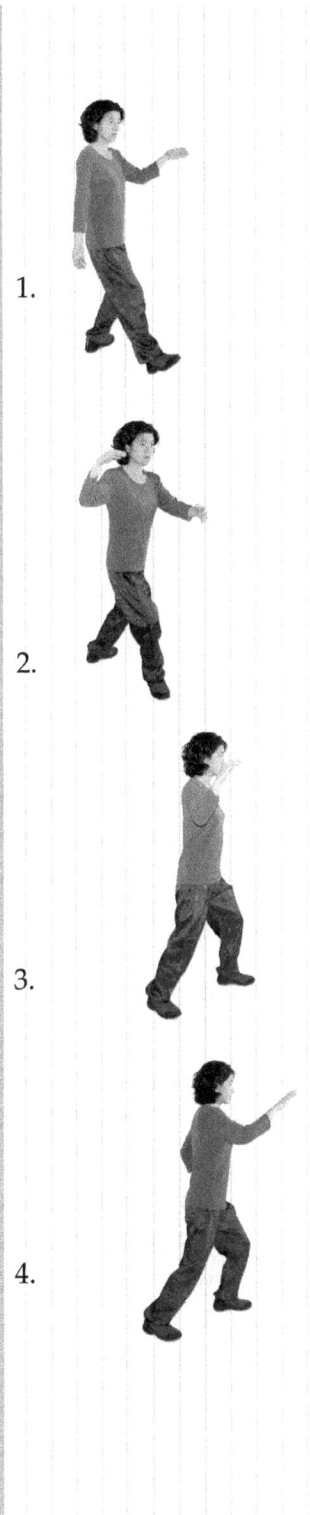

17. Play Guitar

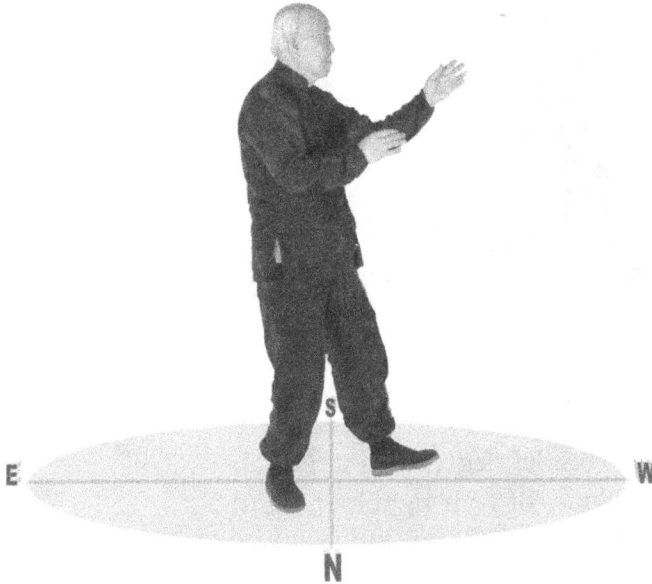

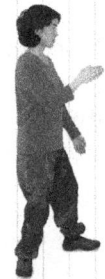

1.

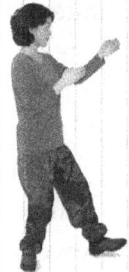

2.

During the counts of:

1. Shift your weight all the way forward onto your left leg and pick up your right foot. Turn it out 45 degrees to the right so that the toes are pointing north and place it back down (approximately in the same place).

2. Shift your entire weight onto your right foot and pick up your left foot, bringing it sideways to the right and place it down on the heel in line with your right heel. At the same time your arms create a scissors-like action with your left hand coming up and your right hand, palm facing south, coming down to a position opposite your left elbow. Your left palm faces north with the fingers pointing west in line with your mouth and the left elbow remains slightly bent. This position simulates playing a harp (or the Chinese intrument called the pipa).

18. Step Forward and Brush Knee (left)

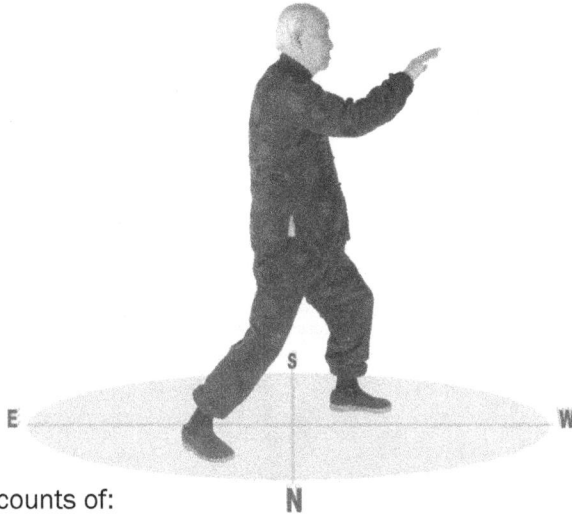

During the counts of:

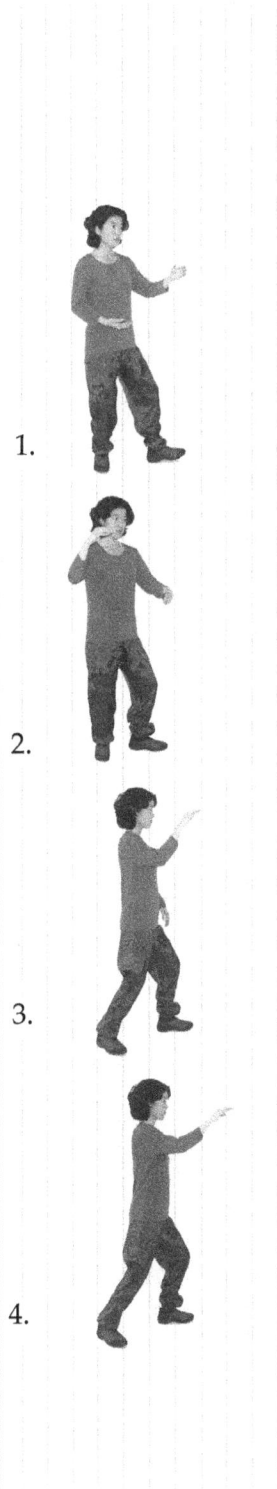

1. | Turn your torso slightly to the right and at the same time turn your right hand palm up, and let it begin to drop down in a counterclockwise motion.

2. | Continue to turn your torso to the right until it is facing northwest (45 degrees) with your right hand continuing its counterclockwise motion until it comes full circle to your right ear with the fingers pointing towards the west and the elbow bent and hanging downwards. During this turning motion of your torso your left hand lowers into a "ward off" position opposite your chest with the fingers pointing north.

3. | Step with your left foot, heel first to the west, so as to form a shoulders' width stance facing west. As you turn your torso to face west brush your left knee with your left hand and let it come to rest in the "position of attention" by your left hip pocket. Your right foot, pivoting on the heel, turns in 45 degrees to point northwest and your weight is now 60% forward on your left leg.

4. | Complete the bow and arrow stance facing west by shifting 10% more of your weight into your left foot. At the same time using your whole body, push forward with your right hand being careful to let your elbow remain relaxed and slightly bent.

19. Chop with Fist

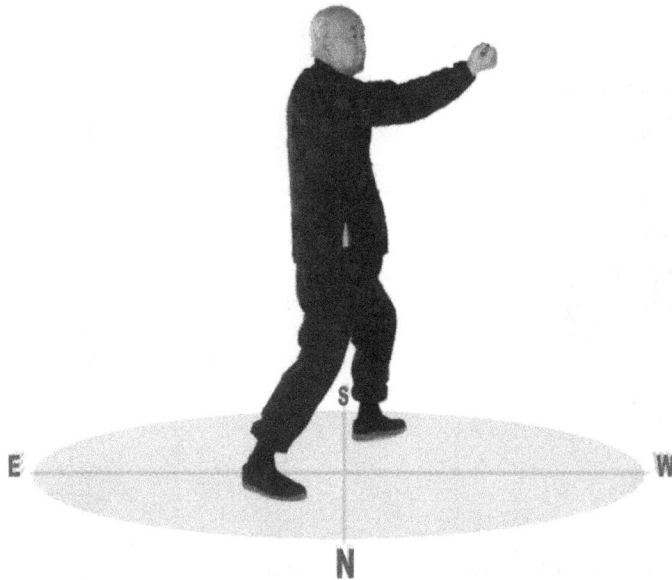

During the counts of:

1. Draw your body back onto your right foot and turn your torso and left foot, pivoting on your heel, to point southwest. At the same time both hands, palms down, swing back so the fingers point southeast.

2. Shift your weight about 70% onto your left foot. When your weight becomes more than 50% on your left leg turn your torso to face northwest. Use this turning motion to chop with the back of your right fist, in an overhand arch, to the northwest corner at about eye level (as though you are chopping to the bridge of the nose of your imaginary opponent).

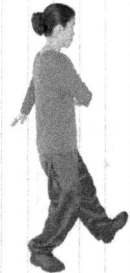

1.

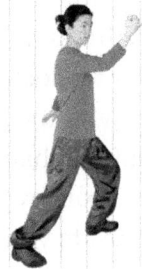

2.

20. Step Forward, Deflect Downward, Intercept and Punch

1. Shift your weight back onto your right foot and turn your torso to face southwest. At the same time extend both hands at waist level to the southwest. Your palms are facing each other as though holding a ball.

2. Shift your weight forward onto your left foot.

3. Turning your waist to the west, raise your right foot and step forward diagonally to the right. At the same time make a fist with your right hand and circle it clockwise around to the right side of your waist and attach it to your right hip, palm side facing up. In unison with this motion your left hand circles clockwise upward and forward in front of your face. Your left elbow remains relaxed and down.

4. Facing west, shift your weight to your right foot (toes pointing to the north/northwest) and simultaneously bring your left hand forward, deflecting downward to the level of your stomach, palm facing the floor.

5. Step directly forward, to maintain a shoulders' width stance, with your left foot and shift 60% of your weight onto it. At the same time extend or intercept with your left hand forward and to the left. The left hand is open with the fingers pointing west and the palm is facing north. With this motion your right foot turns inwards, pivoting on the heel, so that the toes are pointing northwest.

6. Complete the bow and arrow stance facing west by shifting 10% more of your weight into your left foot. At the same time, using your whole body (not just your arm), punch forward with your right fist, "tiger's mouth" (the space between your thumb and forfinger) facing up. As your right hand is punching forward, let your left hand come over and cover the inner wrist of your right hand.

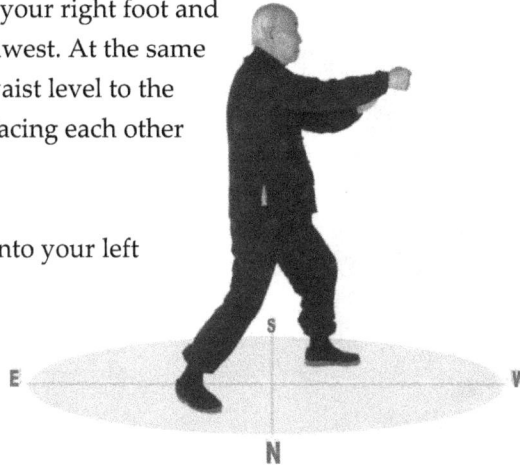

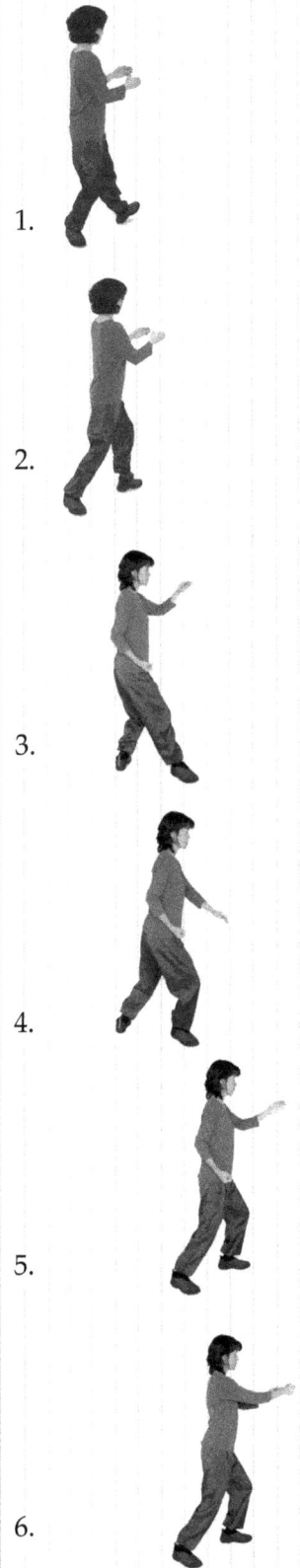

21. Withdraw and Push

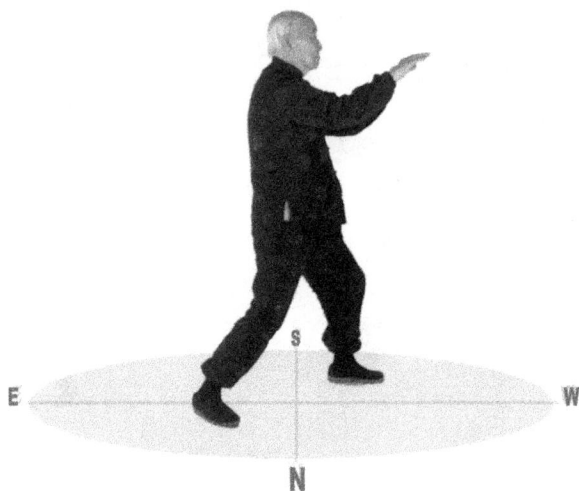

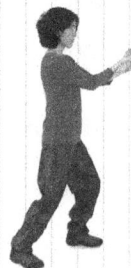

1.

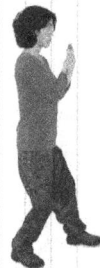

2.

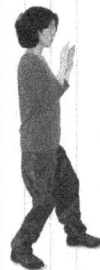

3.

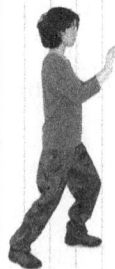

4.

During the counts of:

1. | Slide your left hand, palm up, under your right wrist and open the right fist so that both palms are now open and facing upwards with your hands crossed at the wrists.

2. | Shift your weight back onto your right foot and draw both hands back with your palms facing your chest. Separate your hands ...

3. | ... and then turn both palms outward to face west. Without moving your hands and arms separately from your body, push forward by shifting your weight forward onto your left leg. The push is coming from the forward movement of your body - not your arms.

4. | Complete the bow and arrow stance by shifting an additional 10% of your weight into your left foot. At the same time slightly raise your fingertips so that the intention of the push is coming from your palms.

22. Crossing Hands

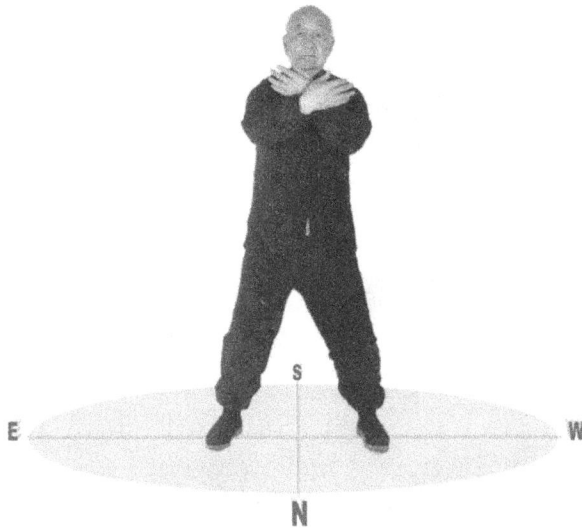

During the counts of:

1. Keep your back straight and shift your weight back onto your right leg, and as you do this, let your arms straighten out.

2. Turn your torso to face north and, bending at your elbows, circle your hands in front of your face with both palms facing out to the north. Your right hand is slightly higher than your left.

3. Shift your weight back onto your left foot and circle both hands out and down.

4. Step back with your right foot and place it down a shoulders' width distance from your left foot and parallel to it. At the same time bring your hands (your right hand outside the left) up in front of your face, crossing them at the wrists with both palms facing to the south. Your eyes gaze just over the fingertips. Your weight shifts slightly more than 50% onto your left leg.

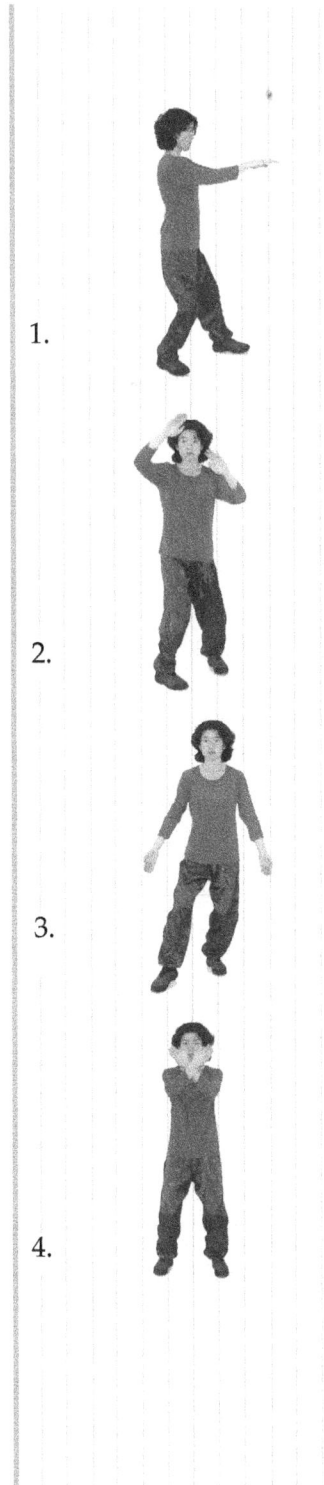

1.

2.

3.

4.

23. Embrace the Tiger to Return to the Mountain

During the counts of:

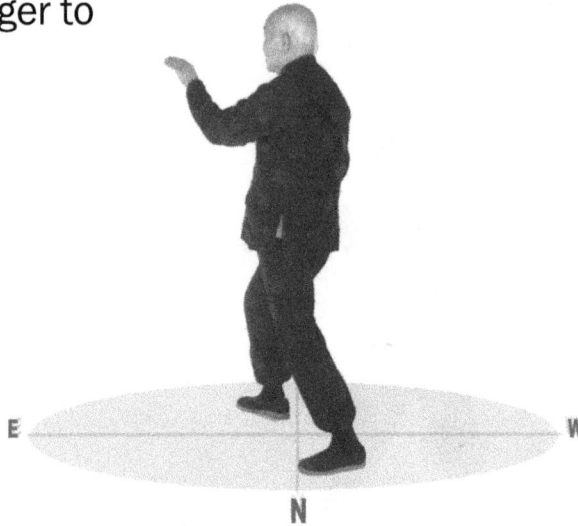

1. Turn your torso clockwise to your right to face northeast. Keep your wrists crossed and lower your hands parallel to the ground while turning your right hand palm down and leaving your left hand palm up. At the same time turn your right foot, pivoting on the toes, to point notheast.

2. Pick your right foot up and step to the southeast corner. At the same time separate your hands. Your right hand (palm facing down) moves to the southeast corner together with your right foot. Your left hand moves back to the north with the palm facing up.

3. Place your right foot, heel down first, in a shoulders' width stance facing southeast. As you shift 60% of your weight onto it, withdraw your right hand, turning your palm to face upwards, beside your right thigh. Circle your left hand, palm up, in a clockwise motiontowards your left ear with palm and fingers facing forward and the elbow lowered. Turn your torso to face southeast and at the same time turn your left foot clockwise, pivoting on the heel, to point east.

4. Complete the bow and arrow stance facing southeast by shifting 10% more of your weight into your right foot. In conjunction with this shifting of your weight, use your whole body to push forward with your left hand. The left elbow remains slightly bent with the fingers pointing forward and diagonally upward.

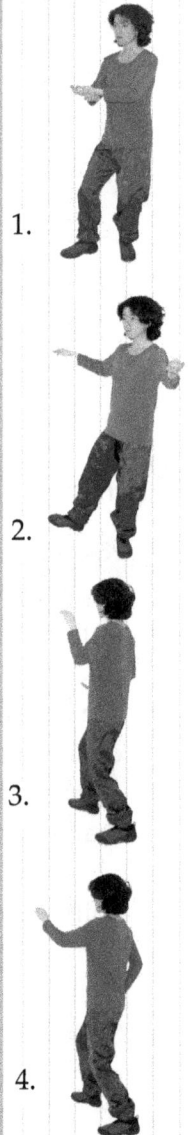

24. Roll Back

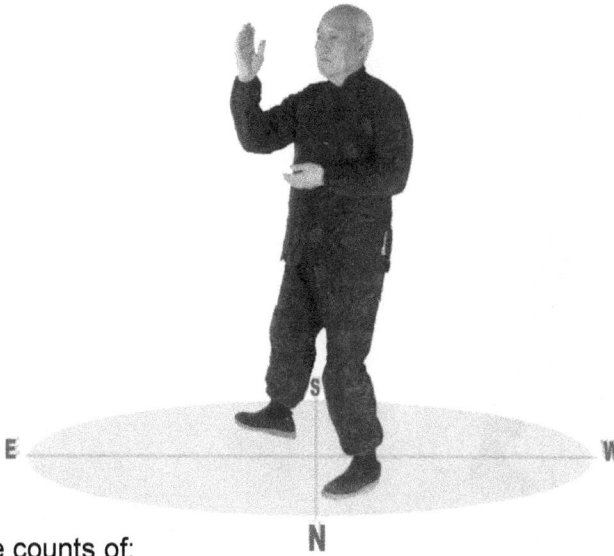

During the counts of:

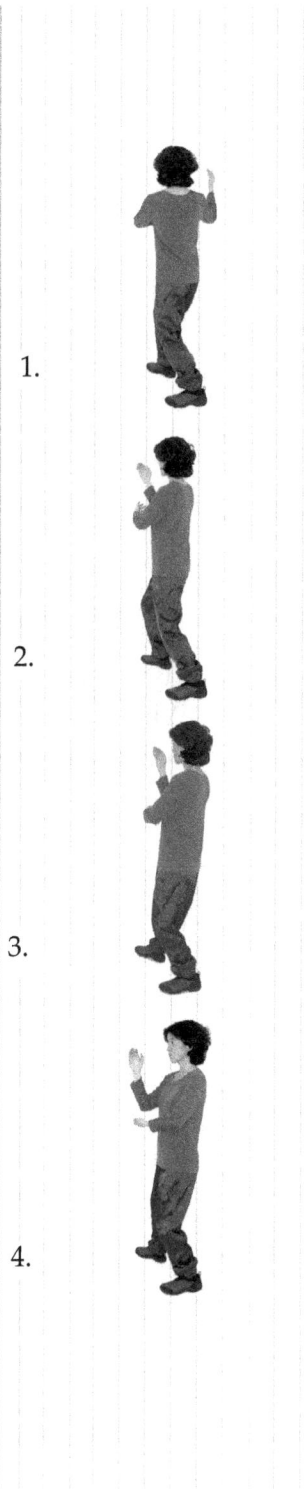

1.   Turn your torso to your right 45 degrees and bring your right forearm up virtically and perpendicular to your body. At the same time bring your left forearm across in front of the chest with your left palm facing your chest and the fingers almost touching your right elbow.

2.   Keeping your weight on your right leg, as one unit, turn your torso to your left to face southeast again. Your upper body, arms and hands move together as one unit.

3.   Keep your torso facing southeast while you withdraw your weight back onto your left foot.

4.   Turn your torso to the left 45 degrees. At the same time turn your left palm upwards. You are now facing east.

25. Press

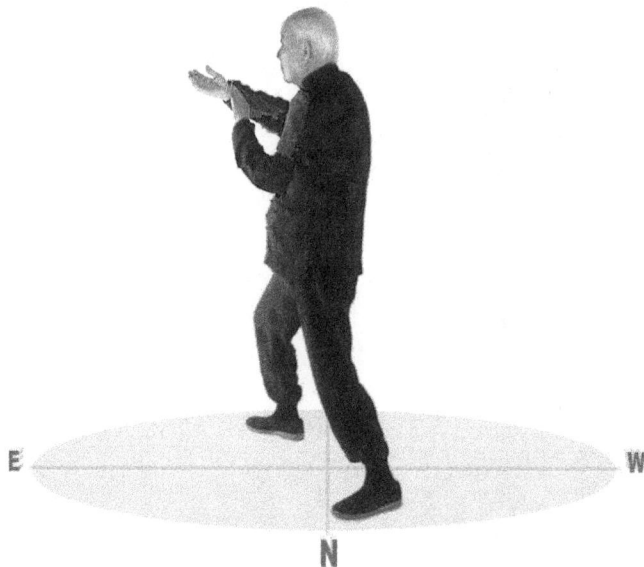

During the counts of:

1. | Turn your torso 45 degrees to your left to face northeast. With the momentum of this turn let your left hand drop down and circle around (without lifting the elbow), heading up toward your left ear.

2. | As your left hand is passing by your ear, turn your torso back 90 degrees to your right to face southeast and lightly attach your left fingers to the inside of your right wrist (as though you're feeling your pulse). Your right forearm drops slightly down into a diagonal position in front of your upper chest with the left elbow lowered.

3. | Without letting your hands and arms move separately from your body, shift your weight onto the right leg and press forward with your right forearm. It's important here to move your whole body as one unit and not let your hands and arms move independently or initiate any movement.

4. | Continue to press forward and slightly upwards until your right leg bears about 70% of your weight.

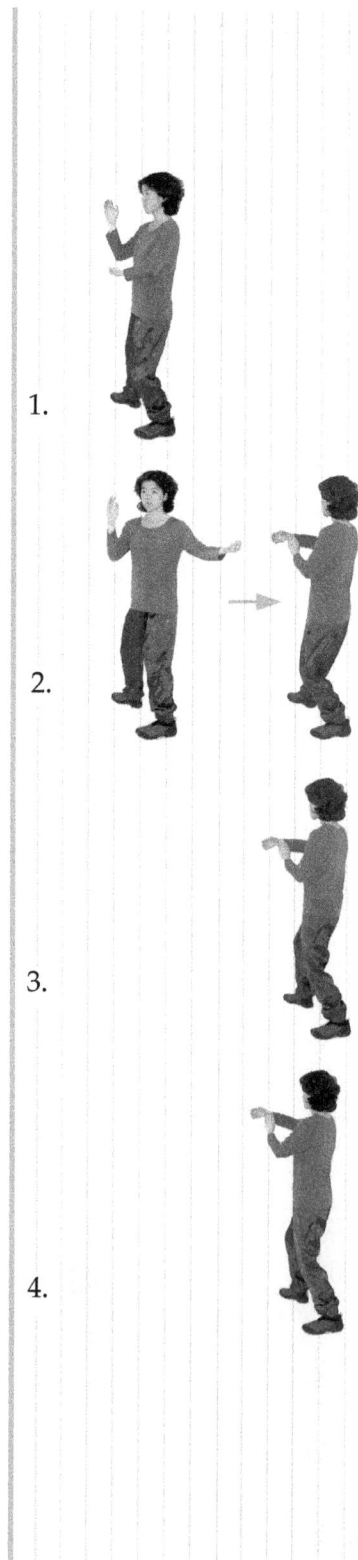

26. Push

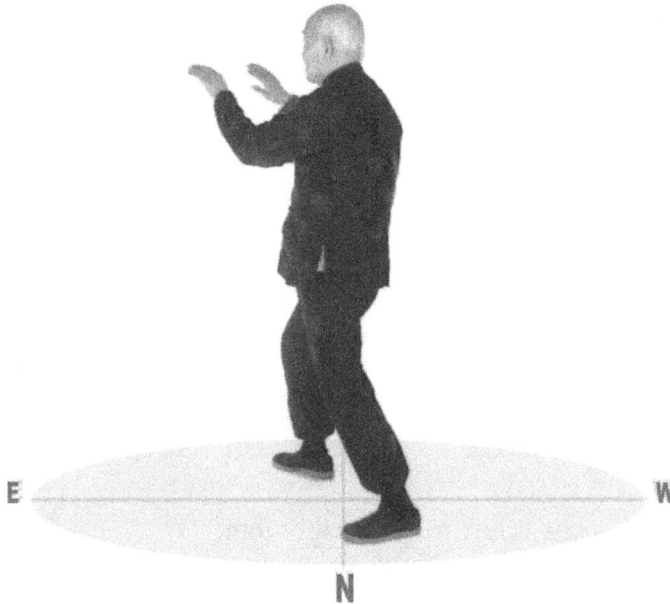

During the counts of:

1. Seperate your hands, palms down, at the level of your shoulders.

2. Keeping your back straight, shift your weight back onto your left leg and simultaneously withdraw your hands slightly towards your upper chest. The fingers of both hands point forward and the elbows remain relaxed and bent downwards.

3. Without moving your hands and arms separately from your body, shift your weight onto your right leg . The push is coming from the forward movement of your whole body - not your arms.

4. Complete the bow and arrow stance by shifting an additional 10% of your weight into your right foot. At the same time slightly raise your fingertips so that the intention of the push is coming through your palms and directed to the southeast corner.

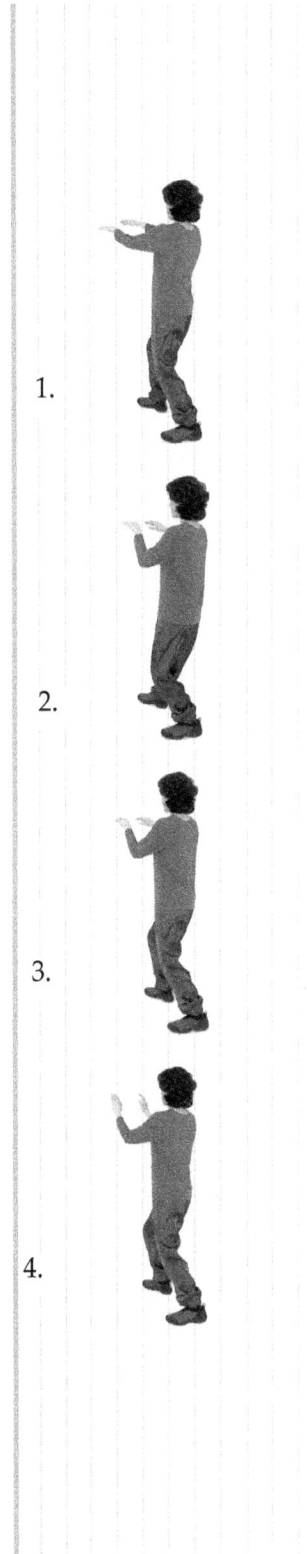

27. Slanting Single Whip

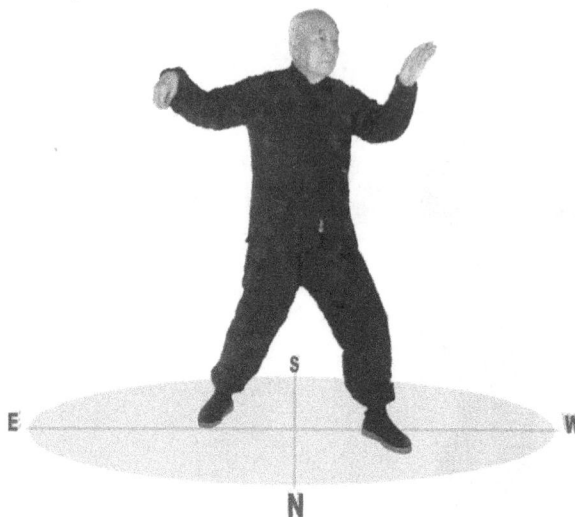

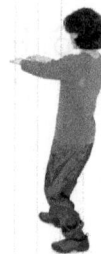

1.

During the counts of:

1. | Shift your weight back onto your left foot and let your arms stretch out slightly with your palms facing downward.

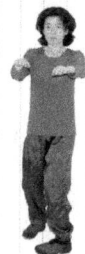

2.

2. | Turn your torso to the left until it faces north and at the same time turn your right foot, pivoting on the heel, so that the toes point northeast. (If you look down at your feet they should appear "pigeon-toed.")

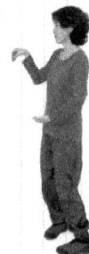

3.

3. | Shift your weight back to your right leg as you turn your torso to face east. Simultaneously withdraw both hands; your left hand comes down opposite the navel with its palm facing up and your right hand forms a hook (the fingers pointing downward with all 5 digits touching at the fingertips) near your right armpit.

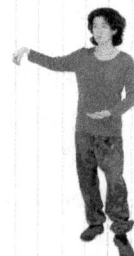

4.

4. | Turn your torso back to face the northeast corner. Let this movement simultaneously pivot your left foot on the toes to point north and strike to the east with your right hand "hook."

5. | Continue to turn your torso to face northwest and step with your left foot, heel first, so as to form a shoulders' width stance facing northwest. The turning movement of your torso brings your left hand, palm facing in, around in front of your body at face level as well as initiating the turning of your right foot, pivoting on the heel, to point north. The right hand "hook" does not move.

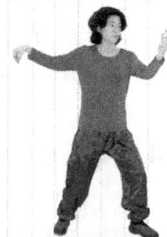

5.

6. | Complete the bow and arrow stance facing northwest by shifting an additional 10% of your weight into your left foot. At the same time turn your left hand palm outward being careful to leave the elbow slightly bent. Your eyes gaze just over and past the fingertips.

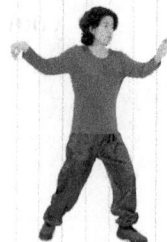

6.

28. Punch Under Elbow

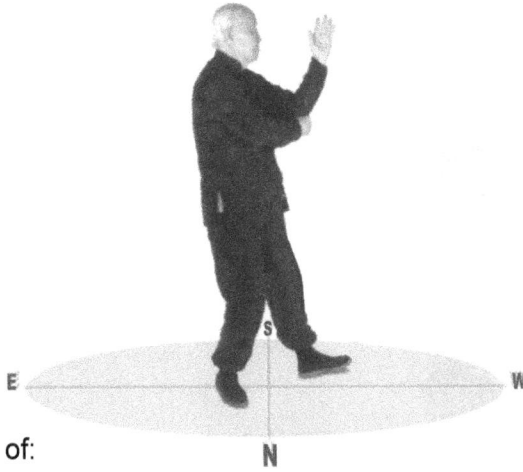

During the counts of:

1. Shift your weight back to your right leg and, as you do, let your left arm straighten out slightly.

2. Pick up the left foot and, as one unit, turn your torso counter-clockwise to the left so that your waist is facing west. Place your left foot down, heel first, with the toes pointing west. At the same time open the "hook" of your right hand so that the palm is facing down.

3. Shift your weight forward onto your left foot.

4. Step with your right foot slightly forward to the northwest and then, as you shift your weight onto it, turn your torso to face south. With this turning motion your left foot pivots on the toes to point south and your arms extend outward so that your right hand is pointing west and your left hand is pointing east. Both palms are facing down.

5. Turn your torso back to face west and circle your left hand downward and forward to the west.

6. Continue to circle your left hand up and inside your right forearm until the fingers are pointing upward. At the same time take a step with your left foot diagonally to the west, letting only your heel touch down in front of and in line with your right heel. When your heel touches the ground make a fist with your right hand turning it so that the "tiger's mouth" is facing up and attach it lightly just beneath your left elbow. Your weight remains on your right leg.

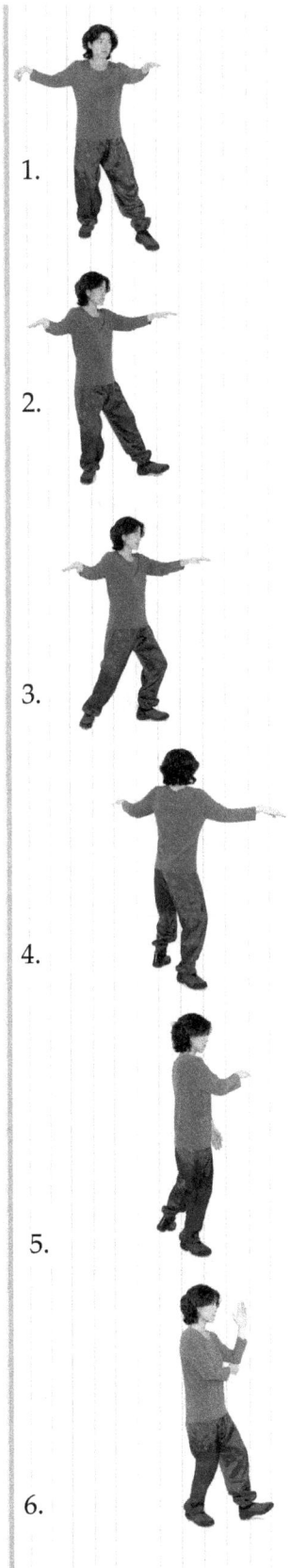

1.

2.

3.

4.

5.

6.

29. Step Back to Repulse the Monkey (right) style)

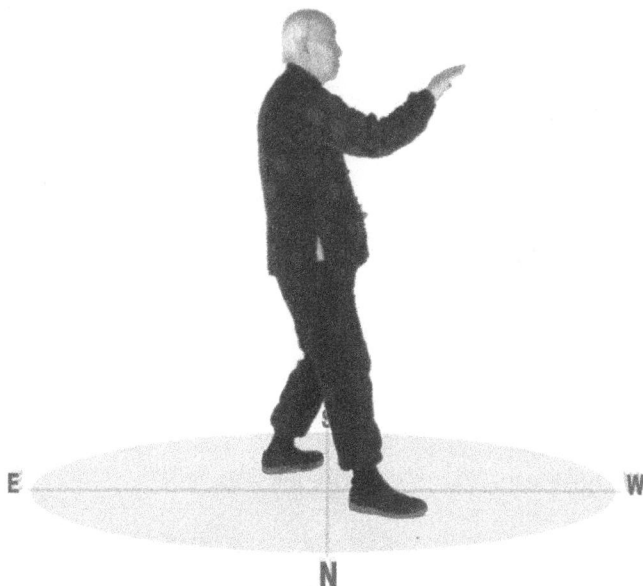

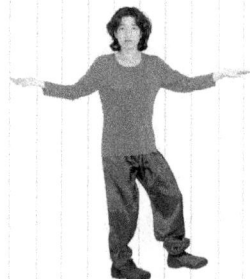

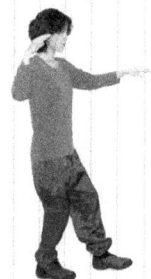

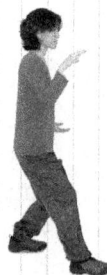

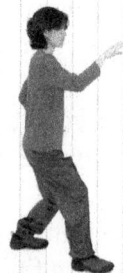

During the counts of:

1. Keep your weight on your right leg and turn your torso to the right to face north. With this movement, extend both hands at shoulder level to the east and west. Your right hand circling to the east, palm open and facing up. Your left hand to the west, its palm open and facing down.

2. Turn your torso back to the left to face west and bring your right hand forward beside your right ear with palm and fingers pointing slightly forward.

3. Turn your left hand palm up and draw it back and down to your left thigh. At the same time step back with your left foot with the toes pointing straight ahead to the west and shift your weight back onto it. Your right foot, pivoting on the heel, turns inward so that both feet are parallel and pointing west.

4. Sink your weight into your left foot and push forward or issue with your right hand.

30. Step Back to Repulse the Monkey (left)

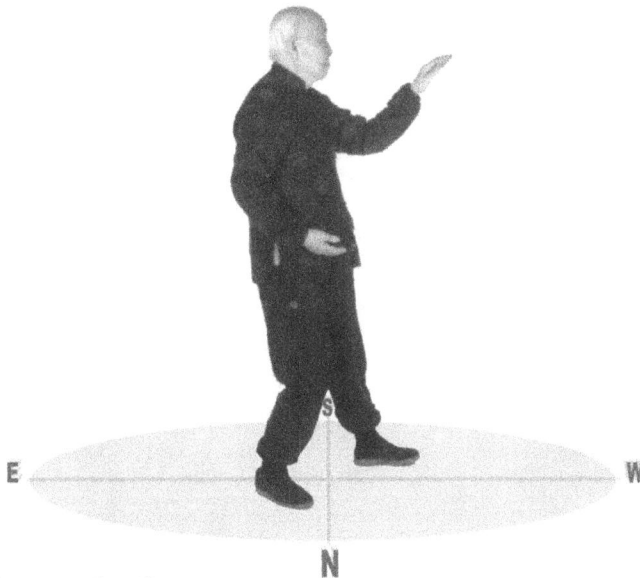

During the counts of:

1. Keep your weight on your left leg and turn your torso to your left to face south. With this movement, extend both hands at shoulder level to the east and west. Your left hand circling to the east, palm open and facing up. Your right hand to the west with its palm open and facing down.

2. Turn your torso back to your right to face west and bring your left hand forward beside your left ear with palm and fingers pointing slightly forward to the west.

3. Turn your right hand palm up and draw it back and down to your right thigh. At the same time step back with your right foot with the toes pointing straight ahead to the west and shift your weight back onto it.

4. Sink your weight into your right foot and push forward (issue) with your left hand.

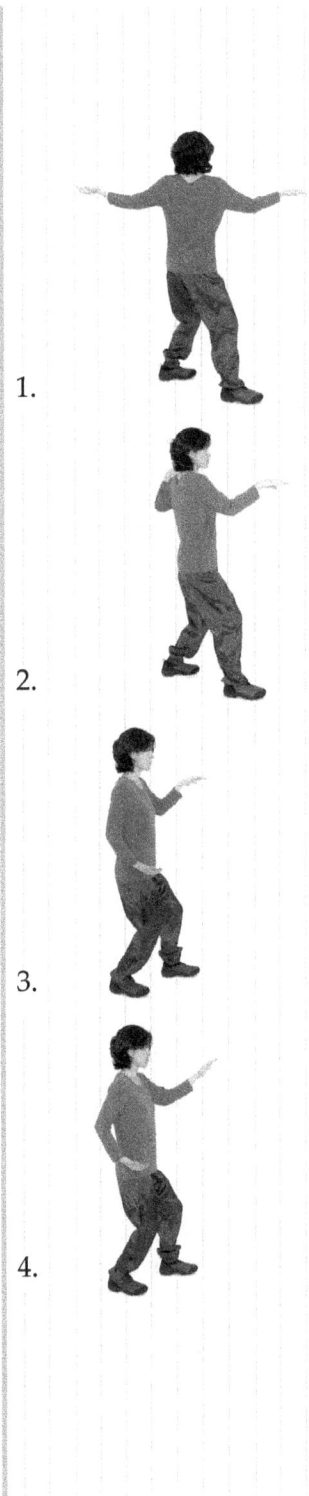

31. Step Back to Repulse the Monkey (right style)

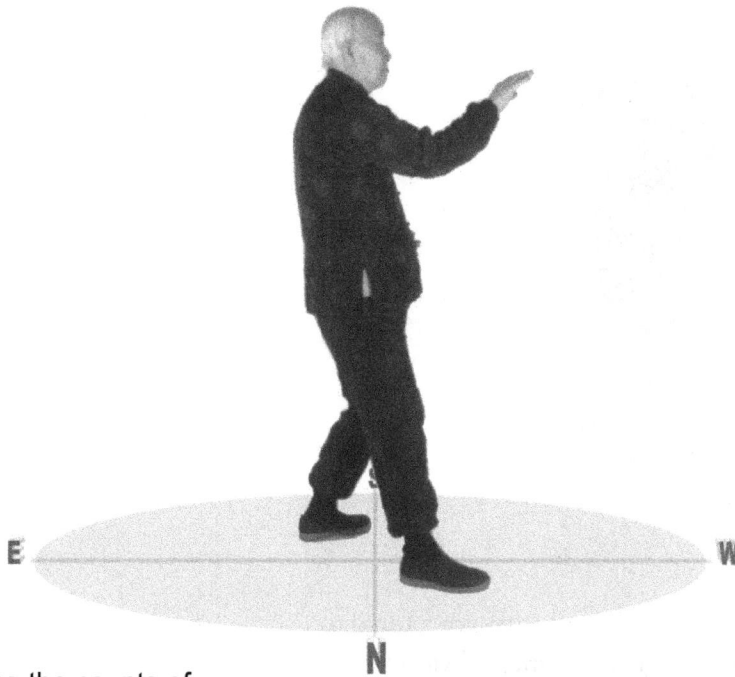

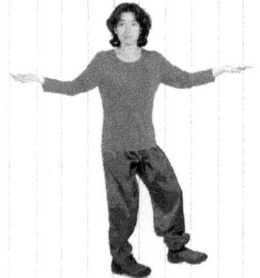

1.

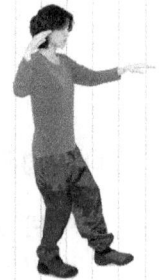

2.

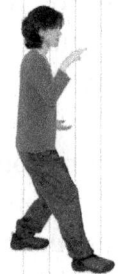

3.

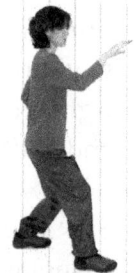

4.

During the counts of:

1. Keep your weight on your right leg and turn your torso to the right to face north. With this movement, extend both hands at shoulder level to the east and west. Your right hand circling to the east, palm open and facing up. Your left hand to the west with its palm open and facing down.

2. Turn your torso back to the left to face west and bring your right hand forward beside your right ear with palm and fingers pointing slightly forward.

3. Turn your left hand palm up and draw it back and down to your left thigh. At the same time step back with your left foot with the toes pointing straight ahead to the west and shift your weight back onto it.

4. Sink your weight into your left foot and push forward (issue) with your right hand.

32. Step Back to Repulse the Monkey (left style)

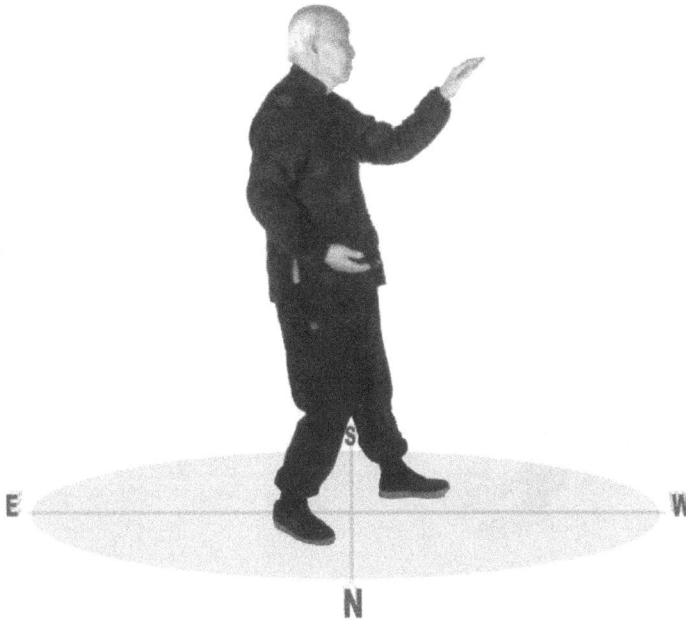

1.

2.

3.

4.

During the counts of:

1. Keep your weight on your left leg and turn your torso to your left to face south. With this movement, extend both hands at shoulder level to the east and west. Your left hand circling to the east, palm open and facing up. Your right hand to the west with its palm open and facing down.

2. Turn your torso back to your right to face west and bring your left hand forward beside your left ear with palm and fingers pointing slightly forward to the west.

3. Turn your right hand palm up and draw it back and down to your right thigh. At the same time step back with your right foot with the toes pointing straight ahead to the west and shift your weight back onto it.

4. Sink your weight into your right foot and push forward (issue) with your left hand.

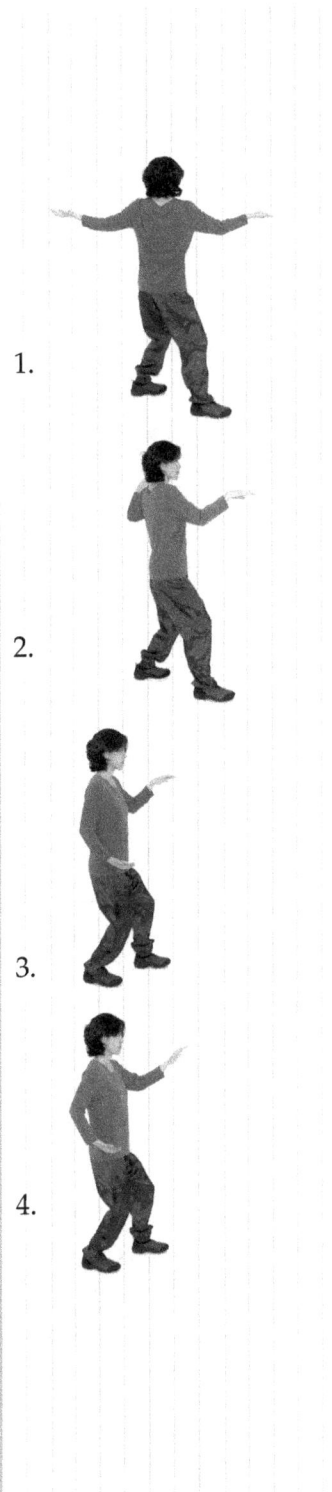

33. Step Back to Repulse the Monkey (right style)

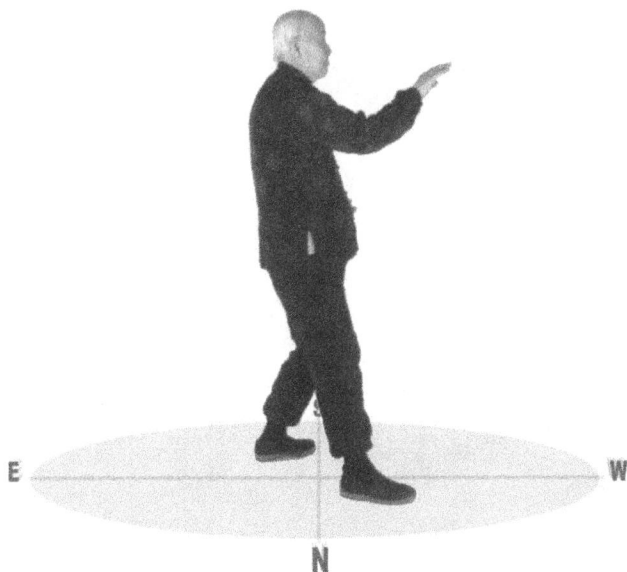

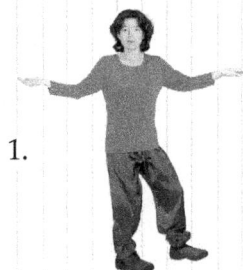

1.

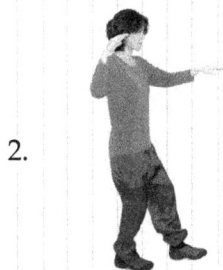

2.

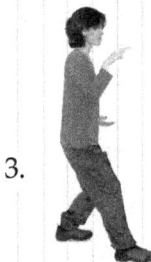

3.

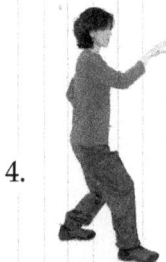

4.

During the counts of:

1. Keep your weight on your right leg and turn your torso to the right to face north. With this movement, extend both hands at shoulder level to the east and west. Your right hand circling to the east, palm open and facing up. Your left hand to the west with its palm open and facing down.

2. Turn your torso back to the left to face west and bring your right hand forward beside your right ear with palm and fingers pointing slightly forward.

3. Turn your left hand palm up and draw it back and down to your left thigh. At the same time step back with your left foot with the toes pointing straight ahead to the west and shift your weight back onto it.

4. Sink your weight into your left foot and push forward (issue) with your right hand.

34. Diagonal Flying Posture

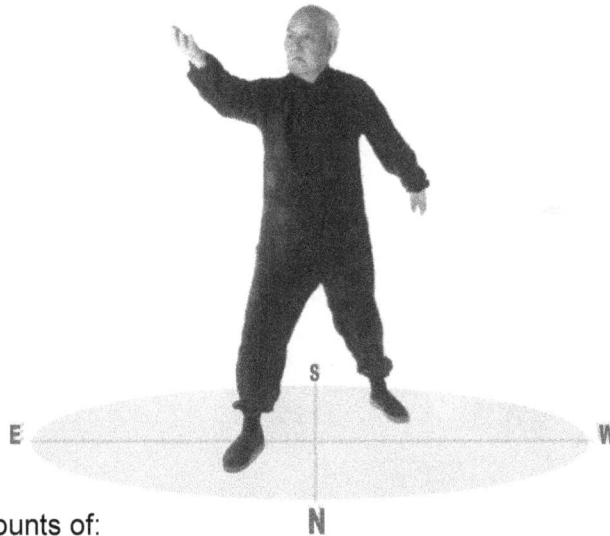

During the counts of:

1. Turn your torso 45 degrees to your left to face southwest. At the same time bring your hands in front of your chest with the palms facing each other as if holding a ball. Your left hand is ontop with the palm facing down and your right hand is on the bottom with the palm facing up.

2. Turn your torso clockwise to your right to face northwest and at the same time bring your right hand inside of your left and place it ontop, crossed at the wrists. Your right palm remains facing up and the left palm facing down.

3. Continue to turn your torso to your right and step with your right foot (almost a backward step) to the northeast with the heel landing first. Keep your right palm facing up and sweep, in a horizontal upward arching motion, your right arm across to the right in conjuncton with the turning of your torso. Shift your weight 60% to your right leg and, with the movement of your torso, turn your left foot in, pivoting on the heel, to point north.

4. Shifting your weight 70% onto your right leg, continue to move your right arm in a diagonal upward motion in conjuction with the torso as it turns to the northeast. At the same time extend your left hand, thumb down, diagonally downward behind your left thigh.

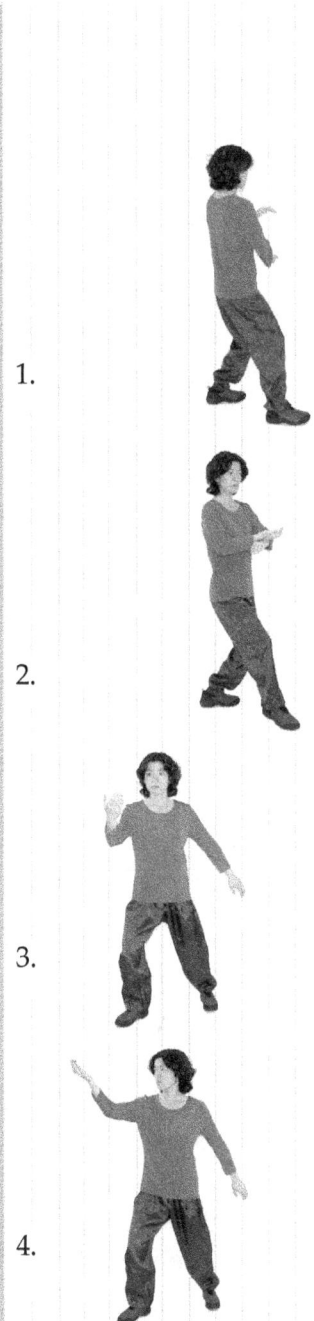

35. Lifting Hands

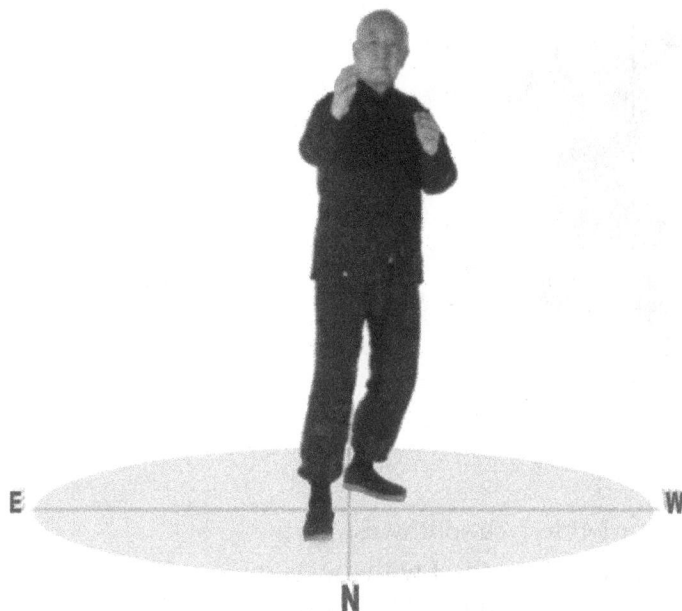

E ———————— W

N

1.

2.

During the counts of:

1. Shift your weight all the way onto your right leg and lift up your left foot and place it back down, adjusting the toes to face northwest.

2. Turn your palms slightly inwards so that they face each other and shift your weight onto your left foot and bring your right foot to the north in front of your body and place it heel down, with the toes slightly off the ground, about 12 inches in front (to the north of) your left heel. Your right leg remains slightly bent. At the same time bring your arms together horizontally, without dropping them down, so that your right arm, with the elbow slightly bent, is aligned over your right leg. Your left hand comes over opposite the inside of your right elbow - about 10" away.

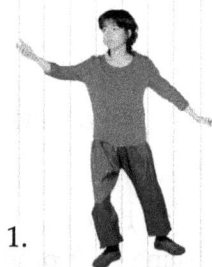

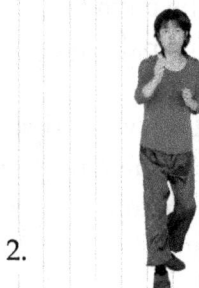

36. Shoulder Stroke

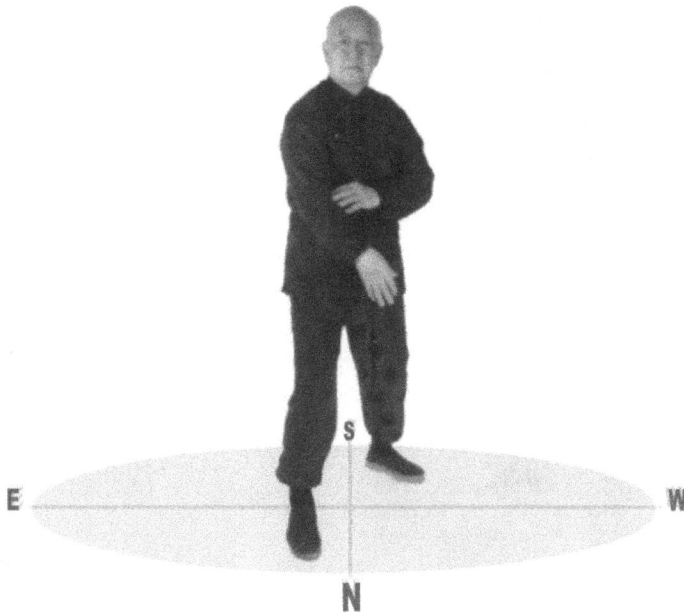

During the counts of:

1. Withdraw your right foot and place it down, heel up, toes touching the ground and pointing north, directly in front of your left heel. At the same time bring your arms down. Your right hand drops to the side of your right thigh with its palm facing backward toward the groin. Your left hand comes down with its palm facing the right palm.

2. Step forward to the north with your right foot (heel touching first and toes pointing very slightly to the northwest). Lightly adhere with your left fingers to the inside of your right forearm and simultaneously shift your weight about 70% forward onto your right foot, striking forward with your right shoulder and side.

1.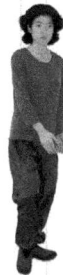

2.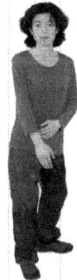

37. White Crane Spreading Wings

During the counts of:

1. Shift your weight to your right foot as you turn to face west, letting the left foot pivot on the toes to point southwest.

2. Raise your body by straightening out your right leg. At the same time bring your left foot forward and place it toes down, heel up, about 14" in front of your right heel. Using this upward momentum, let your right arm come underneath your left and raise it up above your forehead, in a screw motion, to face diagonally outwards, elbow down. Your left hand simultaneously comes to the "position of attention" beside your left hip, palm facing backward.

38. Step Forward and Brush Knee (left)

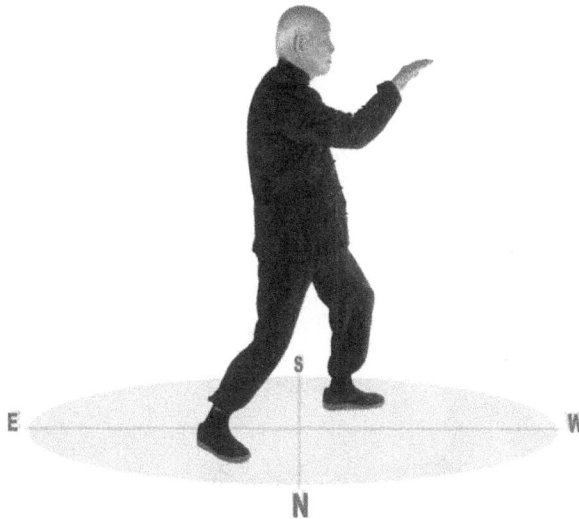

During the counts of:

1. | Lower your body by bending your right knee and turn your torso slightly to the right. At the same time turn your right hand palm up to face you and let it begin to drop down in a counterclockwise motion.

2. | Continue to turn your torso to the right until it is facing northwest (45 degrees) let your right hand continue its counter-clockwise motion until it comes full circle to your right ear with the fingers pointing towards the west and the elbow bent and hanging downwards. During this turning motion of your torso your left hand rises up into a "ward off" position opposite your chest with the fingers pointing north.

3. | Step with your left foot, heel first to the southwest, so as to form a shoulders' width stance facing west. Turn your torso to face west. In conjunction with this turn brush your left knee with your left hand and let it come to rest in the "position of attention" by your left hip pocket. Your right foot, pivoting on the heel, turns in 45 degrees to point northwest and your weight is now 60% forward on your left foot.

4. | Complete the bow and arrow stance facing west by shifting 10% more of your weight into your left foot. At the same, time using your whole body, push forward with your right hand, elbow slightly bent.

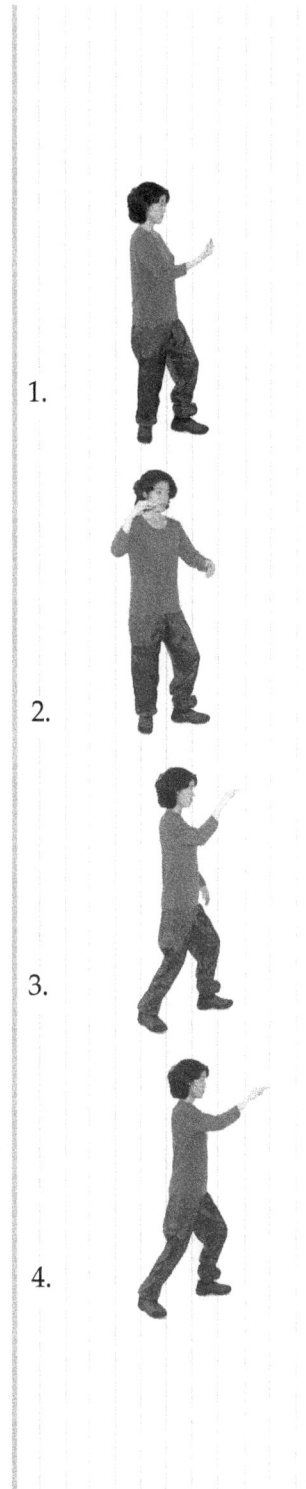

39. Needle at Sea Bottom

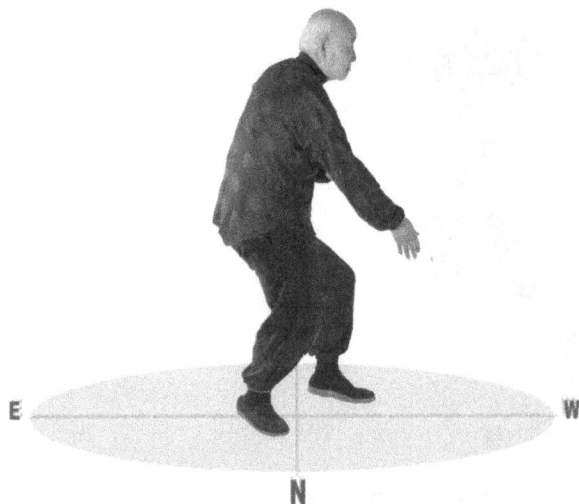

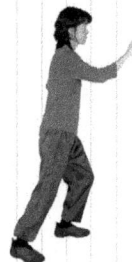

1.

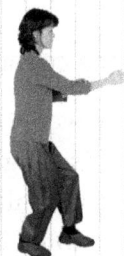

2.

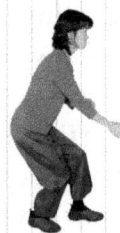

3.

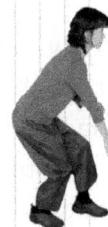

4.

During the counts of:

1. | Shift all of your weight onto your left foot and pick up your right foot and set it down again in the same position - with the toes pointing to the northwest.

2. | Shift your weight onto your right foot and allow your right arm to straighten out slightly. Bring your left hand forward and lightly attach your left hand fingers to the inside of your right forearm. At the same time bring your left foot over and place it about 12" in front of your right heel with only the toes touching the ground.

3. | Keeping your back straight and your weight on your back leg, sink down by bending your right knee.

4. | Without leaning forward too much and your waist facing west, continue to lower your right hand and your body so that your right fingers point directly to the ground in front of your right knee.

40. Fan Penetrates the Back

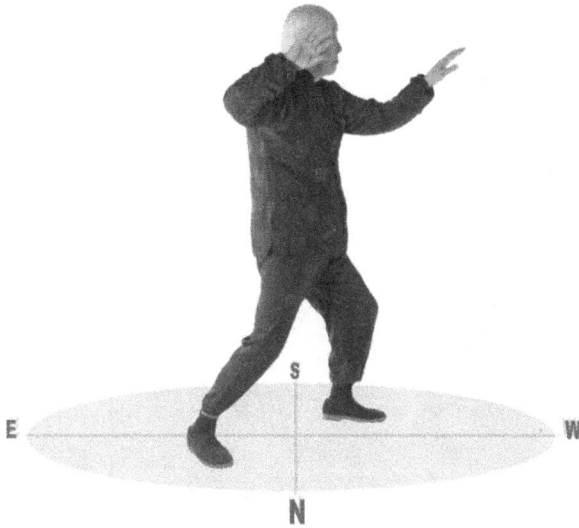

During the counts of:

1. | Raise your body up and raise your right hand to your chest level with the palm facing south and with your left hand still attached to your right forearm.

2. | Withdraw your right hand back near your right ear with the palm outward to the north. At the same time move your left hand forward with palm outward. Let both of your elbows remain bent downwards.

3. | Take a half step forward with your left foot into a bow and arrow stance and shift 60% of your weight onto it.

4. | Push through your left hand by shifting 10% more of your weight onto your left foot.

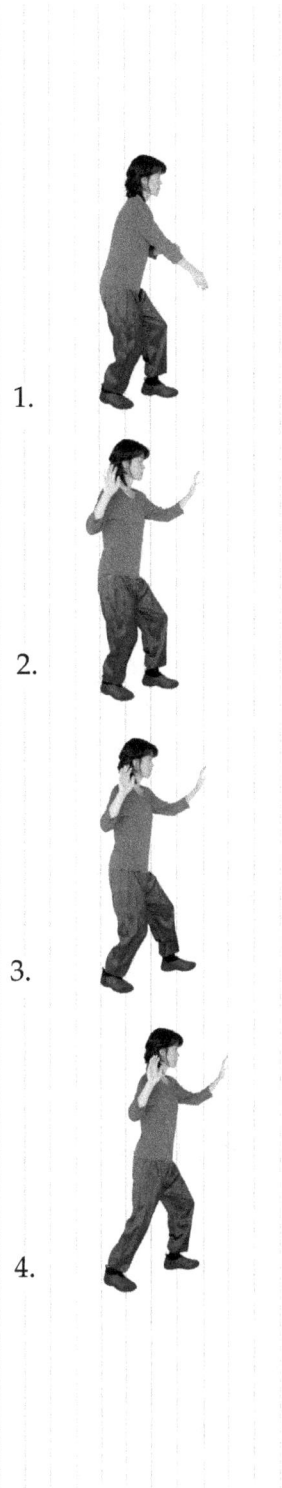

41. Turn Around and Chop

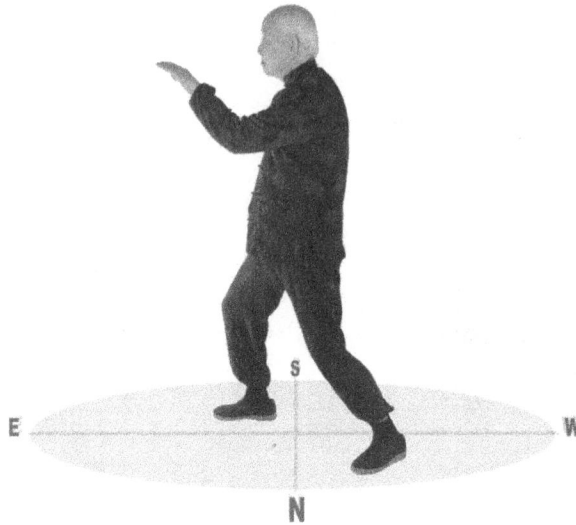

During the counts of:

1. Shift your weight back onto your right foot and as you turn your torso to face north, turn your left foot, pivoting on the heel, so the toes point north. Simultaneously circle your hands, without raising your elbows, in a clockwise motion.

2. While your hands are circling, shift your weight back onto your left leg. Continue to circle your hands clockwise until your left hand is near your left ear, with palm outward and elbow bent, and your right hand, clenched into a fist with the "tiger's mouth" facing your chest, comes under your left elbow. At the same time pivot your right foot on the toes to point north/northeast.

3. Step to the east with your right foot and chop to the east with your right fist. When the arch of your chop is complete, you then shift your weight 60% onto your right foot and bring your right fist back to your right hip. With the turning forward to the east of your torso turn in your left foot, pivoting on the heel, to point northeast.

4. Complete the bow and arrow stance by shifting 10% more of your weight onto your right foot and push forward with your left hand/palm.

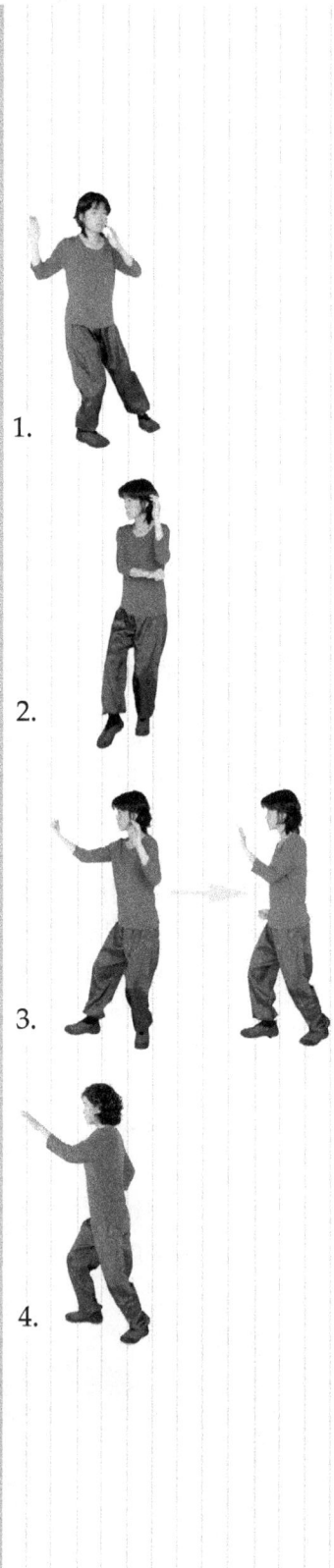

42. Step Forward, Deflect Downward, Intercept and Punch

During the counts of:

1. Shift your weight completely onto your right foot and pick up your left foot and place it back down, adjusting the toes to point north/northwest.

2. Shift your weight to your left foot and reach out with both hands at waist level to the northeast. Your palms are facing each other as though holding a ball with your right hand positioned slightly higher than your left.

3. Raise your right foot and take a step diagonally forward to the right. At the same time make a fist with your right hand and circle it clockwise, in a deflecting motion, around to the right side of your waist and attach it to your hip, palm side facing up and tigers mouth facing south. In unison with this motion your left hand circles clockwise upward and forward in front of your face (without raising your elbow too high). This motion is often described as "emptying a bucket."

4. Facing east, shift your weight to your right foot (toes pointing to the south/ southeast) and simultaneously deflect downward with your left hand to the level of your stomach with the palm facing the floor.

5. Step directly forward, to maintain a shoulders' width stance, with your left foot and shift 60% of your weight onto it. At the same time extend or "intercept" with your left hand forward and to the left. The left hand is open with the fingers pointing east and the palm is facing south. With this motion your right foot turns inwards, pivoting on the heel, so that the toes are pointing southeast.

6. Complete the bow and arrow stance facing west by shifting 10% more of your weight into your left foot. At the same time, using your whole body behind it, punch forward with your right fist ("tiger's mouth" facing up). As your right hand is punching forward let your left hand come over and cover the inner wrist of your right hand.

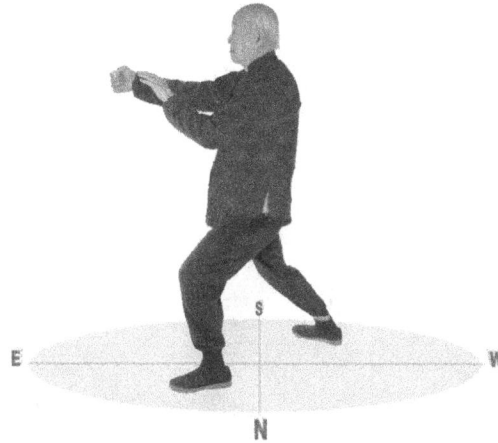

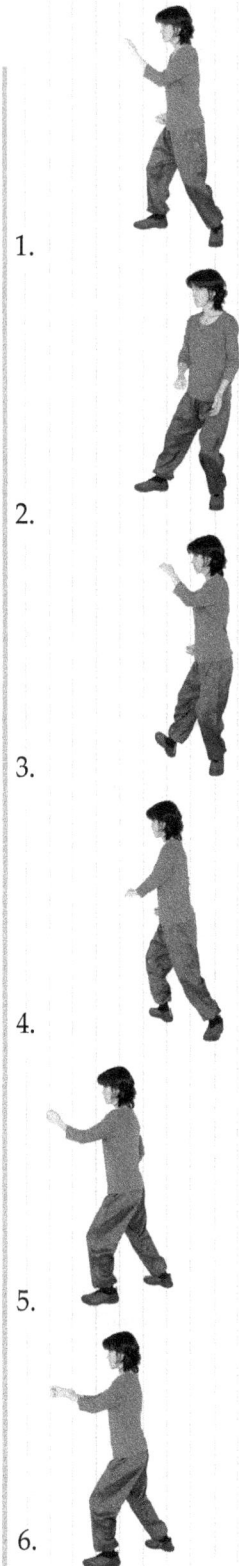

107

43. Ward Off Right

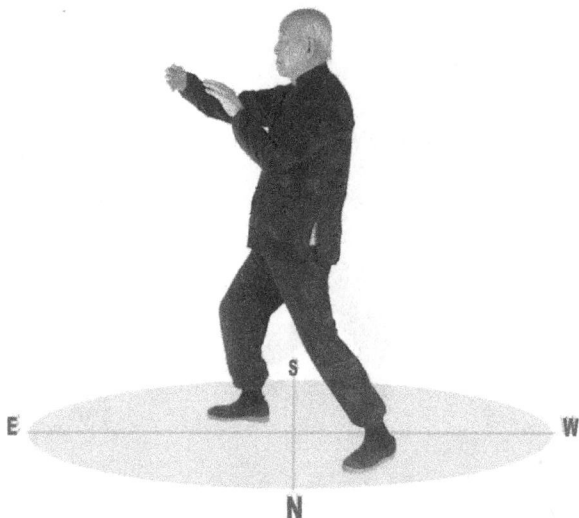

During the counts of:

1. Shift your weight back onto your right leg while turning your torso to face northeast and turning your palms to face each other. At the same time turn your left foot, pivoting on the heel, to point north/northeast.

2. Shift your weight onto your left foot ...

3. ... and step forward to the east into a bow and arrow stance with your right foot. Shift your weight 60% onto your right leg as you turn your torso to face east. Simultaneously pivot on your left heel, turning your left foot inward so the toes are pointing to the northeast. During this count, bring your right hand up in front of your chest/neck with the palm facing in. Your left hand faces your right palm, as if holding a small ball. Your right arm remains rounded out and your left elbow is lowered.

4. Complete the bow and arrow stance facing east by shifting an additional 10% of your weight onto your right foot. At the same time, using your whole body, push forward with the back of your right hand, both elbows remaining slightly bent.

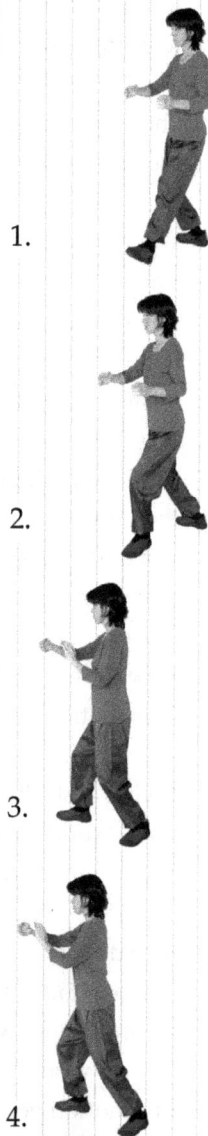

44. Roll Back

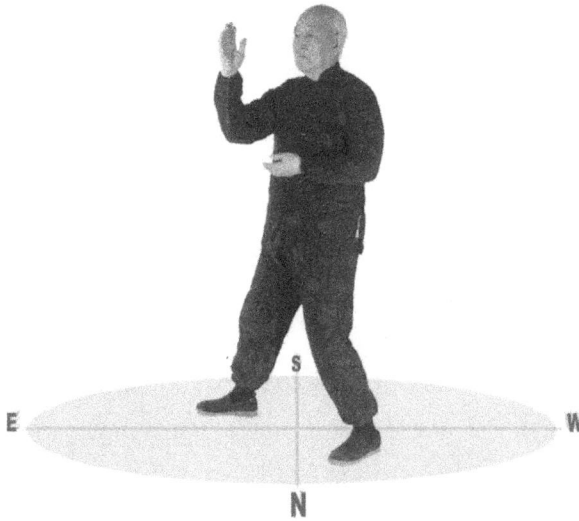

During the counts of:

1. Turn your torso to the right 45 degrees and bring your right forearm up vertically and perpendicular to your chest. At the same time bring your left forearm across in front of the chest with your left palm facing in and the fingers almost touching your right elbow.

2. Keeping your weight on the right foot, turn your upper torso back to the left 45 degrees to face east again. Your waist, upper body, arms and hands move together as one unit.

3. With your torso facing straight ahead to the east, withdraw your weight back onto your left foot.

4. Turn your torso to the left 45 degrees to face northeast. At the same time turn your left palm upwards.

1.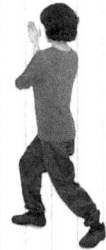

2.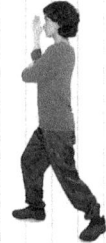

3.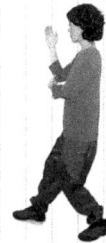

4.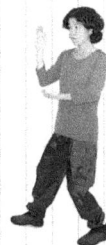

45. Press

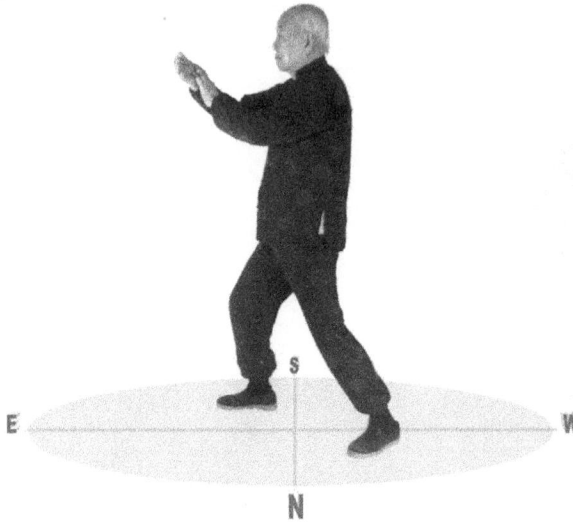

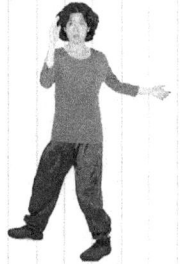

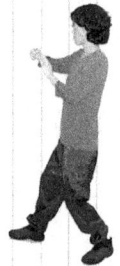

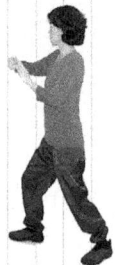

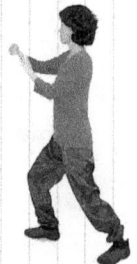

During the counts of:

1.   Turn your torso 45 degrees to your left to face north. With the momentum of this turn let your left hand drop down and circle around (without lifting the elbow), heading up toward your left ear.

2.   As your left hand is passing by your ear, turn your torso back 90 degrees to your right to face east and lightly attach your left fingers to the inside of your right wrist (as though you're feeling your pulse). Your right forearm drops slightly down into a diagonal position in front of your upper chest with the left elbow lowered.

3.   Without letting your hands and arms move separately from your body, shift your weight onto the right leg and press forward with your right forearm. It's important here to move your whole body as one unit and not let your hands and arms move independently or initiate any movement.

4.   Continue to press forward and slightly upwards until your right leg bears about 70% of your weight.

46. Push

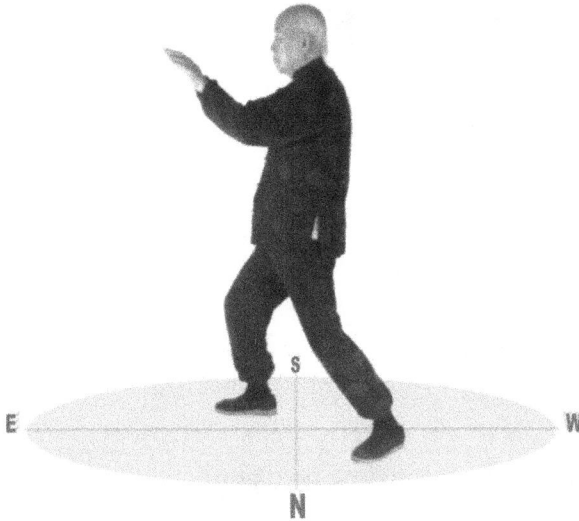

During the counts of:

1. Separate your hands, palms down, at the level of your shoulders.

2. Keeping your back straight, shift your weight back onto your left leg and simultaneously withdraw your hands slightly towards your upper chest. The fingers of both hands point forward and the elbows remain relaxed and bent downwards.

3. Without moving your hands and arms separately from your body, shift 60% of your weight onto your right leg again. The push is coming from the forward movement of your whole body - not your arms.

4. Complete the bow and arrow stance by shifting about 10% more of your weight into your right foot. At the same time slightly raise your fingertips so that the intention of the push is coming through your palms and directed to the east.

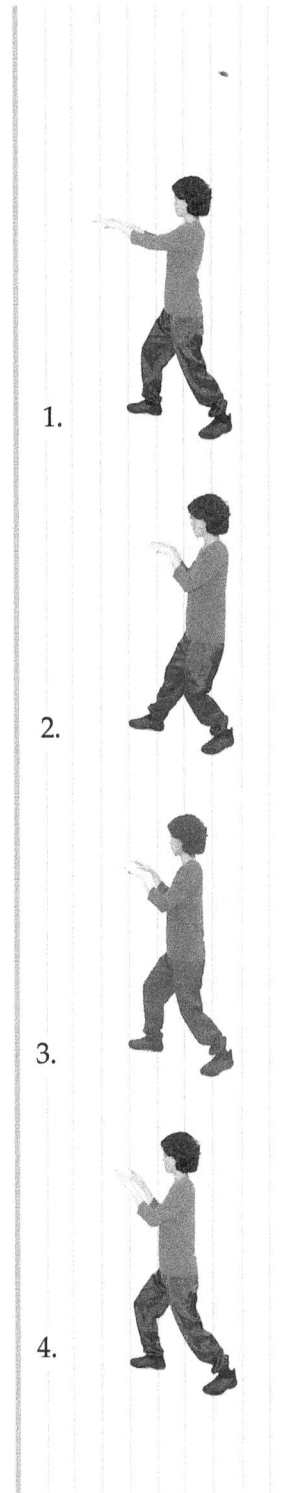

1.

2.

3.

4.

47. Single Whip

During the counts of:

1. Shift your weight back onto your left foot and let your arms stretch out slightly with the palms of the hands facing downward.

2. Turn your torso to the left until it faces northwest and at the same time turn your right foot, pivoting on the heel, so that the toes point north.

3. Shift your weight back to your right leg as you turn your torso to face northeast. Simultaneously withdraw both hands. The left hand comes down opposite the navel with its palm up and the right hand forms a "hook" (all 5 digits are touching at the tips and pointing downward) near your right armpit.

4. Turn your torso counterclockwise back to the northwest corner. With this movement strike to the northeast corner with your right hand "hook" and simultaneously pivot the left foot on the toes to point northwest.

5. Continue to turn your torso to face west and step with your left foot, heel first, so as to form a shoulders' width stance facing west with 60% of your weight on your left foot. The movement of your torso brings your left hand, palm facing in, up in front of your body at face level. At the same time let this movement turn your right foot, pivoting on the heel, to point northwest. The right hand "hook" does not move.

6. Complete the bow and arrow stance facing west by shifting your weight about 70% onto your left foot. At the same time turn your left hand palm outward being careful to leave your arm slightly bent. Your eyes gaze just over and past the fingertips.

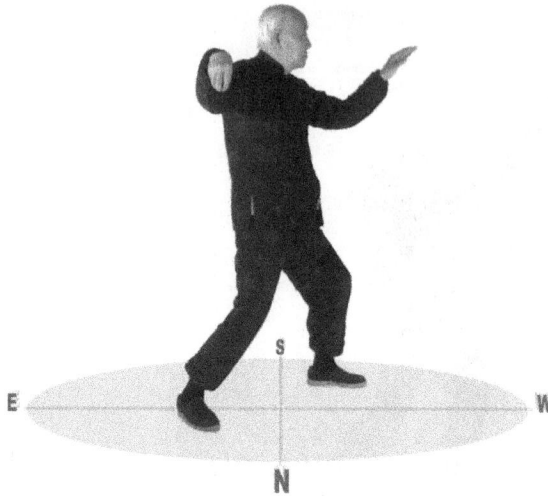

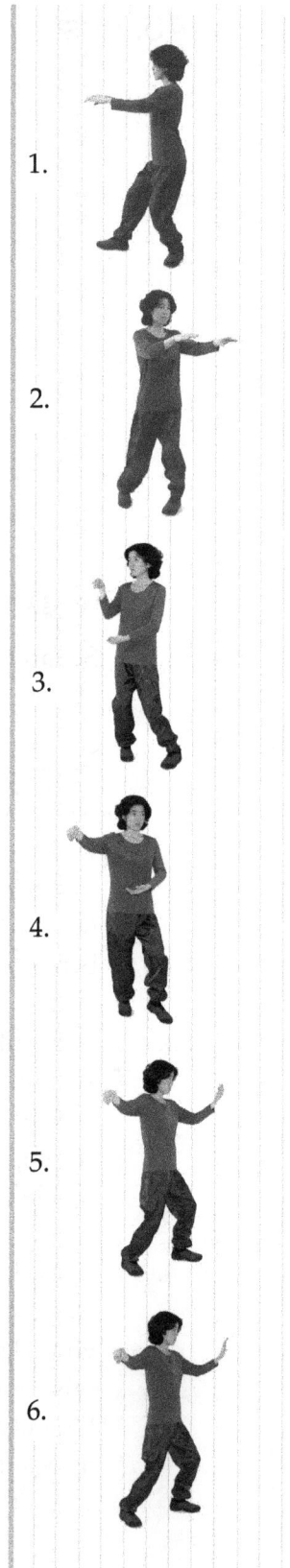

48. Wave Hands in Clouds (left)

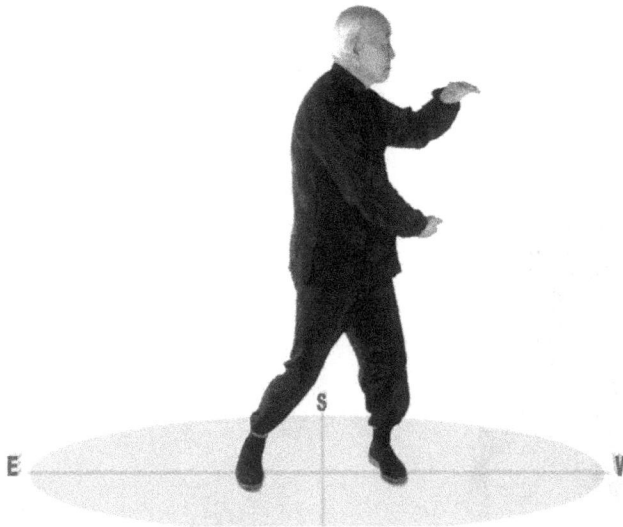

During the counts of:

1. Shift your weight completely onto your right leg as you turn your torso to face northeast and your left foot, pivoting on the heel, to face north. At the same time open your right hand so that the palm is facing down and bring your left hand, palm facing up, in front of your waist so as to simulate holding a ball in front of your chest.

2. Turn both palms in to face your body and simultaneously bring your right hand down to your waist level and bring your left hand up to the level of your neck. The right hand passes on the inside of the left.

3. Turn your torso and hands as one unit to the left as you begin shifting your weight onto your left leg. On this beat your waist is now facing north.

4. Shift 80% of your weight onto your left foot as you turn your torso to face west. Then turn both palms to face each other so that they are in a position of holding a ball in front of your chest.

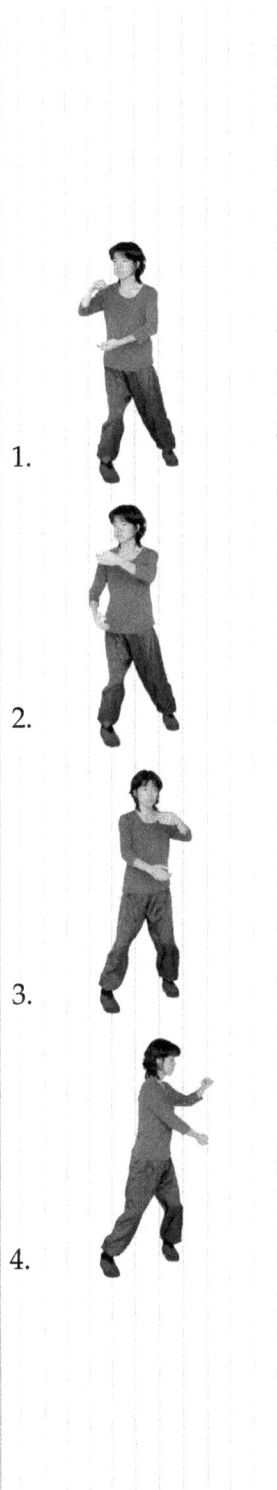

1.

2.

3.

4.

49. Wave Hands in Clouds (right)

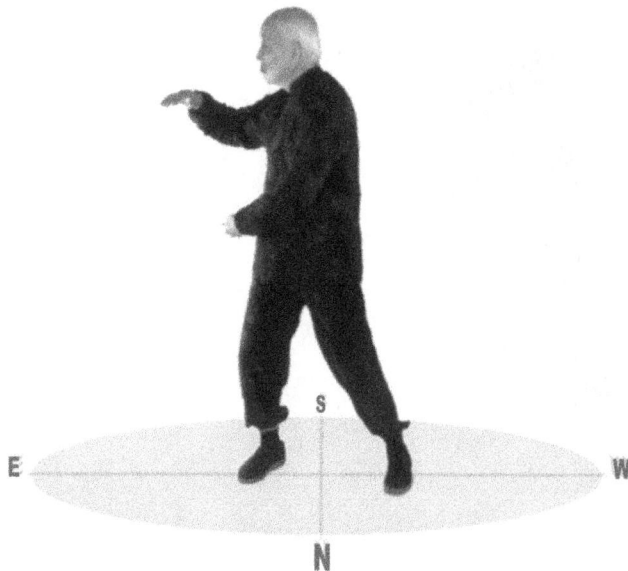

During the counts of:

1. Bring your left hand down to your waist level and simultaneously bring your right hand up to your neck level as you turn both palms to face inward. Your left hand passes on the outside of your right hand as they exchange positions.

2. Turn your torso clockwise to your right as you step backwards and to the east with your right foot, placing it parrallel to your left foot so that there is about 10" between them (less than a shoulders' width).

3. Continue to shift your weght onto right foot as you turn your torso and hands as one unit to the right. On the count of three you are facing directly north (not in picture).

4. Continue to turn your torso and hands to the right until you're facing east with 80% of your weight on your right leg. Your right hand now turns palm down and your left hand turns palm up. Again you are simulating holding a ball in front of your chest.

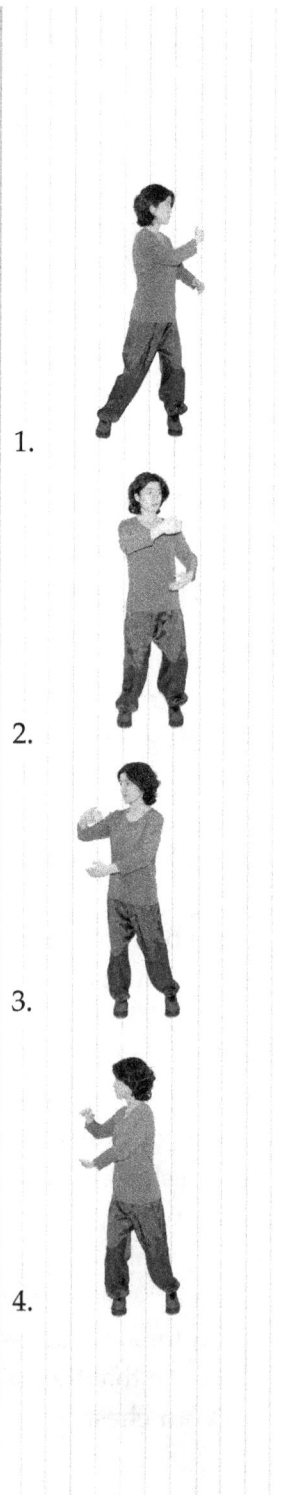

50. Wave Hands in Clouds (left)

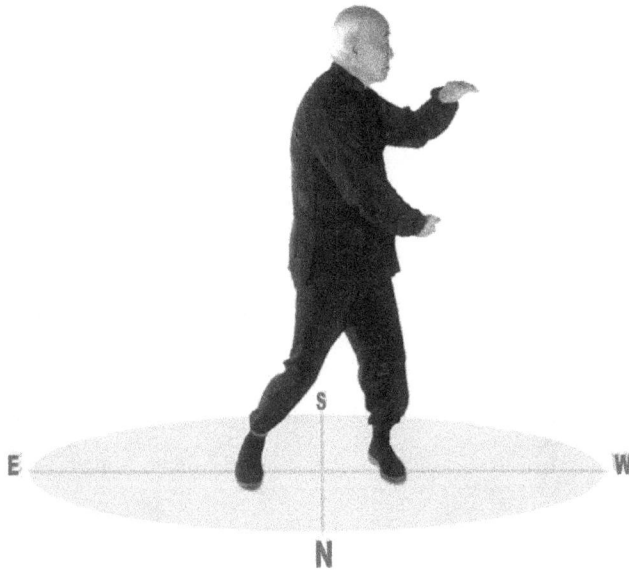

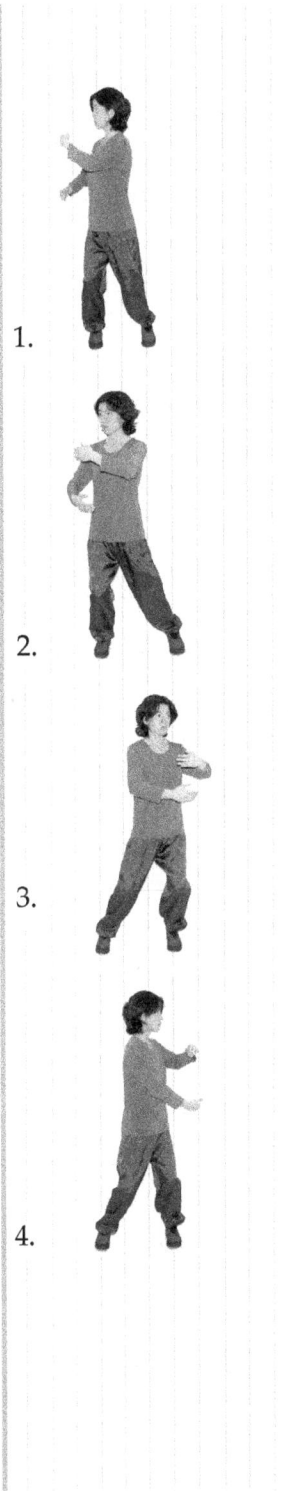

1.

2.

3.

4.

During the counts of:

1. Passing on the outside, bring your right hand down to your waist level and simultaneously bring your left hand, on the inside, up to your neck level as you turn both palms to face inwards.

2. As you turn your torso to your left, step and to the west with your right foot, placing it parallel to your left foot so that there is about 18" between them (more than a shoulders' width).

3. Continue to shift your weight onto your left foot as you turn your torso and hands as one unit to the left.

4. Continue to turn your torso and hands to the left until you're facing west with 80% of your weight on your left leg. Your left hand now turns palm down and your right hand turns palm up. Again you are simulating holding a ball in front of your chest.

51. Wave Hands in Clouds (right)

1.

2.

3.

4.

During the counts of:

1. Bring your left hand down to your waist level and simultaneously bring your right hand up to your neck level as you turn both palms to face inwards. Your left hand passes on the outside of your right hand as they exchange positions.

2. As you turn your torso to your right, step to the east with your right foot, placing it parrallel to your left foot so that there is about 8 to 10" between them (less than a shoulders' width).

3. Continue to shift your weght onto your right foot as you turn your torso and hands as one unit to the right. On the count of three you are facing directly north (not in picture).

4. Continue to turn your torso and hands to the right until you're facing east with 80% of your weight on your right leg. Your right hand now turns palm down and your left hand turns palm up. Again you are simulating holding a ball in front of your chest.

52. Wave Hands in Clouds (left)

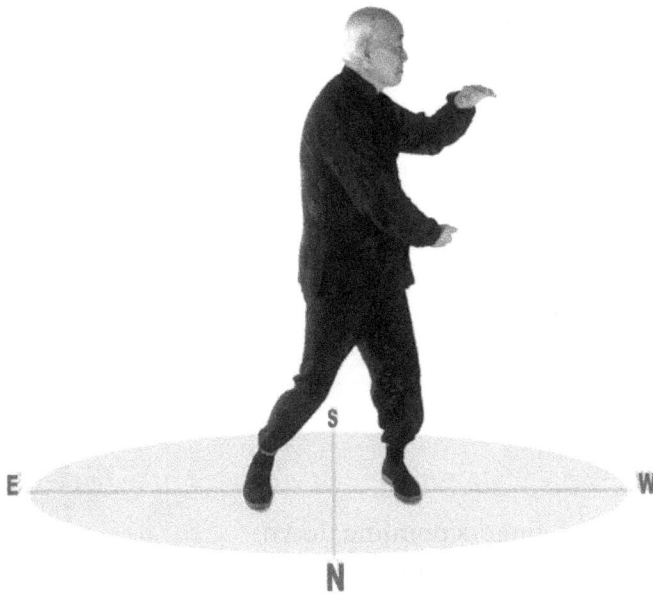

During the counts of:

1. Passing on the outside, bring your right hand down to your waist level and simultaneously bring your left hand, on the inside, up to your neck level as you turn both palms to face inwards.

2. As you turn your torso to your left, step and to the west with your right foot, placing it parralel to your left foot so that there is about 18″ between them (more than a shoulders' width).

3. Continue to shift your weight onto your left foot as you turn your torso and hands as one unit to the left.

4. Continue to turn your torso and hands to the left until you're facing west with 80% of your weight on your left leg. Your left hand now turns palm down and your right hand turns palm up. Again you are simulating holding a ball in front of your chest.

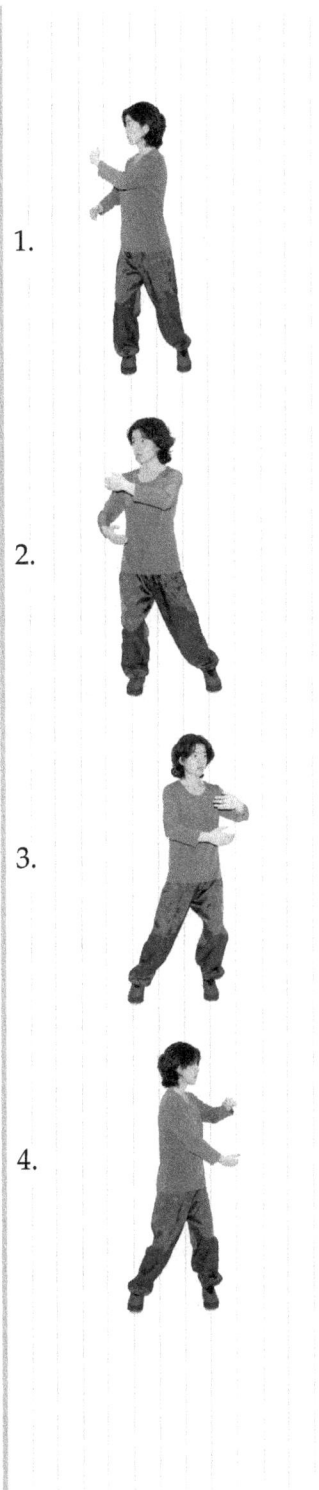

53. Single Whip

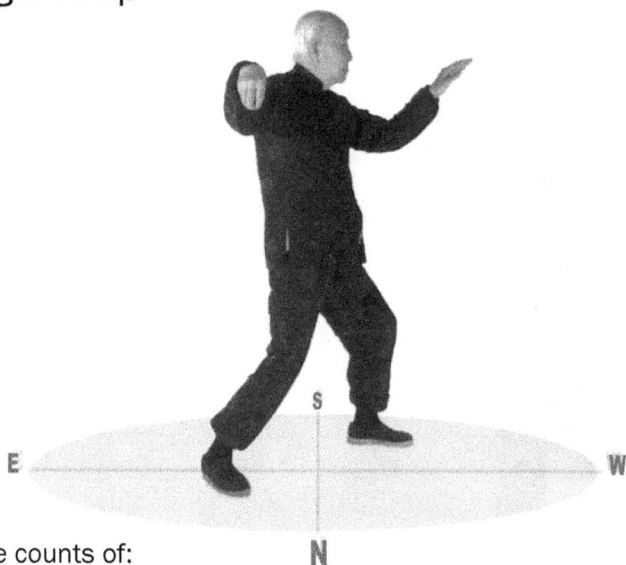

During the counts of:

1. Form a "hook" with your right hand, fingers pointing down, and strike out with it in a diagonal direction upwards to the northeast corner, as you take a step with your right foot in this same direction. At the same time lower your open left hand, palm up, in front of your stomach.

2. Shift your weight completely onto your right foot and turn your torso to the left facing northwest. Let this turning motion turn your left foot, pivoting on the toes to face west.

3. Continue to turn your torso to face west and step with your left foot, heel first, so as to form a shoulders' width stance facing west. The movement of your torso brings your left hand, palm facing in, up in front of your body at face level. At the same time let this movement turn your right foot, pivoting on the heel, to point northwest. The right hand "hook" does not move.

4. Complete the bow and arrow stance facing west by shifting your weight 70% into your left foot. At the same time turn your left hand palm outward being careful to leave your arm slightly bent. Your eyes gaze just over and past the fingertips.

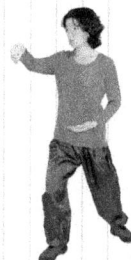

1.

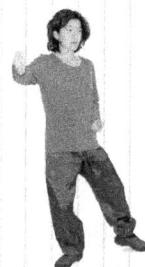

2.

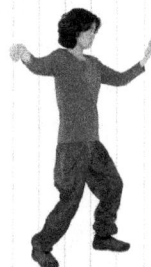

3.

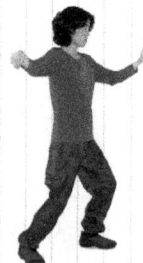

4.

54. High Pat on Horse

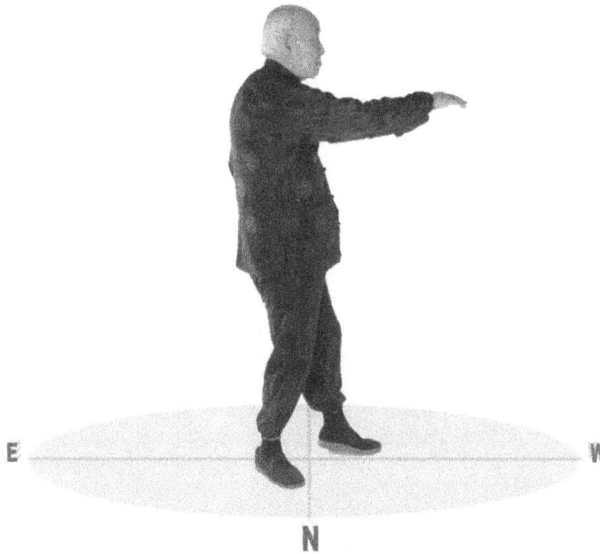

During the counts of:

1. Pick up your right foot, readjust it, and then place it back down with the toes once again pointing northwest.

2. Shift your weight back onto your right foot and place the toes of your left foot down about 12" in front of your right heel facing west. As soon as the toes touch the ground open your right hand so that the palm is facing the floor.

3. Bring your right hand over, palm still facing down, and cover your left inner elbow. At the same time turn your left hand so that the palm is facing up.

4. Withdraw your left hand, palm up, down to your left pocket and simultaneously strike forward with your right hand at neck level, palm facing down.

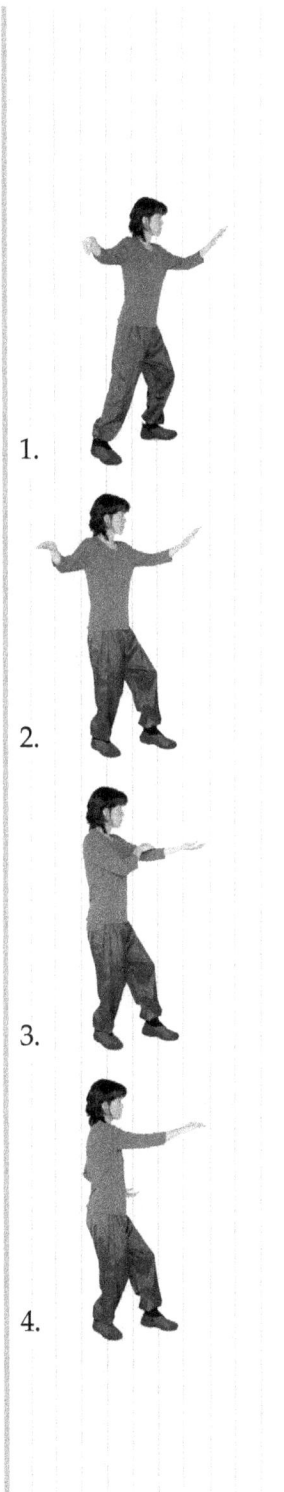

1.

2.

3.

4.

55. Separating Right Foot

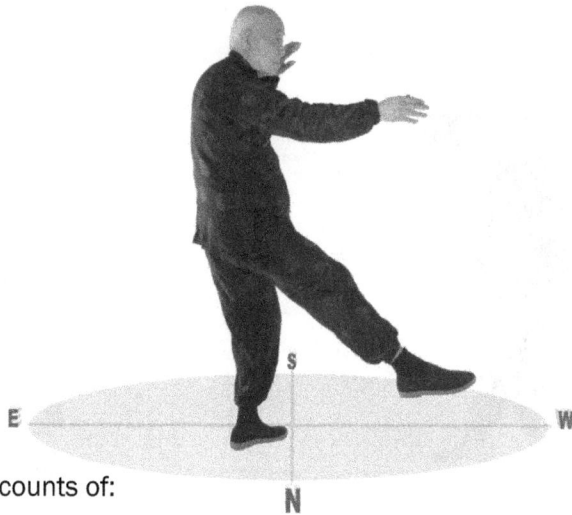

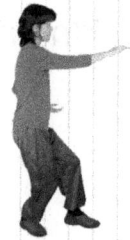

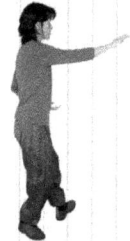

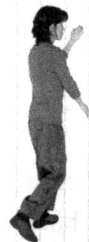

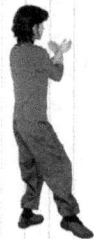

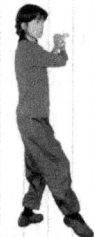

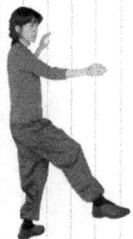

During the counts of:

1. Bending your right knee, sink your weight down ...

2. ... and then turn your torso and step with your left foot toward the southwest corner.

3. Begin to shift your weight onto your left foot as you start to circle your hands in a figure eight motion. Your right hand moves in a clockwise motion, first up and to your right, and then down. Your left hand, also in a clockwise motion, first moves down and to the left and then up.

4. Shift your weight entirely onto your left foot and place your right foot, toe down and heel slightly raised, pointing northwest in a "T" formationto your left foot . Your hands continue to circle in a figure eight until they join at the wrists with the right hand outside of the left hand and both palms facing inward.

5. Turn your palms outward to face southwest as you turn your torso clockwise to your right to face northwest..

6. Strike forward with your right hand fingers to the northwest corner. At the same time your left hand moves in the opposite direction ending up near your left ear with the left elbow bent and fingers pointing upward. Without bending your knee, kick forward (or "separate") to the northwest with your right foot, toes pointed forward, about one foot off the ground.

120

56. Separating Left Foot

During the counts of:

1. Bend your right knee and withdraw the right foot so that it is suspended with the toes pointing down. At the same time bring the right hand with palm up back to the belly-button.

2. Step forward with your right foot to the northwest, heel landing first, and begin to shift your weight onto it.

3. As you are transitioning your weight to your right foot turn your body slightly to the left and strike out to the southwest corner with your left hand, palm facing down. Your right hand mirrors the strike with palm facing up. Then circle both hands down in a counterclockwise motion downward...

4. ... and upward until your hands cross, joining at the wrists with your left hand outside of the right hand and both palms facing inward. At the same time shift your weight entirely onto your right foot and place your left foot, toe down, pointing to the southwest corner in a "T" formationto your right foot . You are now facing northwest.

5. Turn your palms outward to face northwest as you turn your torso to the left to face southwest.

6. Strike forward with your left hand fingers to the southwest corner. At the same time your right hand moves in the opposite direction ending up near your right ear with the right elbow bent and fingers pointing upward. Without bending your knee, kick forward (or "separate") to the southwest with your left foot, toes pointed forward, about one foot off the ground.

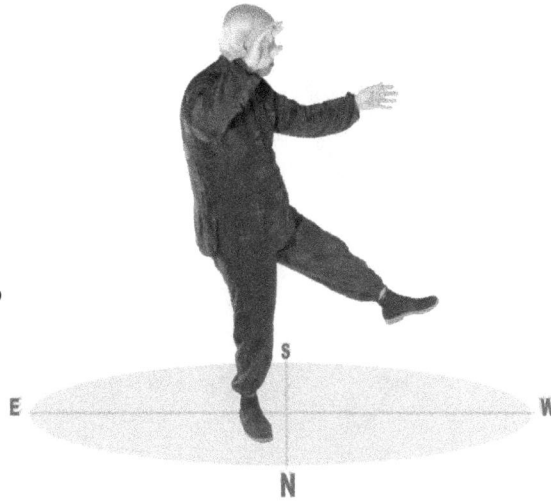

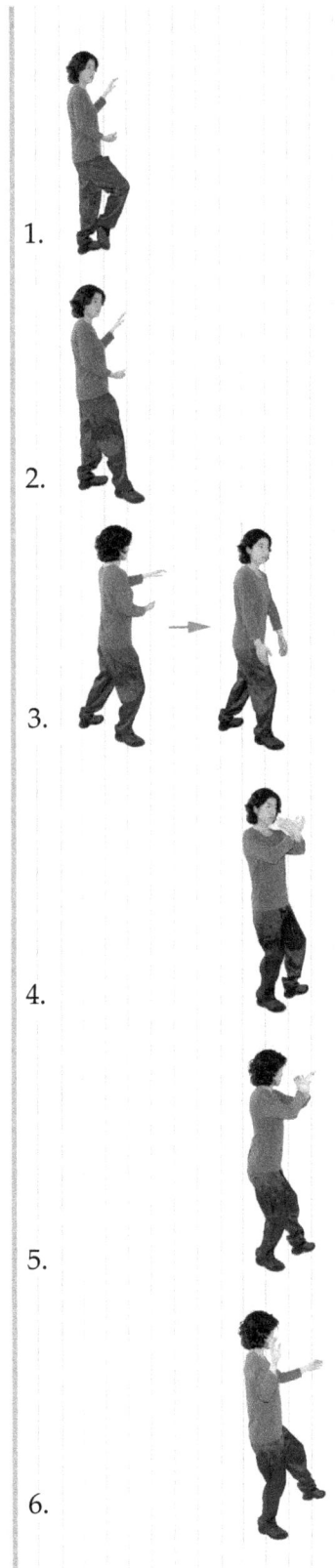

57. Turn Round and Strike with Sole (left foot)

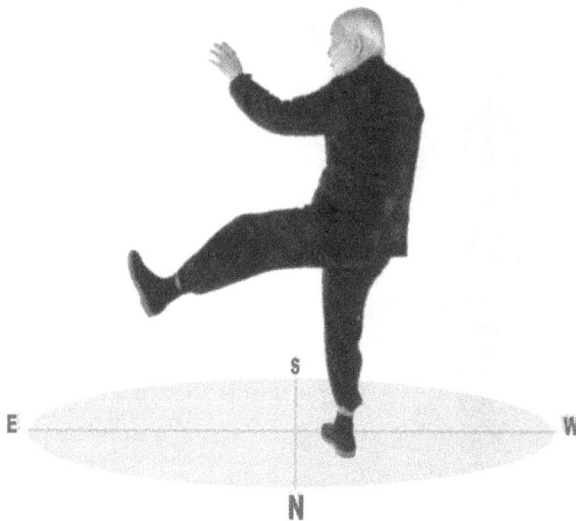

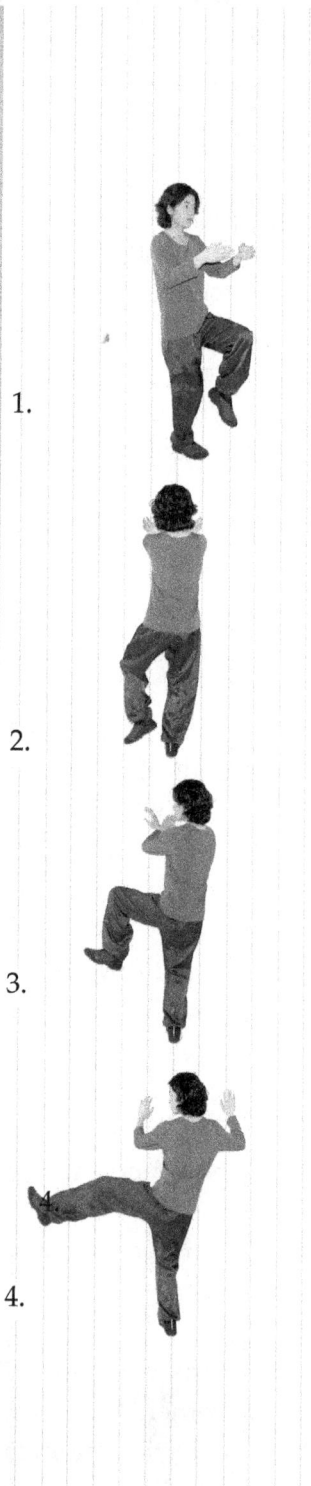

During the counts of:

1. Drop your left foot down so that it is suspended with the toes pointing down. At the same time turn your torso to your right to face northwest and extend your arms and hands in that direction with the palms facing one another.

2. In one motion, swing your whole body counterclockwise, pivoting on your right heel, to the left to face south. Your hands immediately cross at the wrists in front of your face with your left hand on the inside. Both palms face you.

3. Turn your palms outward to the south as you turn your torso to the left to face east. At the same raise your left knee and left toes, exposing the sole of the foot to the east.

4. Kick forward to the east with the sole of your left foot keeping the toes pointing upward. At the same time separate your hands keeping the arms bent at the elbows with the fingers of both hands pointing upward and palms facing south.

58. Step Forward and Brush Knee (left)

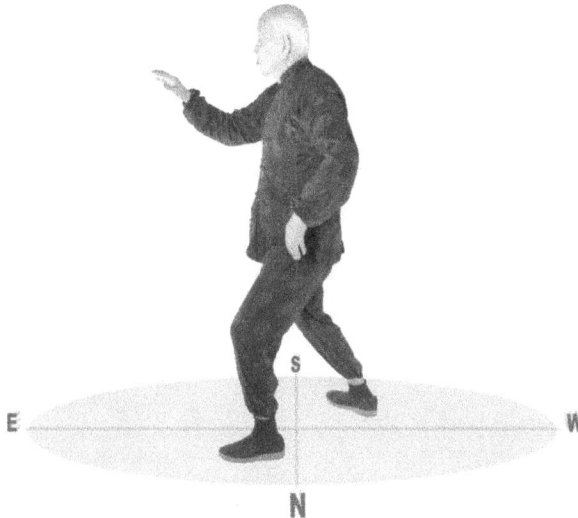

During the counts of:

1. Keep your left knee up and drop your left foot down so that it is suspended with the toes pointing down. At the same time begin to turn your torso to the right. Let your left hand come into a "ward off" position with fingers pointing south, and your right hand begin to circle down to the right in a counterclockwise motion.

2. Turn your torso clockwise to the right until it is facing east. Your right hand continues it's counterclockwise motion until it comes full circle to your right ear with the palm and fingers facing toward the east. Make sure that your right elbow remains relaxed and hanging downward.

3. Step with your left foot, heel first to the east so as to form a shoulders' width stance facing east. Brush your left knee with your left hand and let it come to rest in the "position of attention" by your left hip pocket. Your right foot, pivoting on the heel, turns in 45 degrees to point southeast and your weight is now 60% forward on your left leg.

4. Complete the bow and arrow stance facing west by shifting an additional 10% of your weight into your left foot. At the same time using your whole body, push forward with your right hand being careful to let your elbow remain relaxed and slightly bent.

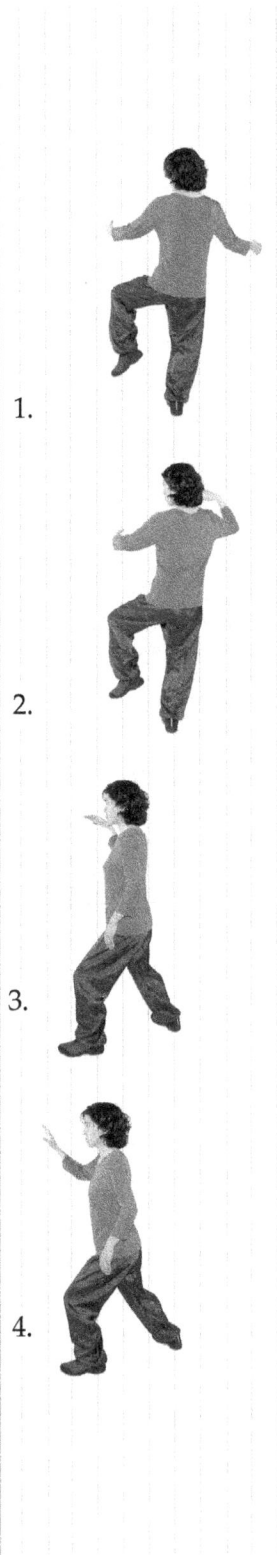

59. Step Forward and Brush Knee (right)

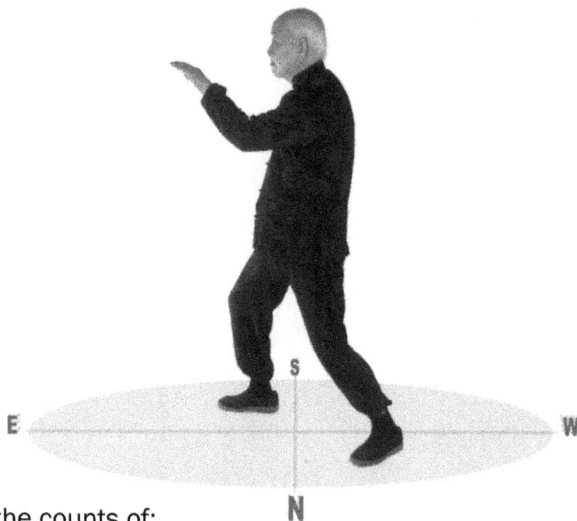

During the counts of:

1. Shifting your weight back onto your right leg, turn your torso slightly to the left and at the same time turn your left hand palm up, and let it circle down in a clockwise motion.

2. Continue to turn your torso to the left until it is facing northeast (45 degrees) and turn the left foot, pivoting on your heel, to point almost to the north. Your left hand continues its counterclockwise motion until it comes full circle to near your left ear with the fingers pointing towards the east and the elbow bent and hanging downwards. During this turning motion of your torso your right hand rises up into a "ward off" position opposite your chest with the fingers pointing north.

3. Step with your right foot, heel first to the east, so as to form a shoulders' width stance facing east. As you turn your torso to face east brush your right knee with your right hand and let it come to rest in the "position of attention" by your right hip pocket. Your left foot, pivoting on the heel, turns in 45 degrees to point northeast and your weight is now 60% forward on your right leg.

4. Complete the bow and arrow stance facing east by shifting 10% more of your weight into your left foot. At the same time using your whole body, push forward with your left hand being careful to let your elbow remain relaxed and slightly bent.

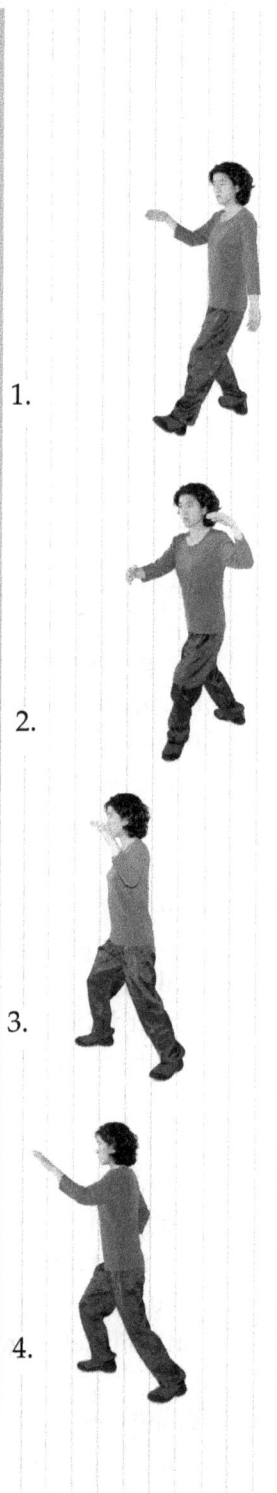

60. Step Forward and Punch Downward

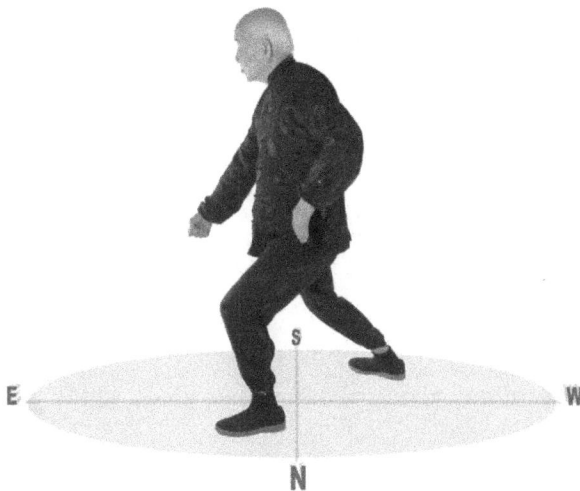

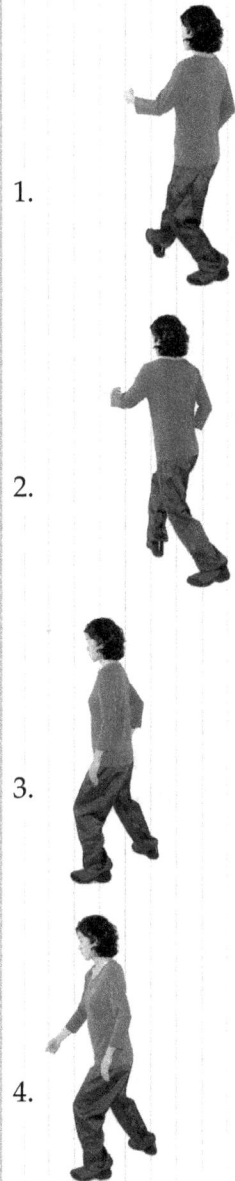

1.

2.

3.

4.

During the counts of:

1. Shift your weight back onto your left foot and turn your torso to the right to face southeast. Pivoting on the right heel, turn your right foot to point southeast and at the same time and let your left hand come into a "ward off" position with fingers pointing south.

2. Shift your weight onto your right foot. Form a fist with your right hand and attach it to your right thigh with the "tiger's mouth" pointing upward.

3. Take a step directly forward into a shoulders' width bow stance with your left foot, heel touching first, and shift your weight 60% onto it. With the turning motion of your torso brush your left knee with your left hand and hold it beside your left thigh with the palm facing backward and turn your right foot inward, pivoting on the heel, to point southeast.

4. Shift an additional 10% of your weight forward into your left foot and punch downward with your right fist.

61. Turn Back and Chop with Fist

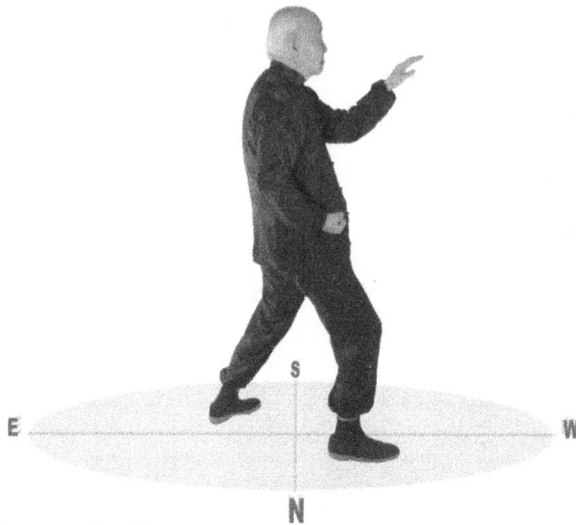

During the counts of:

1. Shift your weight back onto your right foot as you turn your torso to face south and turn your left foot, pivoting on the heel, so the toes point south. Simultaneously begin to circle your hands, without raising your elbows, in a clockwise motion.

2. Shift your weight back onto your left foot and continue to circle your hands clockwise until your left hand is near your left ear, with palm outward and elbow bent, and your right hand, clenched into a fist with the "tiger's mouth" facing your chest, comes under your left elbow. At the same time you pivot with your right foot on the toes to point southwest.

3. Step to the west with your right foot and chop to the west with your right fist. When your chop is complete shift your weight 60% onto your right foot and bring the fist back to your right hip. With the turning forward of your torso to the west, turn in your left foot, pivoting on the heel, to point southwest.

4. Complete the bow and arrow stance by shifting an additional 10% of your weight onto your right foot and push forward with your left hand/palm.

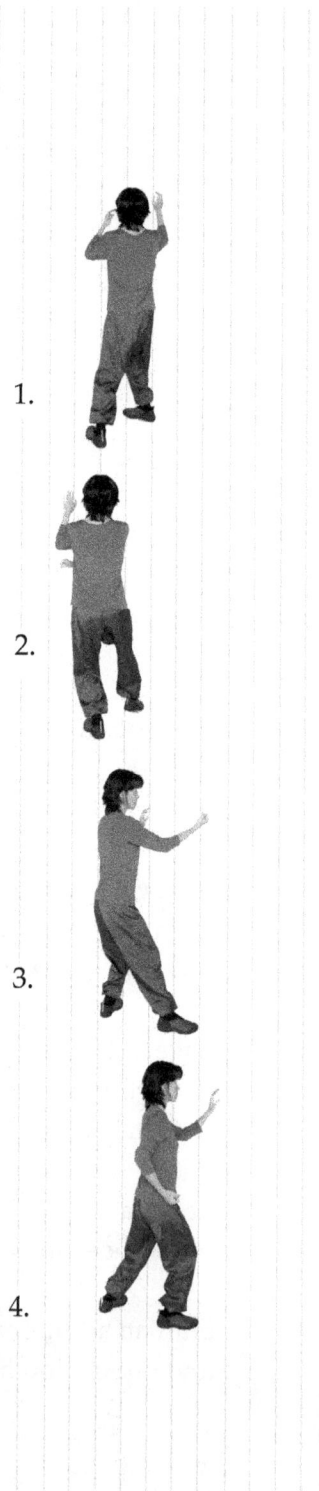

62. Step Forward, Deflect Downward, Intercept and Punch

During the counts of:

1. Pick up your left foot and set it down, heel first, adjusting the toes pointing to the southwest.

2. Shift your weight back onto your left foot and turn your torso to the left to face southwest as you reach out in that direction with both hands. Your palms are facing each other as though holding a ball with your right hand positioned ontop.

3. Raise your right foot and take a step diagonally forward to the right. At the same time make a fist with your right hand and circle it clockwise around to the right side of your waist and attach it to your right hip, palm side facing up with the tigers mouth facing out to the north. In unison with this motion your left hand circles clockwise upward and forward in front of your face. Your left elbow remains relaxed and down.

4. Facing west, shift your weight to your right foot (toes pointing to the north/northwest) and simultaneously bring your left hand forward and down to the level of your stomach, palm facing the floor.

5. Step directly forward, to maintain a shoulder's width stance, with your left foot and shift 60% of your weight onto it. At the same time extend or intercept with your left hand forward and to the left. The left hand is open with the fingers pointing west and the palm is facing north. With this motion your right foot turns inward, pivoting on the heel, so that the toes are pointing northwest.

6. Complete the bow and arrow stance facing west by shifting an additional 10% of your weight onto your left foot. At the same time, using your whole body behind it, punch forward with your right fist (tiger's mouth facing up). As your right hand is punching forward bring your left hand over to cover the inner wrist of your right hand.

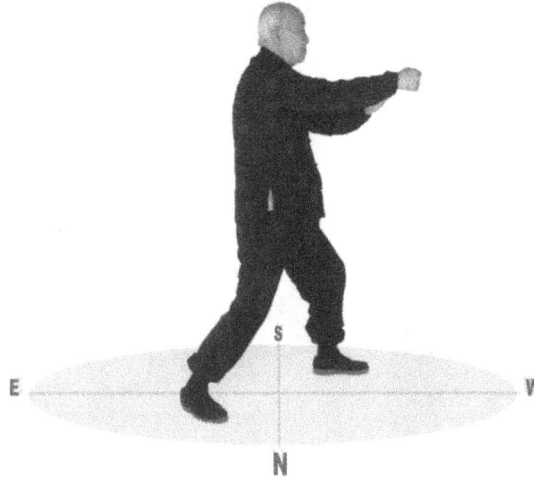

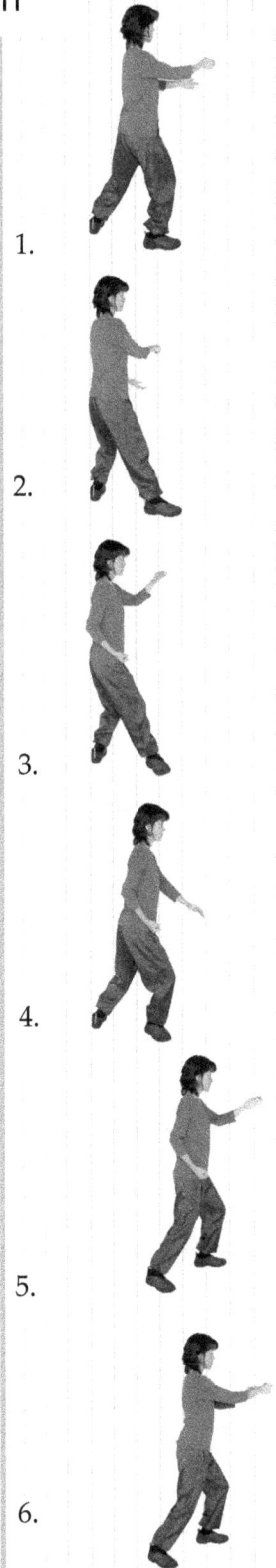

127

63. Kick Upward with Right Foot

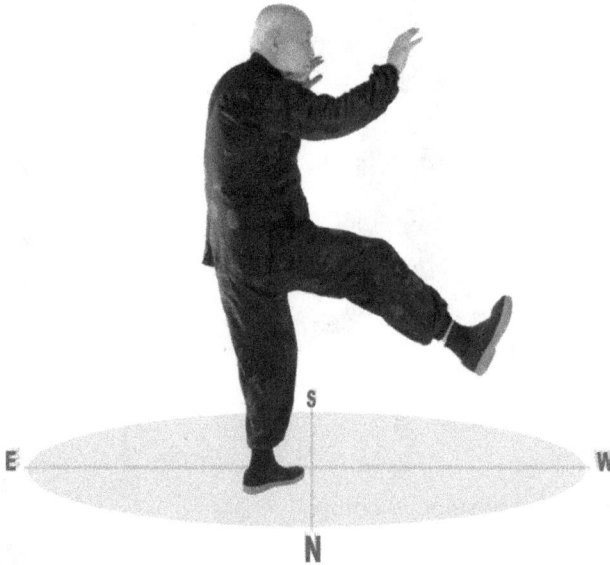

During the counts of:

1. | Shift your weight back onto your right foot and turn your left foot, pivoting on the heel, to point southwest. At the same time open your right fist and separate both hands and begin to circle them out, with palms facing outward, in opposite directions.

2. | Shift your weight forward onto your left foot. At the same time continue to circle your hands downward and up until they cross diagonally at the wrists, right hand on the inside with both palms facing in. Bring your right foot up to form a "T" with the toes touching the ground and pointing northwest.

3. | Turn both palms outward to face southwest and turn your torso clockwise to the right to face northwest.

4. | Separate your hands, bringing your forearms into a vertical position with the elbows down and relaxed. At the same time kick upwards with your right foot.

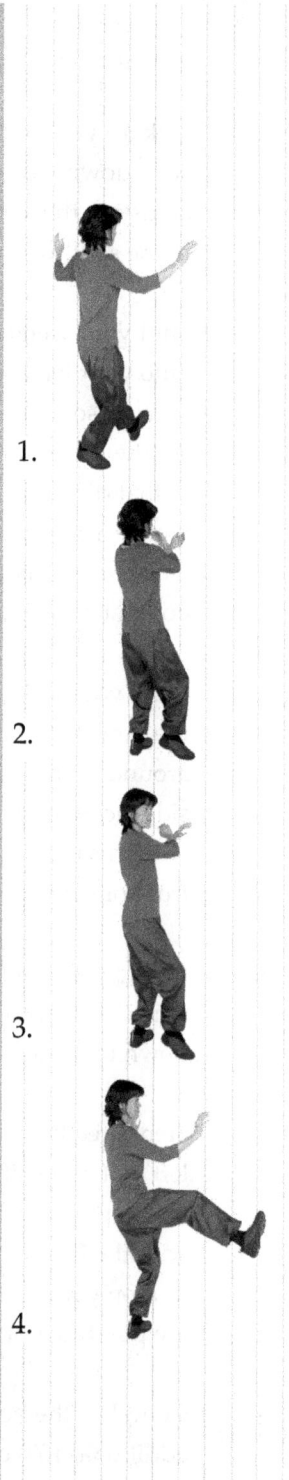

64. Strike Tiger Left

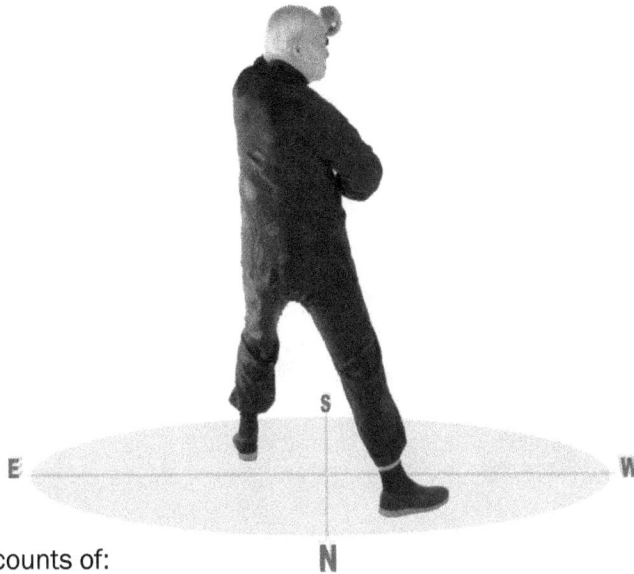

During the counts of:

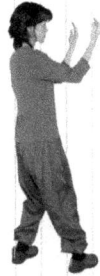

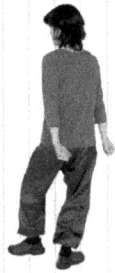

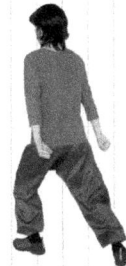

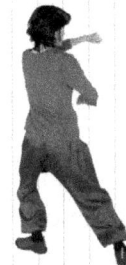

1. Lower your right foot and place it down about 10" in front of your left foot with the toes pointing southwest. Lower your arms and turn both palms facing up.

2. Shift your weight onto your right leg and continue to bring your hands downward to your hips. Then turn your torso to face southeast and turn your left foot, pivoting on the toes, to point southeast as well. Form two fists with the "tiger mouths" facing in and the knuckles pointing down.

3. Take a step with your left foot to the southeast (heel landing first) and shift your weight 60% onto it. Turn your right foot, pivoting on the heel so that the toes point south.

4. Shift your weight 10% more onto your left foot and turn your torso back to the southwest corner. Bring your left fist above the forehead with the palm facing out and the "tiger's mouth" facing down. Simultaneously bring your right fist around to opposite your solar plexus with the palm facing down and the "tiger's mouth" facing in.

65. Strike Tiger Right

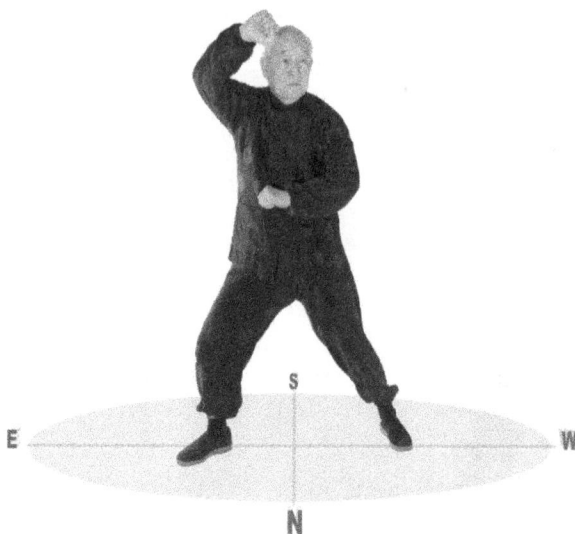

During the counts of:

1. Turn your torso to to your right to face west and shift your weight to the right foot as you turn your left foot inward, pivoting on the toes, to point west/southwest. Circle both arms forward to the west with the palms up.

2. Shift your weight onto your left leg and bring your hands downward to your hips. Turn your right foot, pivoting on the toes, to point west as well.

3. Turn your torso to face northeast and form two fists with the "tiger mouths" facing in and the knuckles pointing down. Take a step diagonally with your right foot (heel touching first) to the northwest and shift your weight 60% onto it. Turn your left foot, pivoting on the heel, to point north.

4. Shift an additional 10% of your weight onto your right foot and turn your torso back to the northwest corner. Bring your right fist opposite your forehead with the palm facing out and the "tiger's mouth" facing down. Simultaneously bring your left fist around to a position opposite the level of your solar plexus with the palm facing down and the "tiger's mouth" facing in.

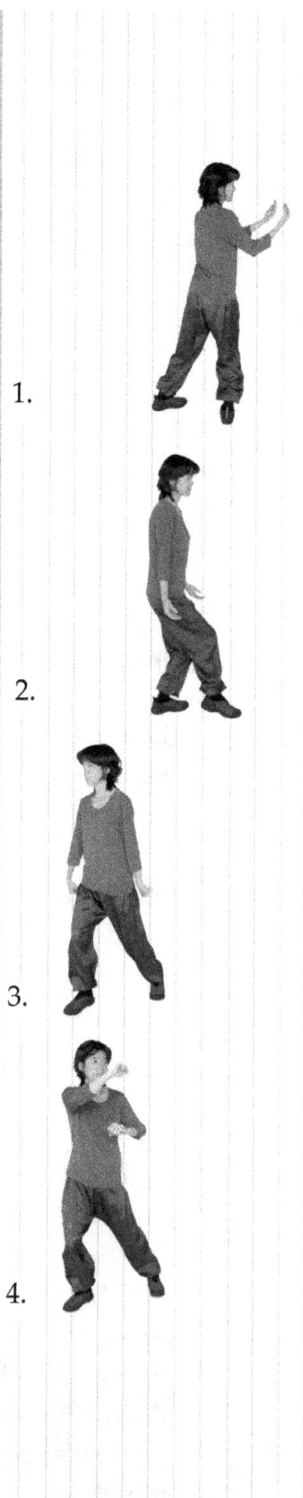

66. Kick Upward With Right Foot

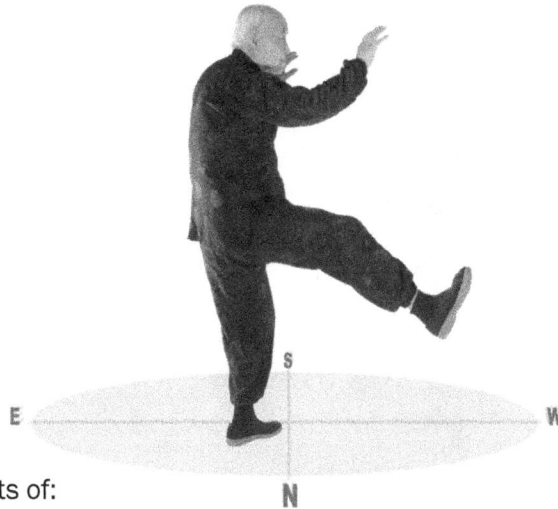

During the counts of:

1. Shift your weight onto your right foot and turn your torso to the left to face southwest. At the same time turn your left foot outward, pivoting on the heel, to point southwest as well. Open your fists and circle your hands upward and out - moving in opposite directions. The right arm circles to the right and the left arm to the left.

2. Shift your weight forward onto your left foot and turn in your right foot, pivoting on the heel, to point northwest. Momentarily shift your weight back onto your right foot and then, shifting all of your weight onto your left foot, bring your right foot up opposite your left foot into a "T" position with the toes touching the ground and pointing northwest. At the same time continue to circle your hands downward and up until they cross diagonally at the wrists, right hand on the inside with both palms facing in.

3. Turn both palms outward to face southwest and turn your torso clockwise to the right to face northwest.

4. Separate your hands bringing your forearms into vertical positions with the elbows down and relaxed. At the same time kick upwards with your right foot.

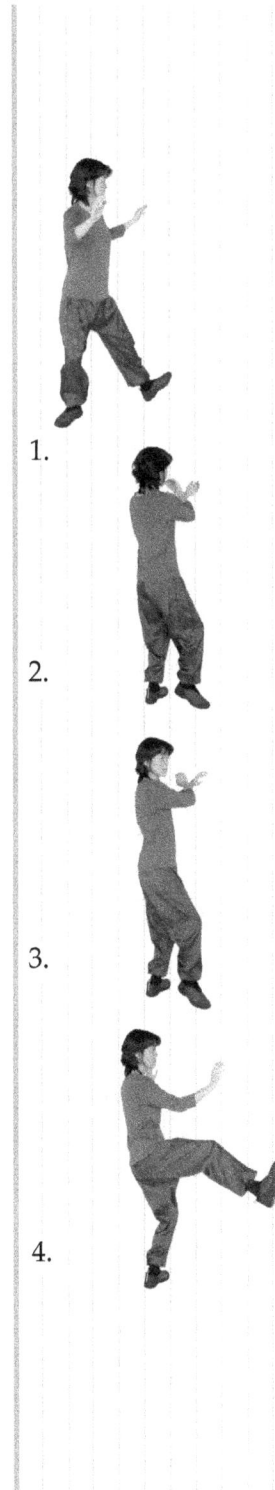

1.

2.

3.

4.

67. Strike with Both Fists

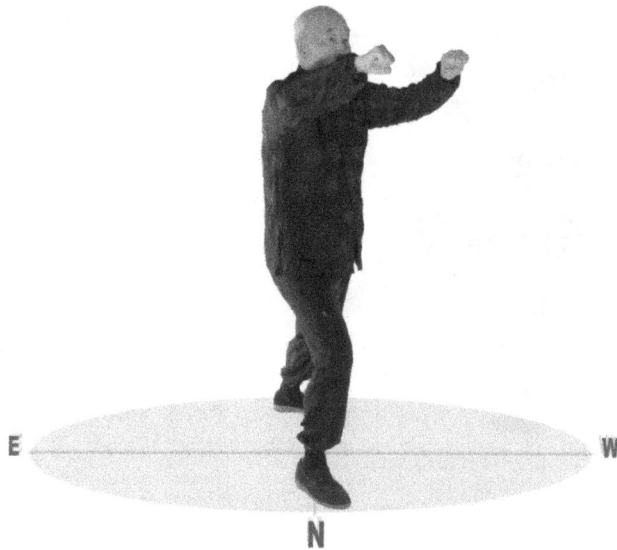

During the counts of:

1. Lower and suspend your right foot with the toes pointing down, and turn your palms to face upward.

2. Keeping your right leg suspended, lower your upturned hands over your right knee down to your hips at pocket level.

3. Step forward with your right foot to the northwest and shift 60% of your weight onto it and turn your left foot in 45 degrees, pivoting on the heel, to point west. At the same time form your hands into lightly held fists with the knuckles pointing down and the "tiger mouths" facing each other.

4. Shift an additional 10% of your weight to your right foot and circle your fists diagonally forward and up so as to strike your imaginary opponent with the "tiger mouths" on either side of his head. Your shoulders remain relaxed and your elbows slightly bent.

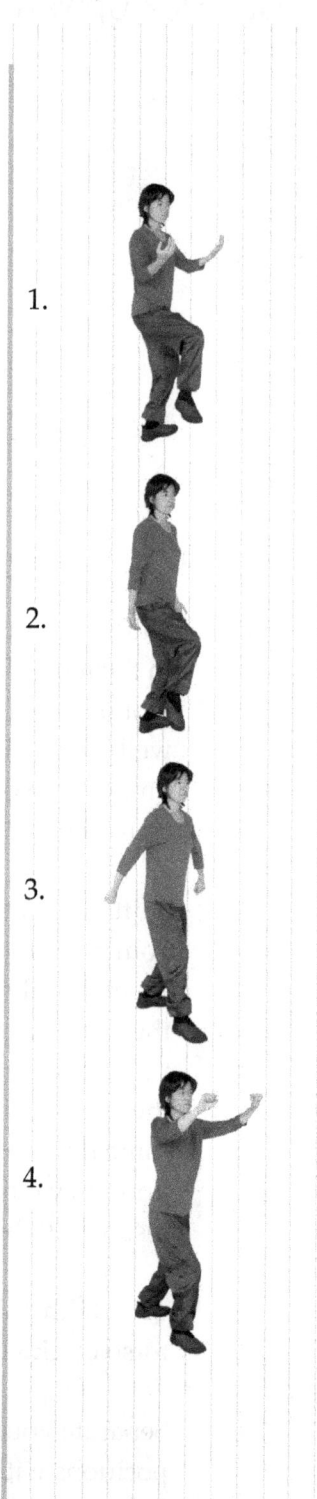

68. Kick Upward With Left Foot

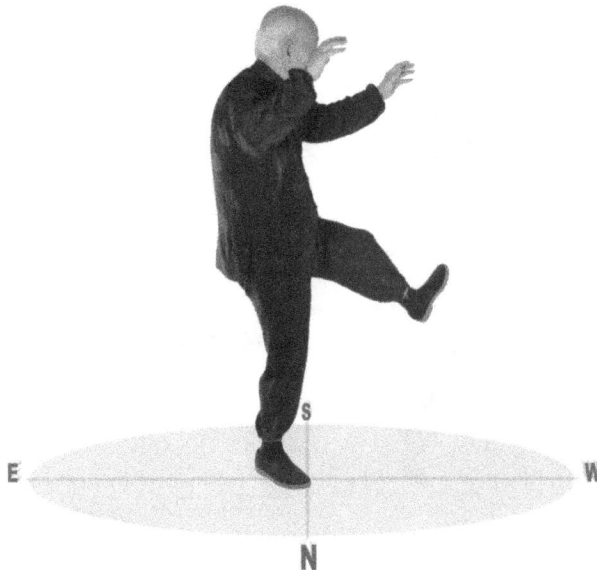

During the counts of:

1. Shift your weight back onto your left foot and open both hands and begin to circle them out, with palms facing outward, in opposite directions.

2. Shift your weight forward onto your right foot. At the same time continue to circle your hands downward and up until they cross diagonally at the wrists, left hand on the inside with both palms facing in. Bring your left foot up to form a "T" with the toes touching the ground and pointing southwest.

3. Turn both palms outward to face northwest and turn your torso counterclockwise to the left to face southwest.

4. Separate your hands by bringing your forearms into a vertical position with the elbows down and relaxed. At the same time kick upwards with your left foot.

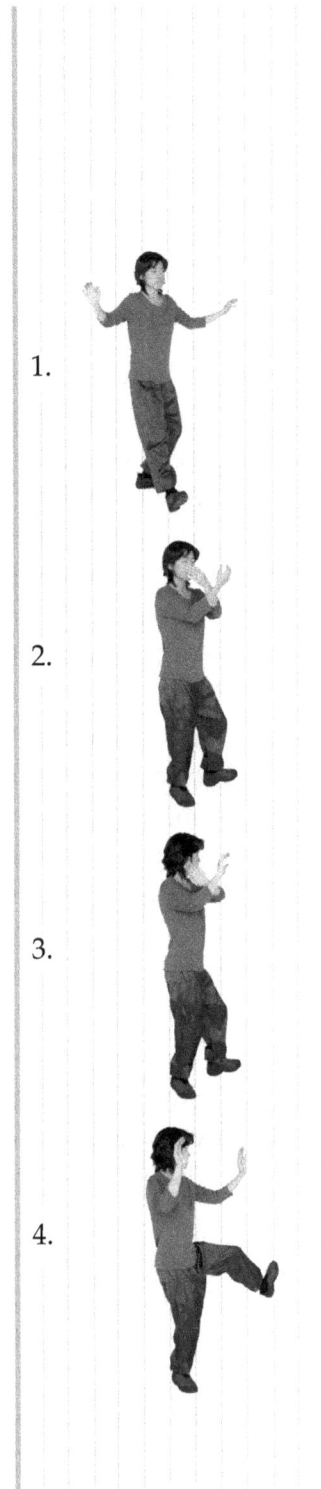

69. Turn Round and Kick with Sole (right foot)

During the counts of:

1. In a windup motion in preparation to turn right, turn your torso in the opposite direction, counterclockwise to your left, as you drop your left foot down (keeping your knee raised). Your hands reach out, palms facing each other, to the southwest corner.

2. Using the momentum of the above movement, turn your torso clockwise, pivoting on the ball of your right foot 315 degrees to face south. Place your left foot down a shoulders' width from your right foot. Both feet point south. Your outstretched arms turn with the torso and your hands turn so the the palms are facing down.

3. Circle your hands up and out in opposite directions as you begin to shift your weight to your left leg.

4. Shift your weight completely onto your left foot and continue to circle your hands around until they cross at the wrists, right hand on the inside, in front of your chest / throat.

5. Turn your palms outward to the south as you turn your torso to the right to face west. At the same time raise your right knee and right toes, exposing the sole of the foot to the west.

6. Kick forward to the west with the sole of your right foot, keeping the toes pointing upward. At the same time separate your hands keeping the arms bent at the elbows with the fingers of both hands pointing upward and palms facing south.

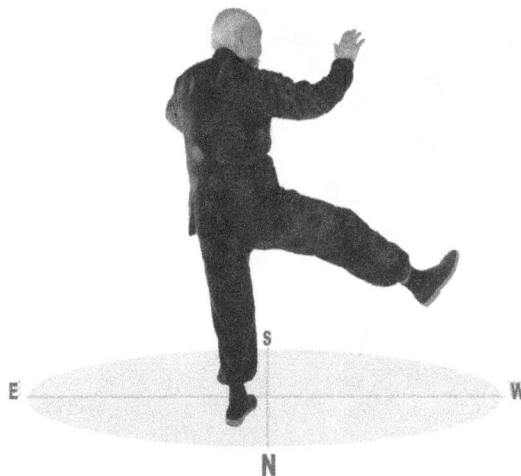

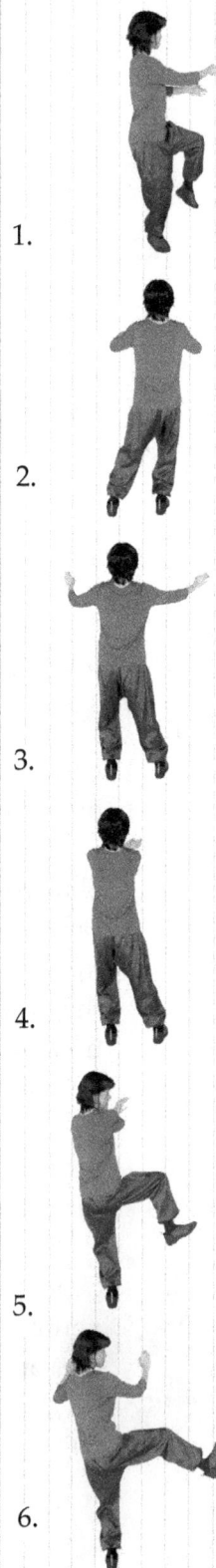

70. Chop with Fist

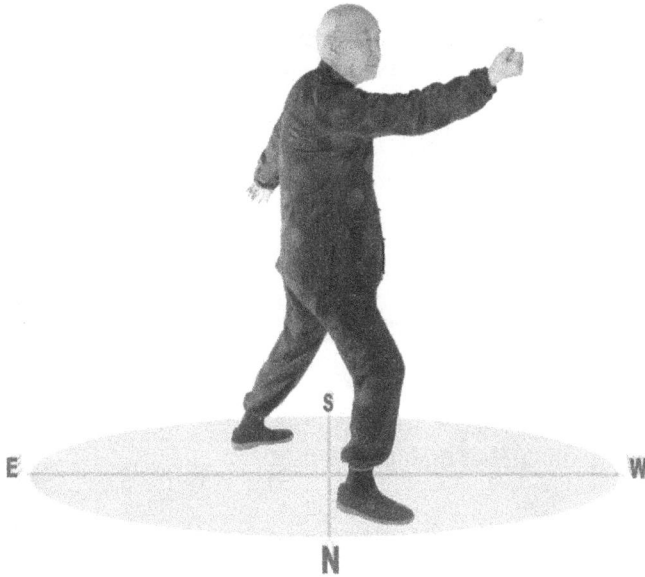

During the counts of:

1. Drop your right foot down (keeping your knee raised) and let your hands swing back to the southeast corner, palms facing down.

2. Step with your right foot to the northwest and, as you shift your weight 70% onto it, turn your torso to the right to face northwest. With the turning of your torso, turn your left foot, pivoting on the heel, so that the toes point west. Use this turning motionto chop with the back of your right fist to the northwest corner at about eye level (as though you are chopping your imaginary opponent ontop of his or her nose). Your left hand remains extended backwards, palm down, to the southeast.

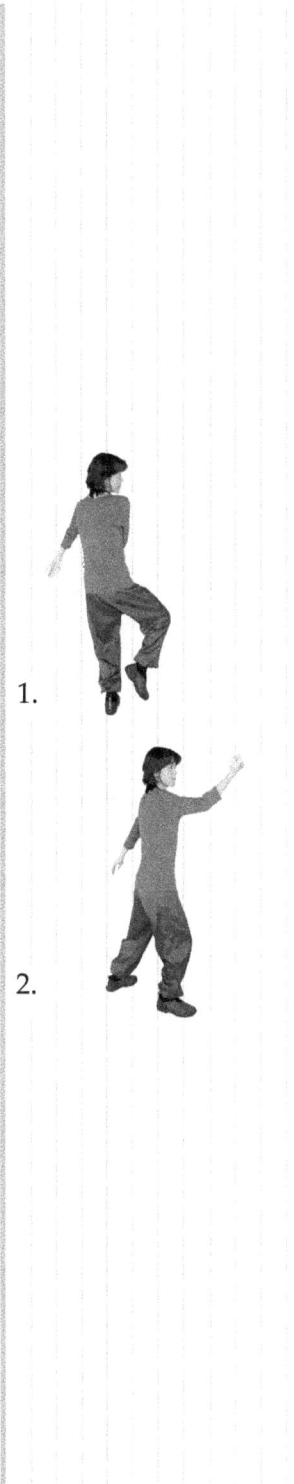

71. Step Forward, Deflect Downward, Intercept and Punch

During the counts of:

1. Pick up your left foot and set it down, heel first, with the toes pointing to the southwest.

2. Shift your weight back onto your left foot and turn your torso to the left to face southwest as you reach out in that direction with both hands. Your palms are facing each other as though holding a ball. Your right hand is slightly higher than your left.

3. Raise your right foot and take a step diagonally forward to the right. At the same time make a fist with your right hand and circle it clockwise around to the right side of your waist (in a deflecting motion) and attach it to your right hip, palm side facing up with the "tiger's mouth" facing out to the north. In unison with this motion your left hand circles clockwise upward and forward in front of your face. Your left elbow remains relaxed and down.

4. Facing west, shift your weight to your right foot (toes pointing to the north/northwest) and simultaneously bring your left hand forward, deflecting downward to the level of your stomach, palm facing the floor.

5. Step directly forward, to maintain a shoulders' width stance, with your left foot and shift 60% of your weight onto it. At the same time extend or intercept with your left hand forward and to the left. The left hand is open with the fingers pointing west and the palm is facing north. With this motion your right foot turns inwards, pivoting on the heel, so that the toes are pointing northwest.

6. Complete the bow and arrow stance facing west by shifting 10% more of your weight into your left foot. At the same time, using your whole body (not just your arm), punch forward with your right fist ("tiger's mouth* facing up). As your right hand is punching forward let your left hand come over and cover the inner wrist of your right hand.

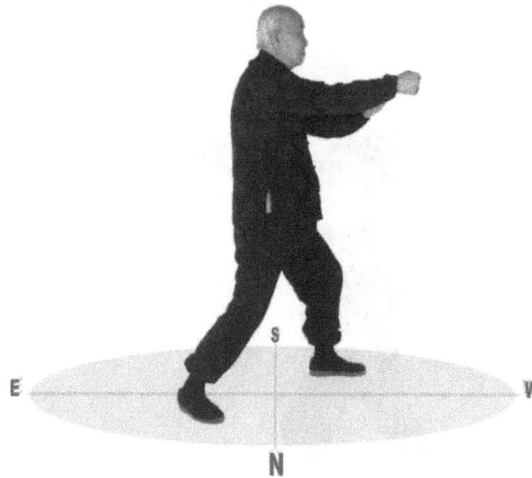

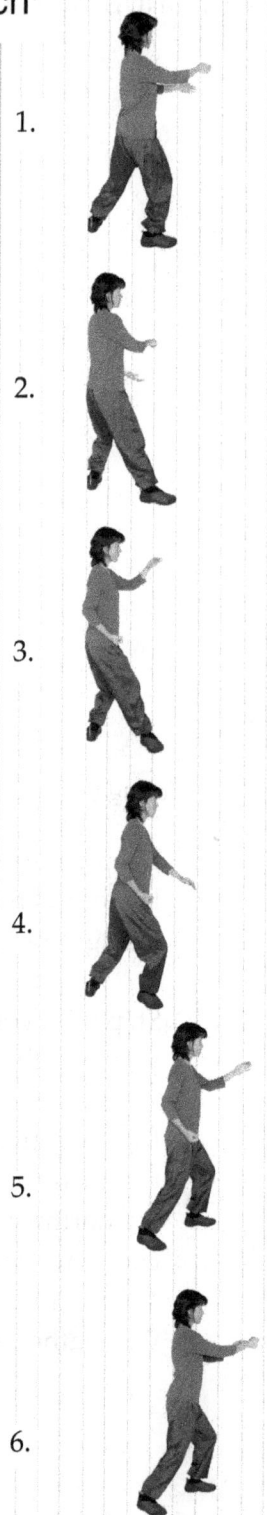

72. Withdraw and Push

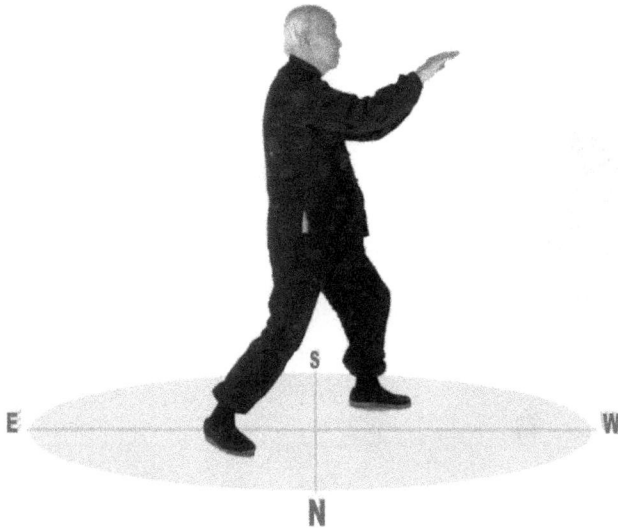

During the counts of:

1.   Slide your left hand, palm up, under your right wrist and open the right fist so that both palms are now open and facing upwards with your hands crossed at the wrists.

2.   Shift your weight back onto your right foot and draw both hands back with your palms facing your chest. Separate your hands ...

3.   ... and then turn both palms outward to face west. Without moving your hands and arms separately from your body, push forward by shifting your weight forward onto your left leg. The push is coming from the forward movement of your body - not your arms.

4.   Complete the bow and arrow stance by shifting an additional 10% of your weight into your left foot. At the same time slightly raise your fingertips so that the intention of the push is coming from your palms.

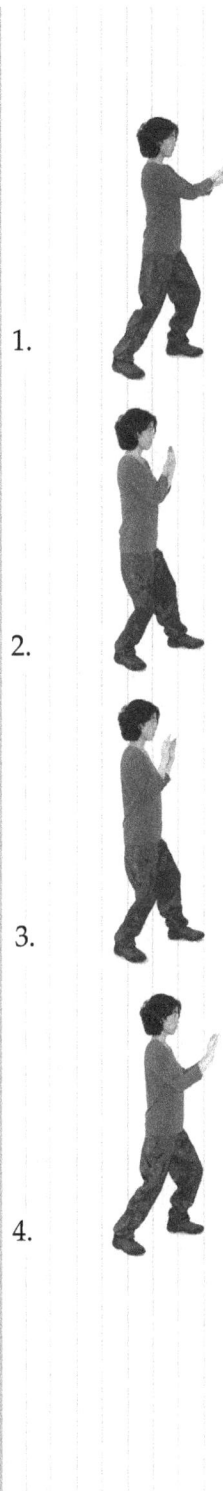

73. Crossing Hands

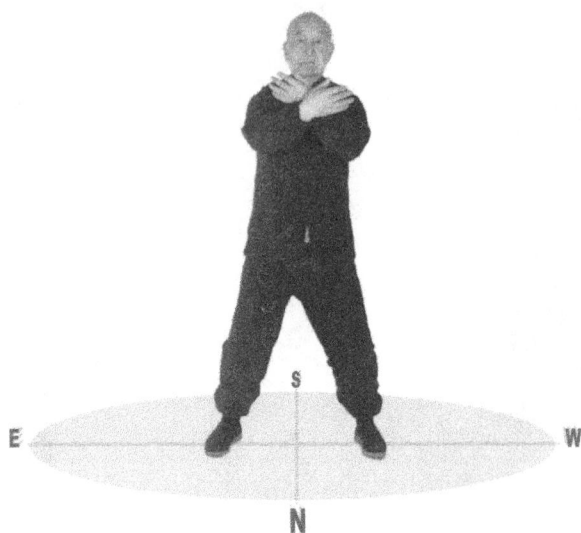

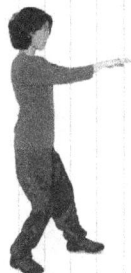

1.

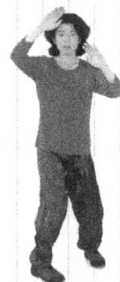

2.

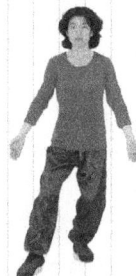

3.

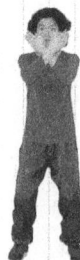

4.

During the counts of:

1. Keep your back straight and shift your weight back onto your right leg, and as you do this, let your arms straighten out.

2. Turn your torso to face north and, bending at your elbows, circle your hands in front of your face with both palms facing out to the north. Your right hand is slightly higher than your left.

3. Shift your weight back onto your left foot and circle both hands out and down.

4. Step back with your right foot and place it down a shoulders' width distance from your left foot and parallel to it. At the same time bring your hands (your right hand outside the left) up in front of your face, crossing them at the wrists with both palms facing to the south. Your weight remains more than 50% on your left leg.

74. Embrace the Tiger to Return to the Mountain

During the counts of:

1. Turn your torso clockwise to your right to face northeast. Keep your wrists crossed and lower your hands parallel to the ground while turning your right hand palm down and leaving your left hand palm up. At the same time turn your right foot, pivoting on the toes, to point notheast.

2. Pick your right foot up and step to the southeast corner. At the same time separate your hands. Your right hand (palm facing down) moves to the southeast corner together with your right foot. Your left hand moves back to the north with the palm facing up.

3. Place your right foot, heel down first, in a shoulders' width stance facing southeast. As you shift 60% of your weight onto it, withdraw your right hand, turning your palm to face upwards, beside your right thigh. Circle your left hand, palm up, in a clockwise motiontowards your left ear with palm and fingers facing forward and the elbow lowered. Turn your torso to face southeast and at the same time turn your left foot clockwise, pivoting on the heel, to point east.

4. Complete the bow and arrow stance facing southeast by shifting 10% more of your weight into your right foot. In conjunction with this shifting of your weight, use your whole body to push forward with your left hand. The left elbow remains slightly bent with the fingers pointing forward and diagonally upward.

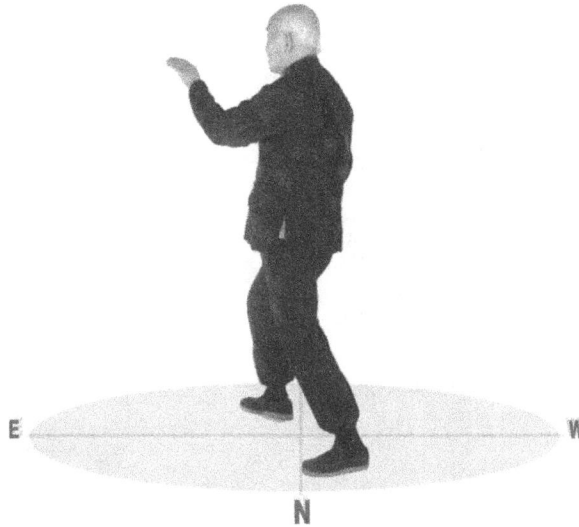

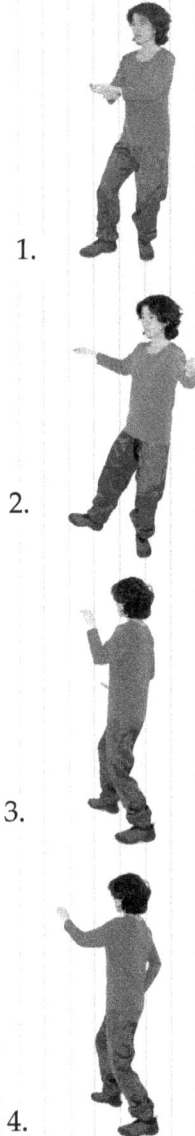

75. Roll Back

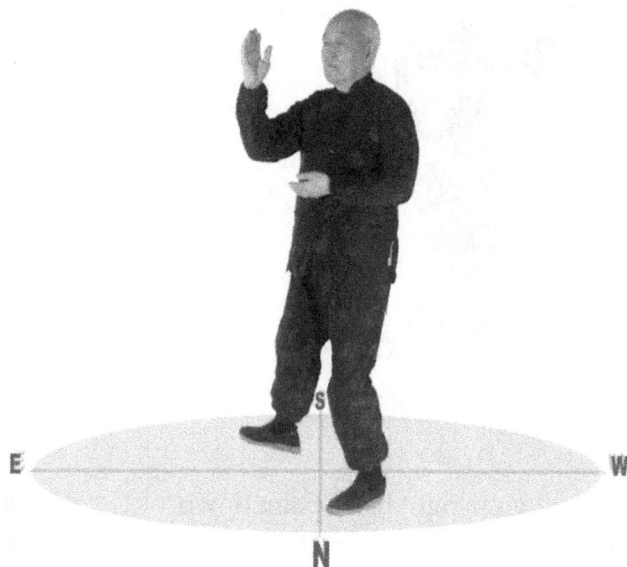

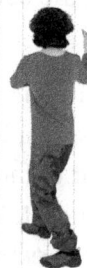

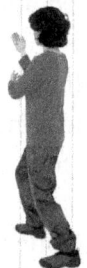

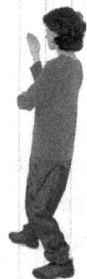

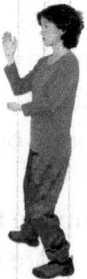

1.

2.

3.

4.

During the counts of:

1. Turn your torso to your right 45 degrees and bring your right forearm up virtically and perpendicular to your body. At the same time bring your left forearm across in front of the chest with your left palm facing your chest and the fingers almost touching your right elbow.

2. Keeping your weight on your right leg, as one unit, turn your torso to your left to face southeast again. Your upper body, arms and hands move together as one unit.

3. Keep your torso facing southeast while you withdraw your weight back onto your left foot.

4. Turn your torso to the left 45 degrees. At the same time turn your left palm upwards. You are now facing east.

76. Press

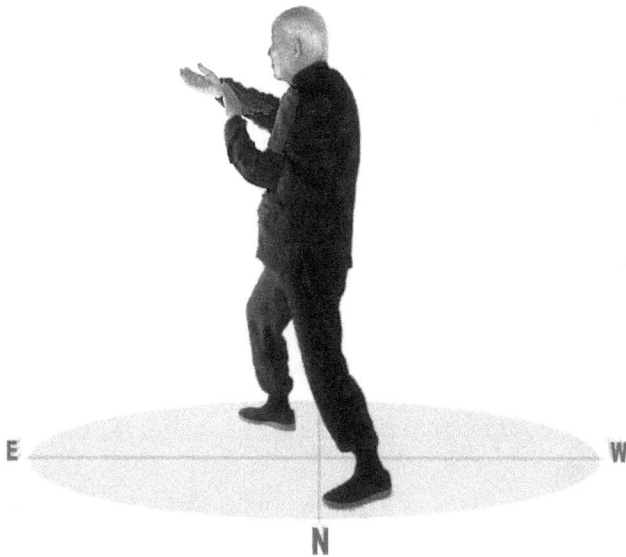

During the counts of:

1. Turn your torso 45 degrees to your left to face northeast. With the momentum of this turn let your left hand drop down and circle around (without lifting the elbow), heading up toward your left ear.

2. As your left hand is passing by your ear, turn your torso back 90 degrees to your right to face southeast and lightly attach your left fingers to the inside of your right wrist (as though you're feeling your pulse). Your right forearm drops slightly down into a diagonal position in front of your upper chest with the left elbow lowered.

3. Without letting your hands and arms move separately from your body, shift your weight onto the right leg and press forward with your right forearm. It's important here to move your whole body as one unit and not let your hands and arms move independently or initiate any movement.

4. Continue to press forward and slightly upwards until your right leg bears about 70% of your weight.

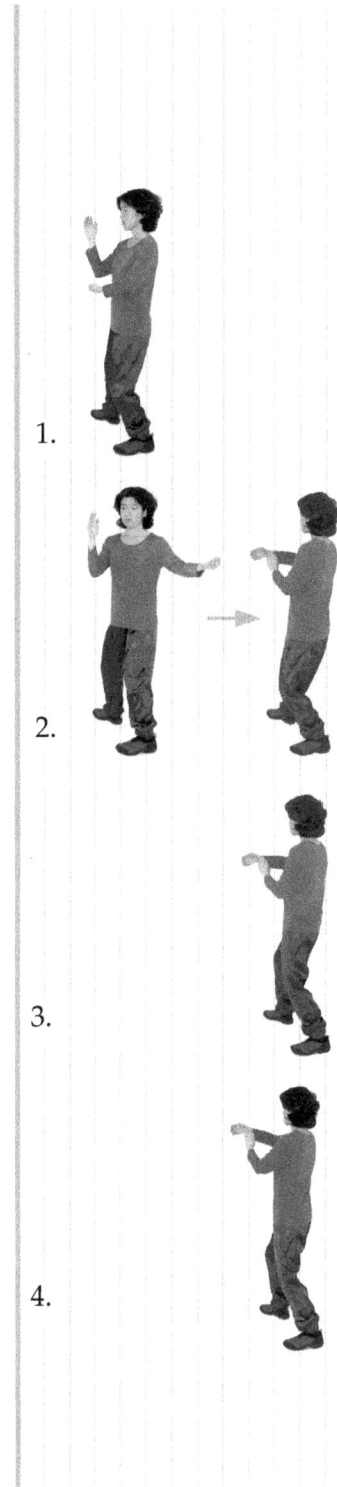

77. Push

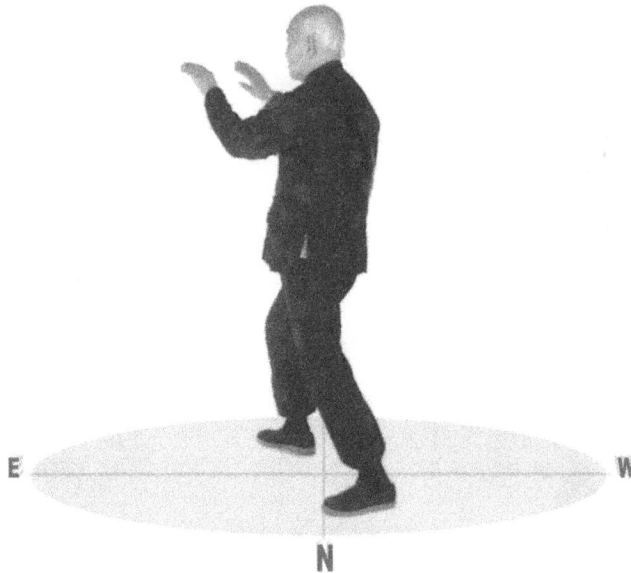

During the counts of:

1. Seperate your hands, palms down, at the level of your shoulders.

2. Keeping your back straight, shift your weight back onto your left leg and simultaneously withdraw your your hands slightly torwards your upper chest. The fingers of both hands point forward and the elbows remain relaxed and bent downwards.

3. Without moving your hands and arms seperately from your body, shift your weight back onto your right leg . The "push" is coming from the forward movement of your whole body - not your arms.

4. Complete the bow and arrow stance by shifting an additional 10% of your weight into your right foot. At the same time slightly raise your fingertips so that the intention of the push is coming through your palms and directed to the southeast corner.

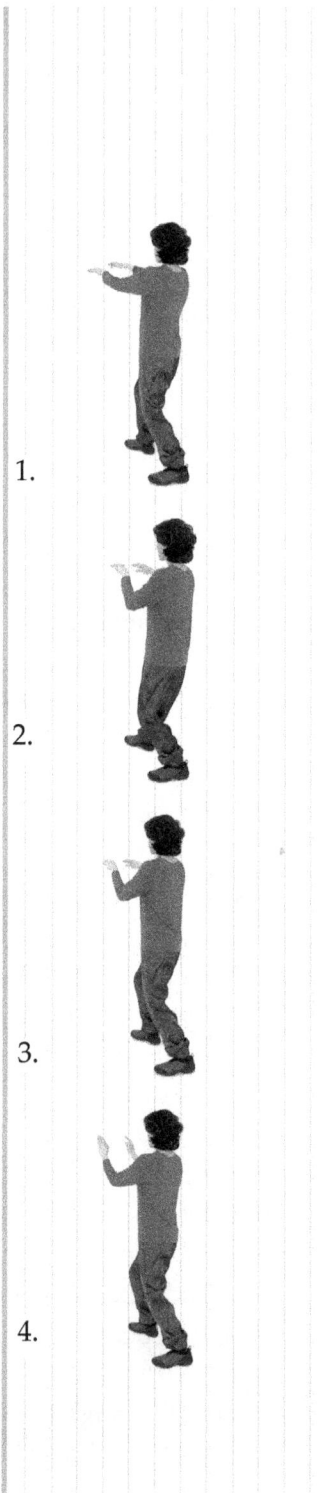

78. Horizontal Single Whip

During the counts of:

1. Shift your weight back onto your left foot and let your arms stretch out slightly with your palms facing downward.

2. Turn your torso to the left until it faces northeast and at the same time turn your right foot, pivoting on the heel, so that the toes point east. (If you look down at your feet they should appear pigeontoed).

3. Shift your weight back to your right leg as you turn your torso to face southeast. Simultaneously withdraw both hands; your left hand comes down opposite the navel with its palm facing up and your right hand forms a "hook" (the fingers pointing downward with all 5 digits touching at the fingertips near your right armpit).

4. Turn your torso back to face the northeast corner. Let this movement simultaneously pivot your left foot on the toes to point north and strike to the southeast with your right hand "hook."

5. Continue to turn your torso to face north and step with your left foot, heel first, so as to form a shoulders' width stance facing north. The turning movement of your torso brings your left hand, palm facing in, around in front of your body at face level as well as turning your right foot, pivoting on the heel, to point northeast. The right hand "hook" does not move.

6. Complete the bow and arrow stance facing north by shifting 10% more of your weight into your left foot. At the same time turn your left hand palm outward while being careful to leave the elbow slightly bent. Your eyes gaze just over and past the fingertips.

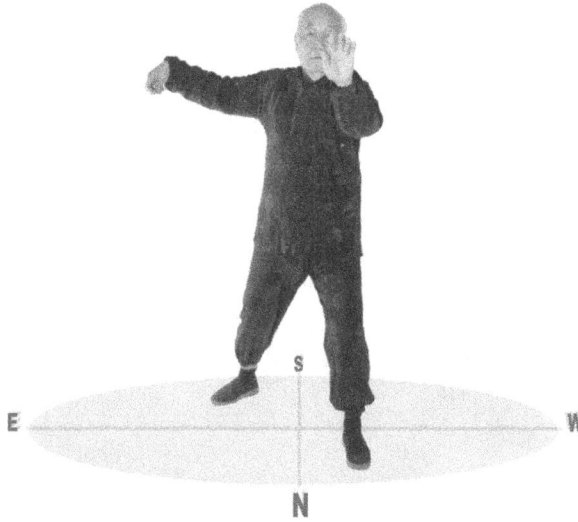

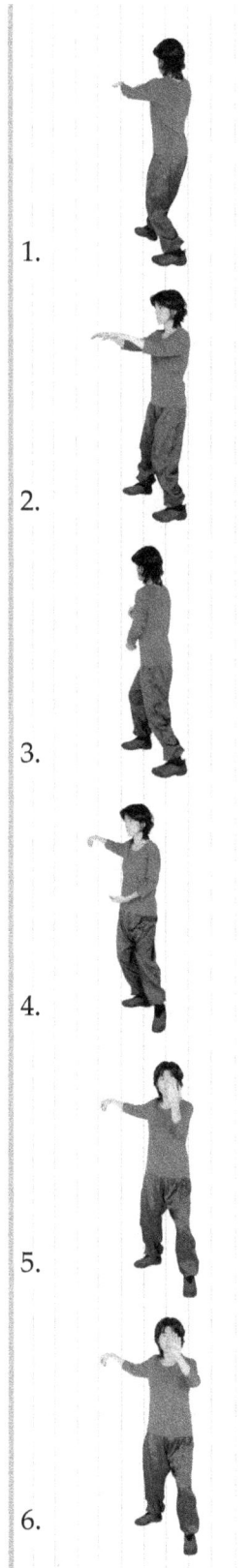

79. Parting Wild Horses Mane (right)

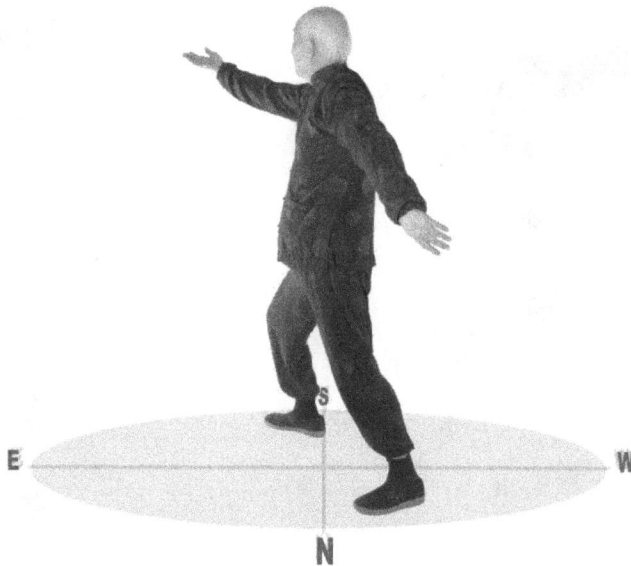

During the counts of:

1. | Shift your weight back onto your right leg and turn your left foot, pivoting on the heel, to point northeast. At the same time bring your hands into a position simulating holding a ball in front of your chest. Your left hand ontop with the palm facing down and the right hand on the bottom with the palm up.

2. | Shift your weight onto your left foot and, in preparation to step, pivot on the right toes.

3. | Step to the southeast corner with your right foot and then shift 60% of your weight onto it. As you turn your torso to face southeast simultaneously turn your left foot, pivoting on the heel, to face east..

4. | Shift 10% more of your weight onto your right foot. Your right hand, palm facing up, moves in a diagonal direction upward to the southeast while your left hand, thumb facing down, moves in the opposite direction diagonally downward to the north/northwest.

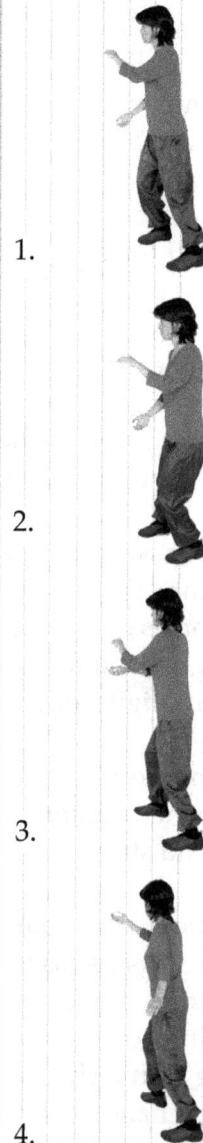

80. Parting Wild Horse's Mane (left)

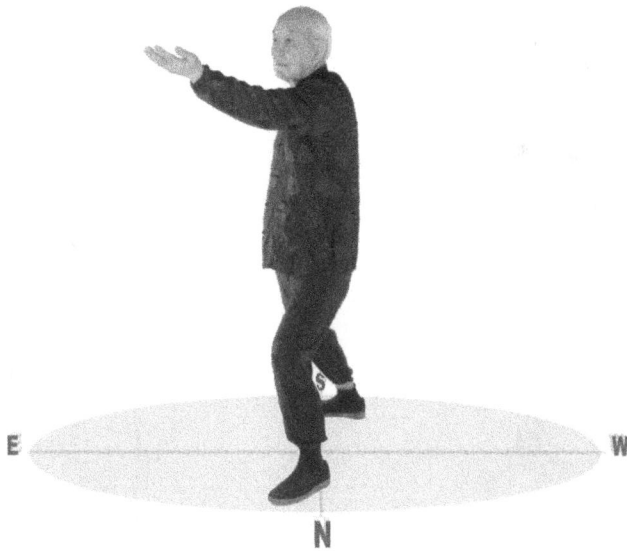

During the counts of:

1. Shift your weight back onto your left leg and turn your right foot, pivoting on the heel, to point south. At the same time bring your hands into a position simulating holding a ball in front of your chest. Your right hand ontop with the palm facing down and your left hand on the bottom with the palm facing up.

2. Shift your weight onto your right foot and, in preparation to step, pivot on the left toes.

3. Step to the northeast corner with your left foot and then shift 60% of your weight onto it. As you turn your torso to face northeast simultaneously turn your right foot, pivoting on the heel, to face east..

4. Shift 10% more of your weight onto your left foot. Your left hand, palm facing up, moves in a diagonal direction upward to the northeast while your right hand, thumb facing down, moves in the opposite direction diagonally downward to the southwest.

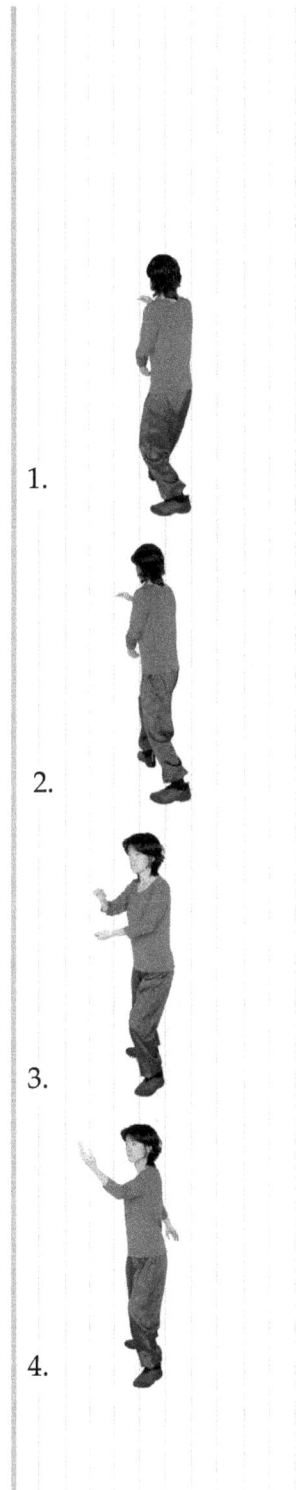

81. Parting Wild Horse's Mane (right)

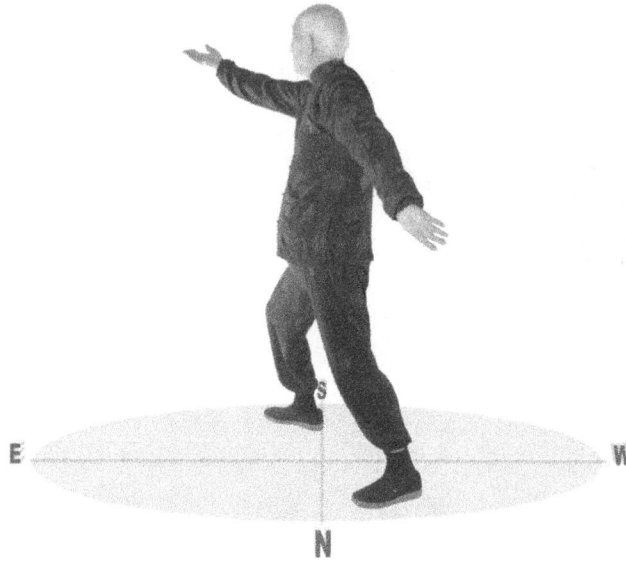

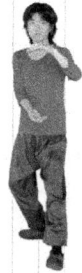

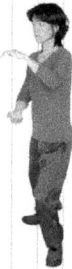

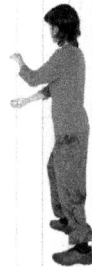

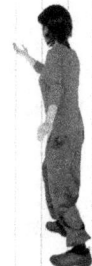

During the counts of:

1. Shift your weight back onto your right leg and turn your left foot, pivoting on the heel, to point north. At the same time bring your hands into a position simulating holding a ball in front of your chest. Your left hand ontop with the palm facing down and the right hand on the bottom with the palm up.

2. Shift your weight onto your left foot and, in preparation to step, pivot on the right toes, turning them to face southeast.

3. Step to the southeast corner with your right foot and then shift 60% of your weight onto it. As you turn your torso to face southeast simultaneously turn your left foot, pivoting on the heel, to face east.

4. Shift 10% more of your weight onto your right foot. Your right hand, palm facing up, moves in a diagonal direction upward to the southeast while your left hand, thumb facing down, moves in the opposite direction diagonally downward to the north/northwest.

82. Ward Off Left

During the counts of:

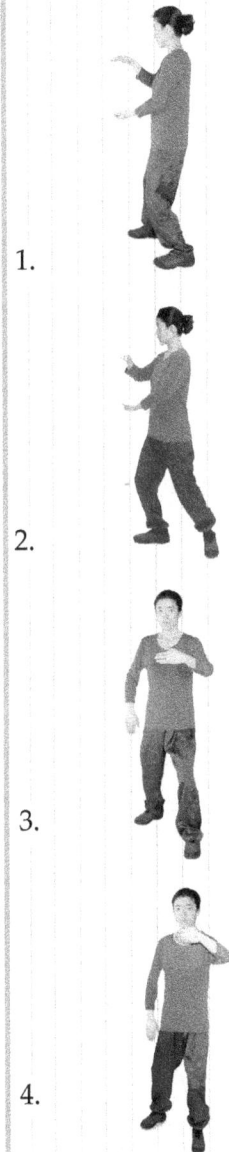

1.   Keeping your back straight, shift your weight to your left leg and turn your right foot, pivoting on the heel to point east. At the same time bring your hands into the position of holding an imaginary beach ball in front of your torso. Your left hand is on the bottom with its palm facing up and your right hand is on the top with its palm facing down. Your arms and elbows are rounded out.

2.   Shifting your weight 100% onto your right foot, turn your torso 45 degrees to the left to face northeast and pivot on your left toes so that they point to the north/northeast.

3.   Step forward to the north with your left foot, placing the heel down in front of where the toes were and point the toes to the north. Shifting your weight 60% onto the left leg, turn your torso to face north and bring your right hand down to the "position of attention" next to your right hip. Simultaneously bring your left hand up into a "ward off" position with your palm facing inward and opposite your neck. With the turning of your torso to face north, turn your right foot, pivoting on your heel, so the toes point to the northeast.

4.   Complete the bow and arrow stance facing north by shifting an additional 10% of your weight onto your left foot. At the same time, using your whole body, push forward with the back of your left hand, elbow slightly bent.

83. Ward Off Right

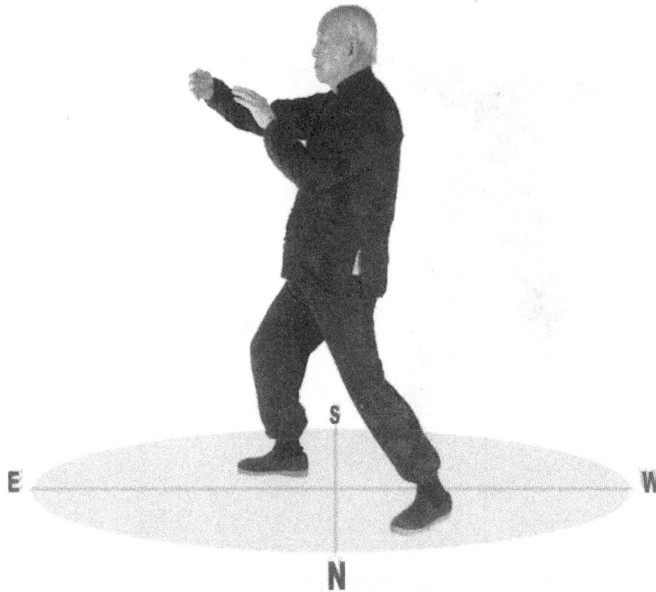

During the counts of:

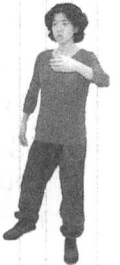

1. | Shift all of your weight to your left leg while turning your torso to face northeast.

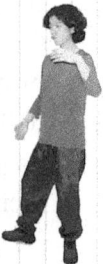

2. | Pivot on your left toes and turn your palms so that they face each other and ...

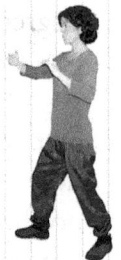

3. | ... step forward with your right foot to the east into a bow and arrow stance. Shift your weight 60% onto your right leg as you turn your torso to face east. Simultaneously pivot on your left heel, turning your left foot inward 45 degrees so the toes are pointing to the northeast. During this count, bring your right hand up in front of your neck with the palm facing in. Your left hand faces your right palm, as if holding an imaginary small ball. Your right arm remains rounded out and your left elbow is lowered.

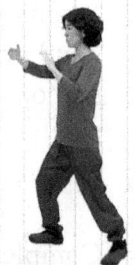

4. | Complete the bow and arrow stance facing east by shifting an additional 10% of your weight onto your right foot. At the same time, using your whole body, push forward with the back of your right hand, both elbows remaining slightly bent.

1.

2.

3.

4.

84. Roll Back

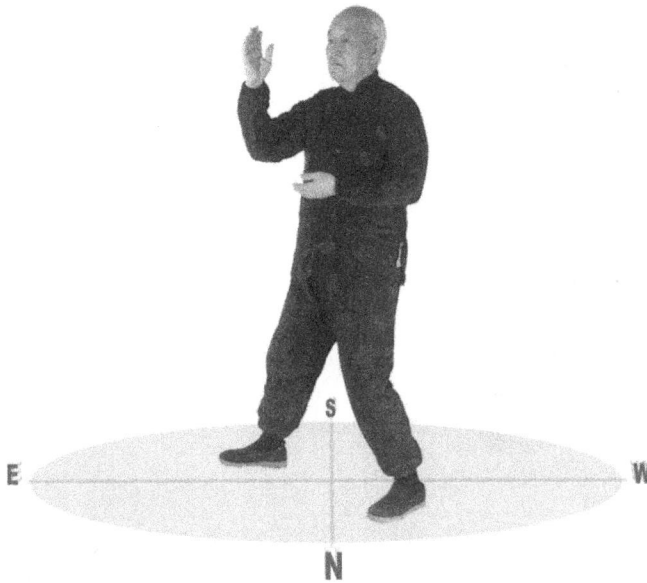

During the counts of:

1. Turn your torso to the right 45 degrees and bring your right forearm up into a 90 degree angle, perpendicular to your body. At the same time bring your left forearm across in front of the chest with your left palm facing in and the fingers almost touching your right elbow.

2. Keeping your weight on the right foot, turn your upper torso back to the left 45 degrees to face east. Your waist, upper body, arms and hands move together as one unit.

3. With your torso facing straight ahead to the east, withdraw your weight back onto your left foot.

4. Turn your torso to the left 45 degrees to face northeast. At the same time turn your left palm upwards.

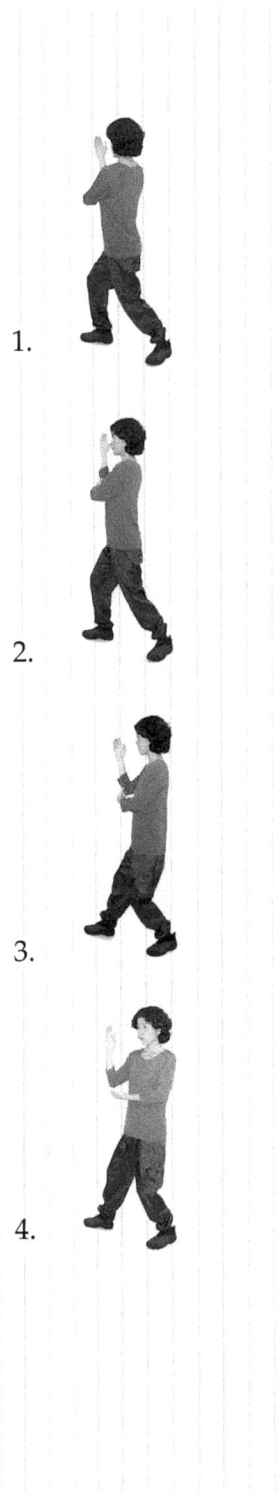

85. Press

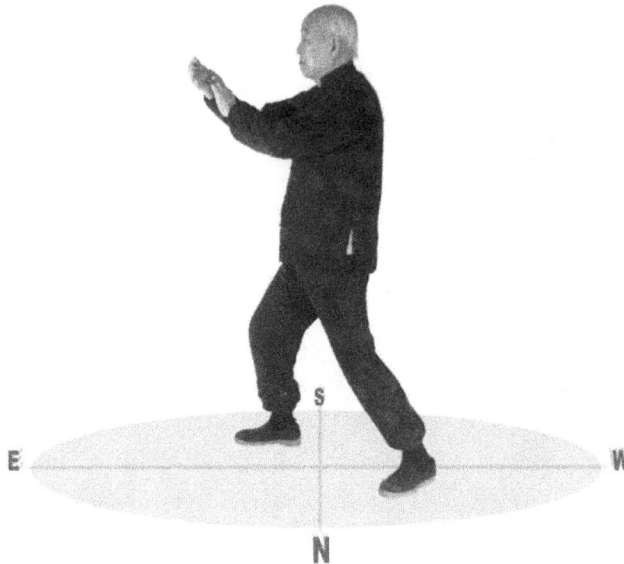

During the counts of:

1. Turn your torso 45 degrees to your left to face north. With the momentum of this turn let your left hand drop down and circle around (without lifting the elbow) heading up toward your left ear.

2. As your left hand is passing by your ear, turn your torso back 90 degrees to your right to face east and lightly attach your left fingers to the inside of your right wrist (as though you're feeling your pulse). Your right forearm drops slightly down into a diagonal position in front of your upper chest with the left elbow lowered.

3. Without letting your hands and arms move separately from your body, shift your weight onto the right leg and press forward with your right forearm. It's important here to move your whole body as one unit and not let your hands and arms move independently or initiate any movement.

4. Continue to press forward and slightly upwards until your right leg bears about 70% of your weight.

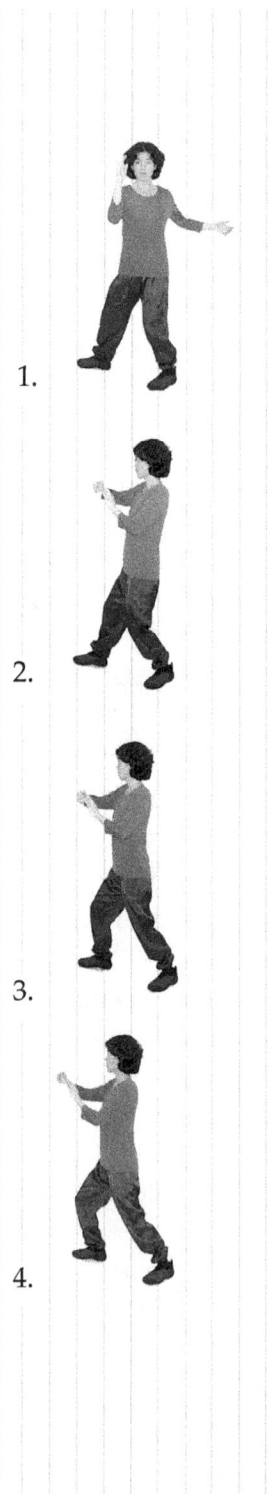

86. Push

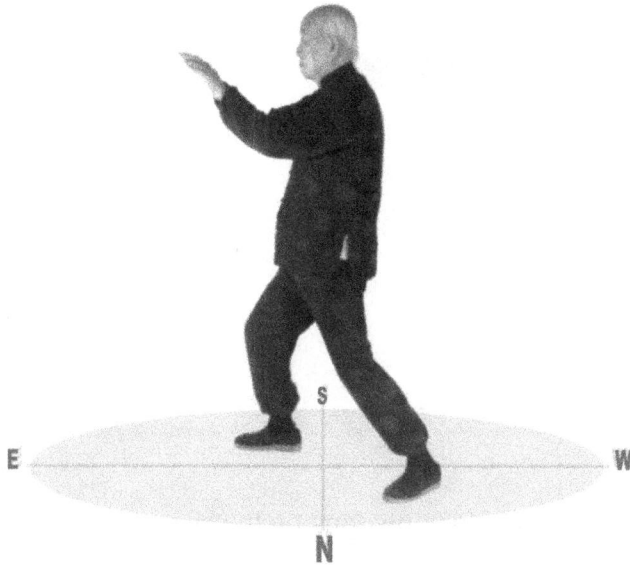

During the counts of:

1. Separate your hands, palms down, at the level of your shoulders.

2. Keeping your back straight, shift your weight back onto your left leg and simultaneously withdraw your hands slightly towards your upper chest. The fingers of both hands point forward and the elbows remain relaxed and bent downwards.

3. Without moving your hands and arms separately from your body, shift 60% of your weight back onto your right leg. The push is coming from the forward movement of your whole body - not your arms.

4. Complete the bow and arrow stance by shifting an additional 10% of your weight into your right foot. At the same time slightly raise your fingertips so that the intention of the push is coming through your palms and directed to the east.

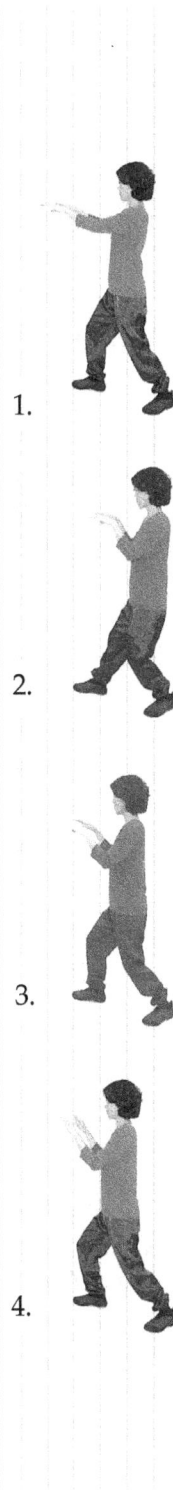

87. Single Whip

During the counts of:

1. Shift your weight back onto your left foot and let your arms stretch out slightly with the palms of the hands facing downward.

2. Turn your torso to the left until it faces northwest and at the same time turn your right foot, pivoting on the heel, so that the toes point north/northwest as well.

3. Shift your weight back to your right leg as you turn your torso to face northeast. Simultaneously withdraw both hands. The left hand comes down opposite the navel with its palm up and the right hand forms a "hook" (all 5 digits are touching at the tips and pointing downward) near your right armpit.

4. Turn your torso counterclockwise back to the northwest corner. With this movement strike to the northeast corner with your right hand "hook" and simultaneously pivot the left foot on the toes to point northwest.

5. Continue to turn your torso to face west and step with your left foot, heel first, so as to form a shoulders' width stance facing west with 60% of your weight on your left foot. The movement of your torso brings your left hand, palm facing in, up in front of your body at face level. At the same time let this movement turn your right foot, pivoting on the heel, to point northwest. The right hand "hook" does not move.

6. Complete the bow and arrow stance facing west by shifting 10% more of your weight onto your left foot. At the same time turn your left hand palm outward being careful to leave your arm slightly bent. Your eyes gaze over and past the fingertips.

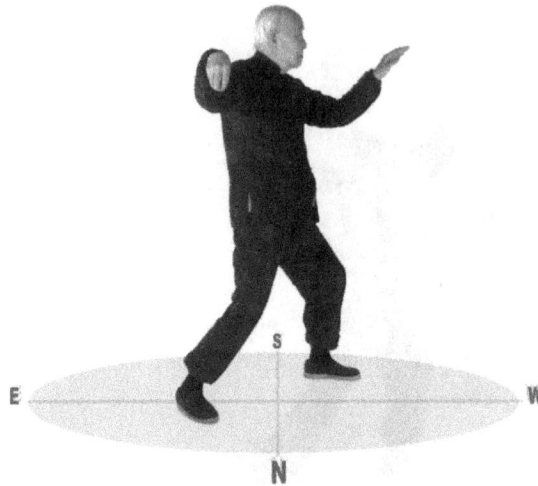

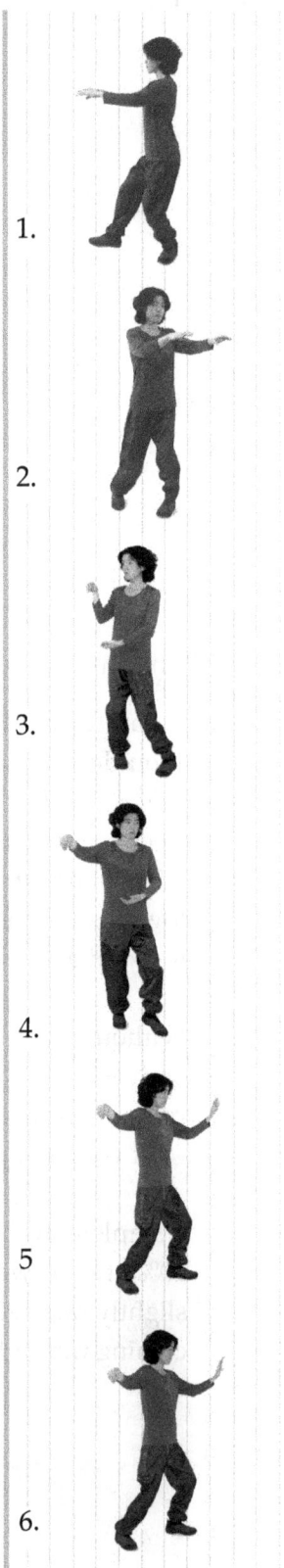

88. Fair Lady Weaving at Shuttles (1)

During the counts of:

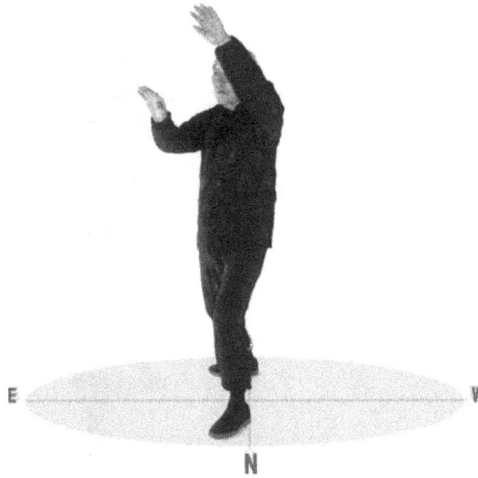

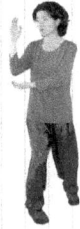

1. Shift your weight back onto the right foot and turn your torso to the right (to face northeast). At the same time turn the left foot inward, pivoting on the heel, pointing the toes north. With the turning of the torso, let the right forearm straighten up vertically and bring your left hand, palm up, to underneath the right elbow.

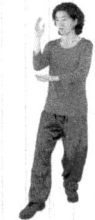

2. Shift your weight to the left foot and turn the right foot, pivoting on the toes to point north/northeast.

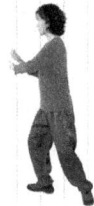

3. Turn your torso and step with your right foot to the southeast. Shift the weight to the right foot and begin circling the right hand down in a counterclockwise motion.

4. Continue circling the right hand in a counterclockwise direction up towards the right ear and pick up the left foot in preparation to step to the northeast corner.

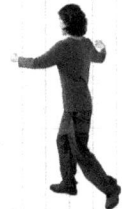

5. Step with your left foot to the northeast corner and shift 60% of your weight onto it. While turning your torso to face northeast, bring the left hand upward, turning the palm out (a screw motion), until it is diagonally slanted to the northeast opposite and above your forehead. The right hand arrives at the right ear with fingers pointing to the northeast. Turn your right foot inward, pivoting on the heel, toes pointing east.

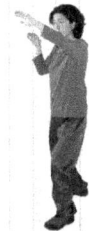

6. Complete the bow and arrow stance facing northeast by shifting 10% more of your weight into the left foot. At the same time, using your whole body, push forward with the right hand, elbow slightly bent, to a position just under and slightly to the rear of the left hand.

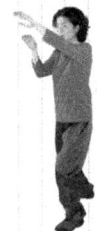

89. Fair Lady Weaving at Shuttles (2)

During the counts of:

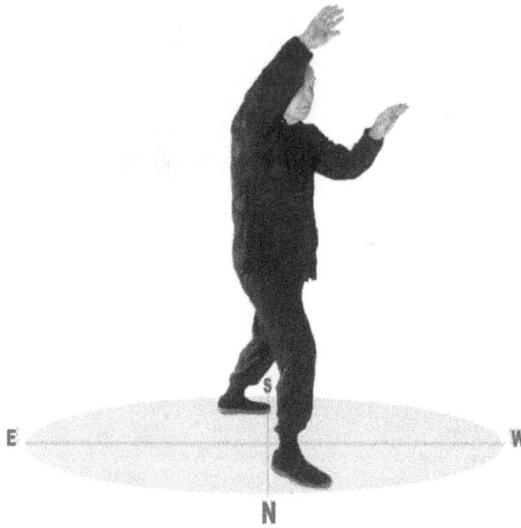

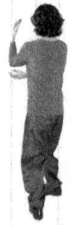

1. Shift your weight back onto your right foot and turn your torso to the right while pivoting on the left heel, turning it, as far as possible to point south. Let your left forearm straighten out vertically while moving to the right with the torso. Bring your right hand, palm up, to underneath the left elbow.

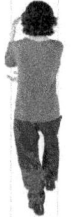

2. Shift your weight back to your left foot and pivot your right foot on the toes to point south.

3. Pick up your right foot in preparation to step to the northwest and begin circling your left hand down in a clockwise motion.

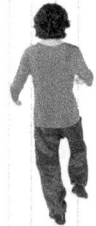

4. Continue circling the left hand in a clockwise wise direction down and up towards the left ear. Turn your torso towards the southwest corner with the right foot moving suspended in the air (above the ground) ready to step.

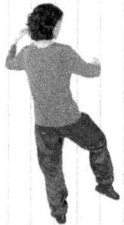

5. Step with your right foot to the northwest corner and shift 60% of your weight onto it. While turning your torso to face northwest, bring the right hand upward, turning the palm out (a screw motion), until it is diagonally slanted to the northwest opposite and above your forehead. The left hand arrives at the left ear with fingers pointing to the northwest. Turn your left foot inward, pivoting on the heel, toes pointing west.

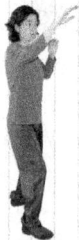

6. Complete the bow and arrow stance facing northwest by shifting another 10% of your weight into the right foot. At the same time, using your whole body, push forward with the left hand, elbow slightly bent, to a position just under and slightly to the rear of the right hand.

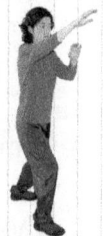

90. Fair Lady Weaving at Shuttles (3)

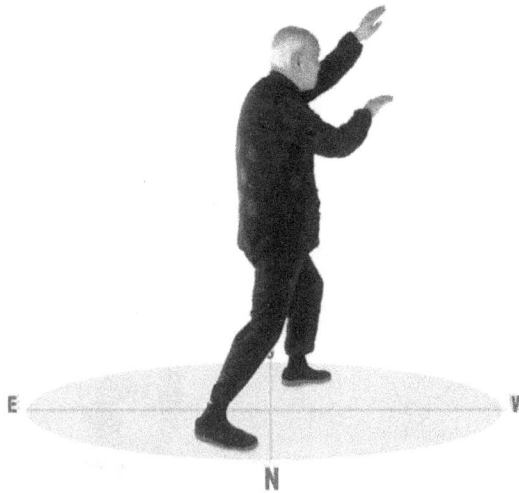

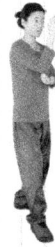

During the counts of:

1. Shift your weight to your left foot. Let the right forearm straighten out vertically and bring your left hand, palm up, to underneath the right elbow.

2. Turn your torso to the slightly to the west and step with your right foot to the northwest. Start to shift the weight to the right foot and begin circling the right hand down, with the palm facing up, in a counterclockwise motion.

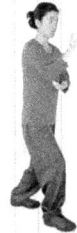

3. Continue circling the right hand in a counterclockwise direction down and upward towards the right ear and pick up the left foot in preparation to step to the southwest corner.

4. Your right hand reaches your right ear and then ...

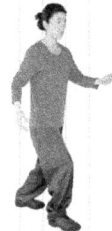

5. ... step with your left foot to the southwest corner and shift 60% of your weight onto it. While turning your torso to face southwest, bring the left hand upward, turning the palm out (a screw motion), until it is diagonally slanted to the southwest opposite your forehead. The right hand arrives at the right ear with fingers pointing to the southwest. Turn your right foot inward, pivoting on the heel, toes pointing west.

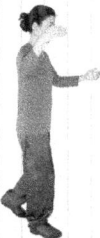

6. Complete the bow and arrow stance facing southwest by shifting an additional 10% of your weight into the left foot. At the same time, using your whole body, push forward with the right hand, elbow slightly bent, to a position just under the left hand.

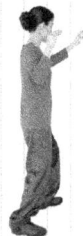

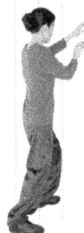

91. Fair Lady Weaving at Shuttles (4)

During the counts of:

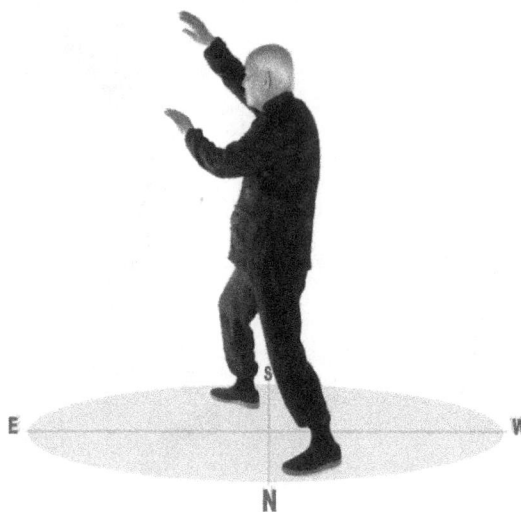

1. Shift your weight back onto the right foot and turn your torso to the right to face north. At the same time turn the left foot inward, pivoting on the heel, pointing the toes north. With the turning of the torso, bring your right hand, palm up, to underneath the left elbow.

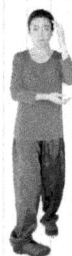
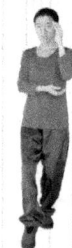

2. Shift your weight to the left foot and turn the right foot, pivoting on the toes to point north.

3. Pick up the right foot in preparation to step to the southwest and begin circling the left hand down in a clockwise motion.

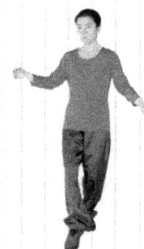

4. Continue circling the left hand in a clockwise direction down and up towards the left ear. Turn your torso towards the southeast corner with the right foot suspended in the air (above the ground) ready to step.

5. Now step with your right foot, heel first, to the southeast corner and shift 60% of your weight onto it. While turning your torso to face southeast, bring the right hand upward, turning the palm out (a screw motion), until it is diagonally slanted to the southeast opposite your forehead. The left hand arrives at the left ear with fingers pointing to the southwest. Turn your left foot inward, pivoting on the heel, toes pointing east.

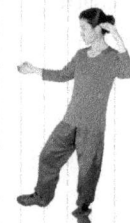

6. Complete the bow and arrow stance facing southeast by shifting an additional 10% of your weight into the right foot. At the same time, using your whole body, push forward with the left hand, elbow slightly bent, to a position just under the right hand.

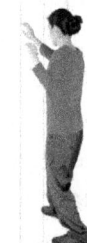
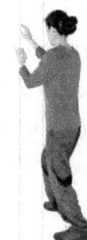

92. Ward Off Left

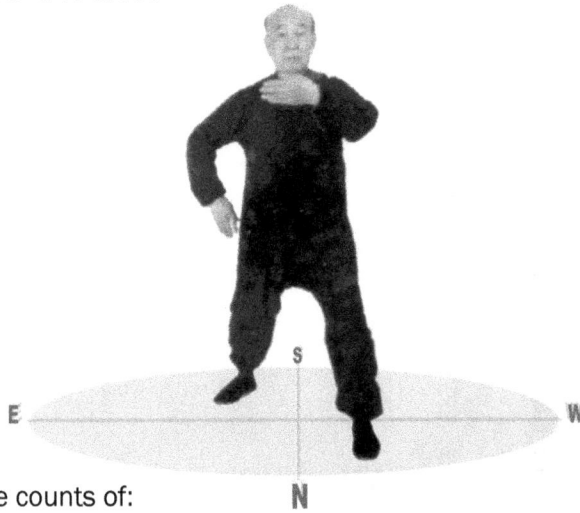

During the counts of:

1. Keeping your back straight, shift your weight to your left leg and turn your right foot, pivoting on the heel to point east. At the same time bring your hands into the position of holding an imaginary beach ball in front of your torso. Your left hand is on the bottom with its palm facing up and your right hand is on the top with its palm facing down. Your arms and elbows are rounded out.

2. Shifting your weight 100% onto your right foot, turn your torso 45 degrees to the left to face northeast and pivot on your left toes so that they point to the north/northeast.

3. Step forward to the north with your left foot, placing the heel down in front of where the toes were and point the toes to the north. Shifting your weight 60% onto the left leg, turn your torso to face north and bring your right hand down to the "position of attention" next to your right hip. Simultaneously bring your left hand up into a "ward off" position with your palm facing inward and opposite your neck. With the turning of your torso to face north, turn your right foot, pivoting on your heel, so the toes point to the northeast.

4. Complete the bow and arrow stance facing north by shifting an additional 10% of your weight onto your left foot. At the same time, using your whole body, push forward with the back of your left hand, elbow slightly bent.

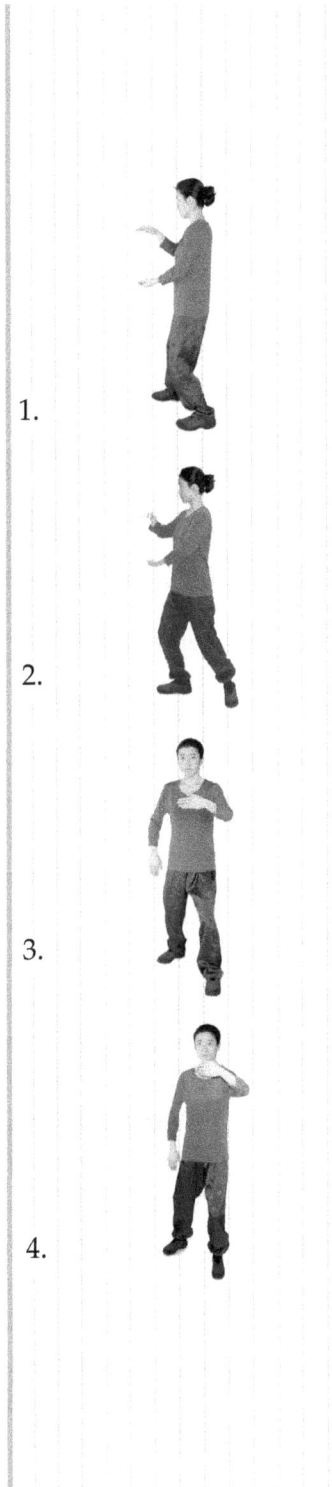

93. Ward Off Right

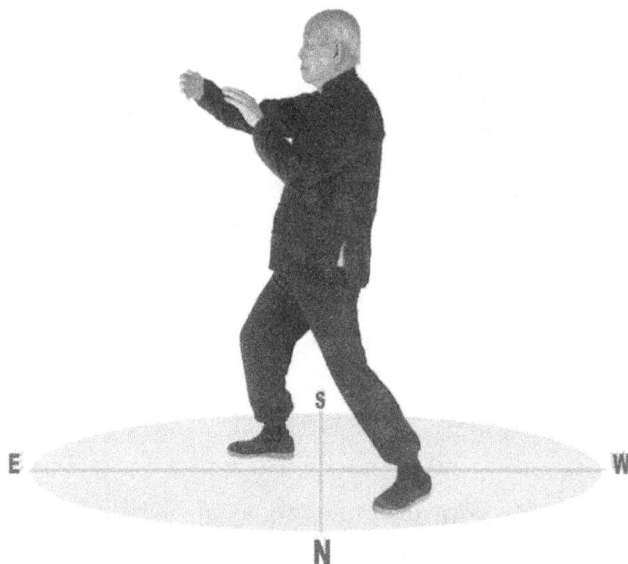

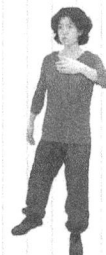

1.

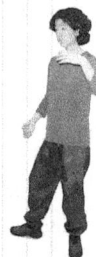

2.

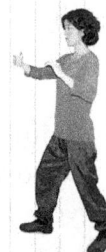

3.

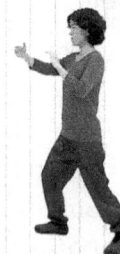

4.

During the counts of:

1. Shift all of your weight to your left leg while turning your torso to face northeast.

2. Pivot on your left toes and turn your palms so that they face each other and ...

3. ... step forward with your right foot to the east into a bow and arrow stance. Shift your weight 60% onto your right leg as you turn your torso to face east. Simultaneously pivot on your left heel, turning your left foot inward 45 degrees so the toes are pointing to the northeast. During this count, bring your right hand up in front of your neck with the palm facing in. Your left hand faces your right palm, as if holding an imaginary small ball. Your right arm remains rounded out and your left elbow is lowered.

4. Complete the bow and arrow stance facing east by shifting an additional 10% of your weight onto your right foot. At the same time, using your whole body, push forward with the back of your right hand, both elbows remaining slightly bent.

94. Roll Back

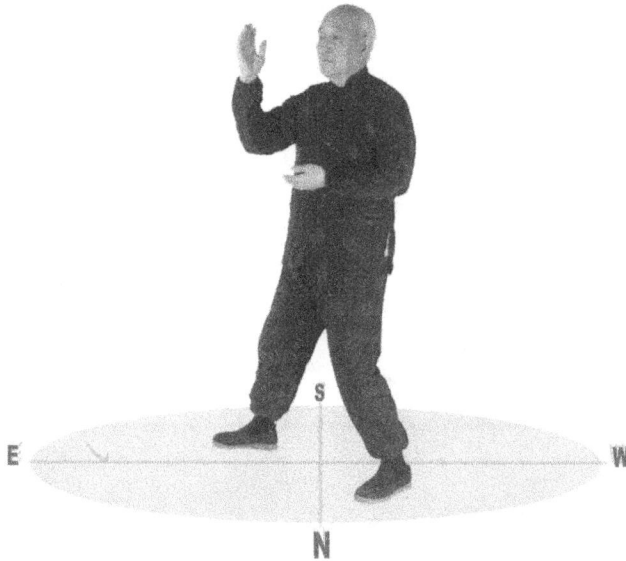

During the counts of:

1. Turn your torso to the right 45 degrees and bring your right forearm up vertically and perpendicular to your body. At the same time bring your left forearm across in front of the chest with your left palm facing in and the fingers almost touching your right elbow.

2. Keeping your weight on the right foot, turn your upper torso back again to the left 45 degrees to face east. Your waist, upper body, arms and hands move together as one unit.

3. With your torso facing straight ahead to the east, withdraw your weight back onto your left foot.

4. Turn your torso to the left 45 degrees to face northeast. At the same time turn your left palm upwards.

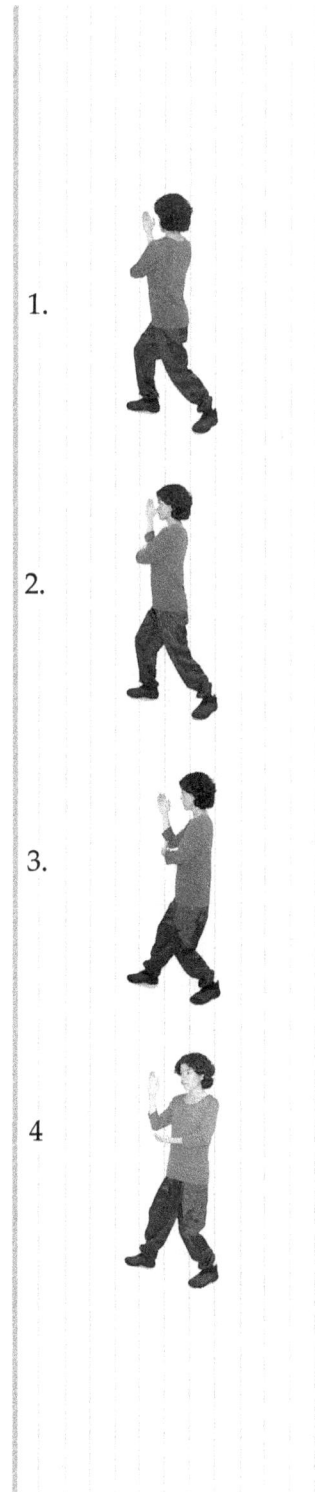

95. Press

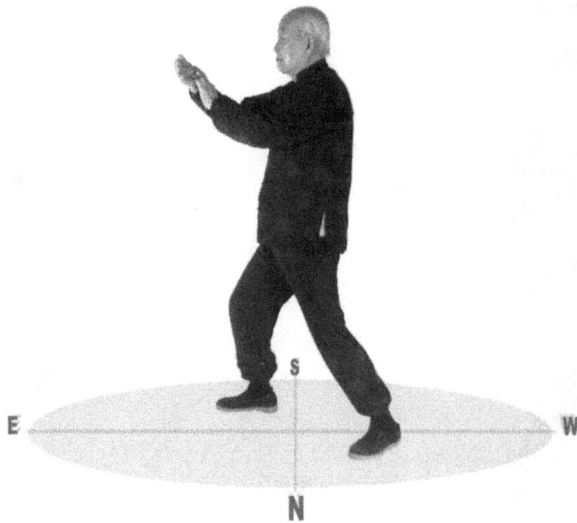

During the counts of:

1. Turn your torso 45 degrees to your left to face north. With the momentum of this turn let your left hand drop down and circle around (without lifting the elbow) heading up toward your left ear.

2. As your left hand is passing by your ear, turn your torso back 90 degrees to your right to face east and lightly attach your left fingers to the inside of your right wrist (as though you're feeling your pulse). Your right forearm drops slightly down into a diagonal position in front of your upper chest with the left elbow lowered.

3. Without letting your hands and arms move separately from your body, shift your weight onto the right leg and press forward with your right forearm. It's important here to move your whole body as one unit and not let your hands and arms move independently or initiate any movement.

4. Continue to press forward and slightly upwards until your right leg bears 70% of your weight.

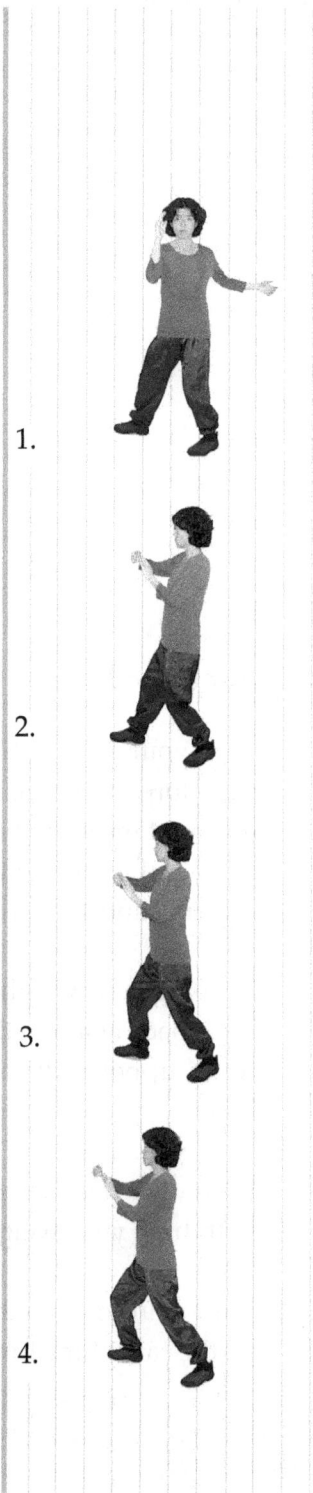

160

96. Push

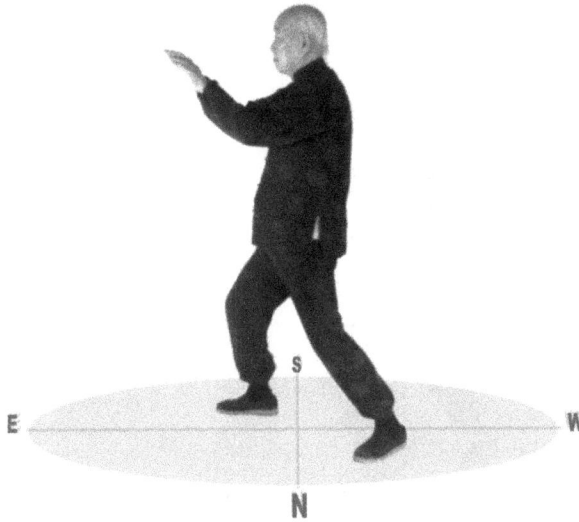

During the counts of:

1.   Separate your hands, palms down, at the level of your shoulders.

2.   Keeping your back straight, shift your weight back onto your left leg and simultaneously withdraw your hands slightly towards your upper chest. The fingers of both hands point forward and the elbows remain relaxed and bent downwards.

3.   Without moving your hands and arms separately from your body, shift 60% of your weight back onto your right leg. The push is coming from the forward movement of your whole body - not your arms.

4.   Complete the bow and arrow stance by shifting an additional 10% of your weight into your right foot. At the same time slightly raise your fingertips so that the intention of the push is coming through your palms and directed to the east.

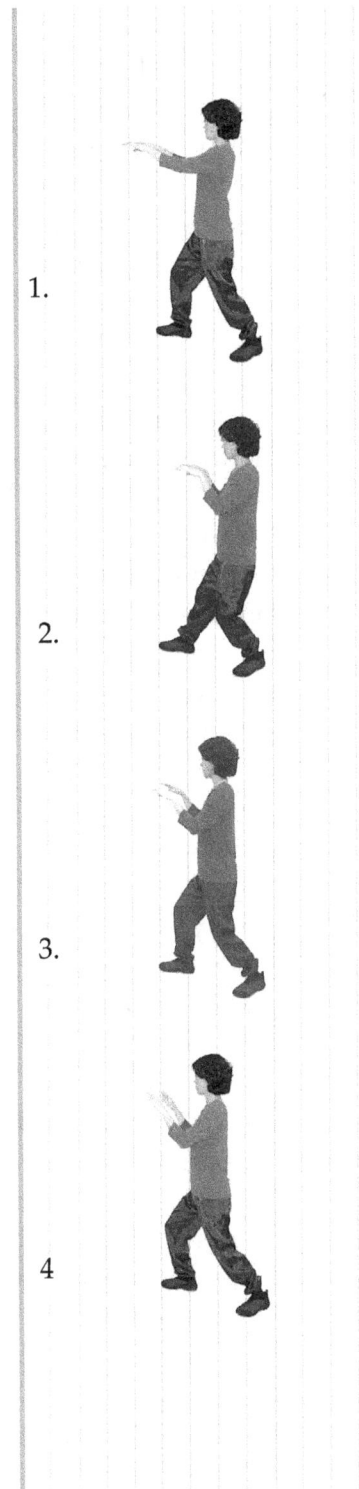

1.

2.

3.

4

97. Single Whip

During the counts of:

1. Shift your weight back onto your left foot and let your arms stretch out slightly with the palms of the hands facing downward.

2. Turn your torso to the left until it faces northwest and at the same time turn your right foot, pivoting on the heel, so that the toes point north/northwest as well.

3. Shift your weight back to your right leg as you turn your torso to face northeast. Simultaneously withdraw both hands. The left hand comes down opposite the navel with its palm up and the right hand forms a "hook" (all 5 digits are touching at the tips and pointing downward) near your right armpit.

4. Turn your torso counterclockwise back to the northwest corner. With this movement strike to the northeast corner with your right hand "hook" and simultaneously pivot the left foot on the toes to point northwest

5. Continue to turn your torso to face west and step with your left foot, heel first, so as to form a shoulders' width stance facing west with 60% of your weight on your left foot. The movement of your torso brings your left hand, palm facing in, up in front of your body at face level. At the same time let this movement turn your right foot, pivoting on the heel, to point northwest. The right hand "hook" does not move.

6. Complete the bow and arrow stance facing west by shifting 10% more of your weight onto your left foot. At the same time turn your left hand palm outward being careful to leave your arm slightly bent. Your eyes gaze over and past the fingertips.

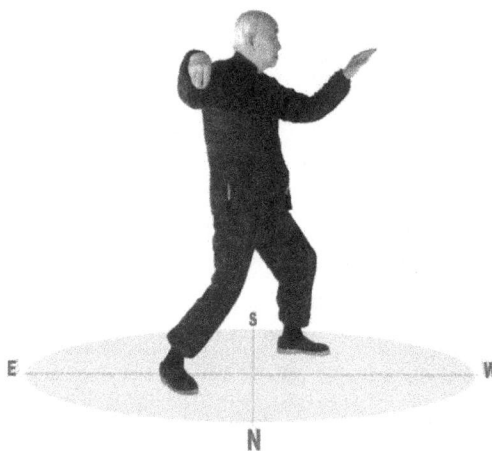

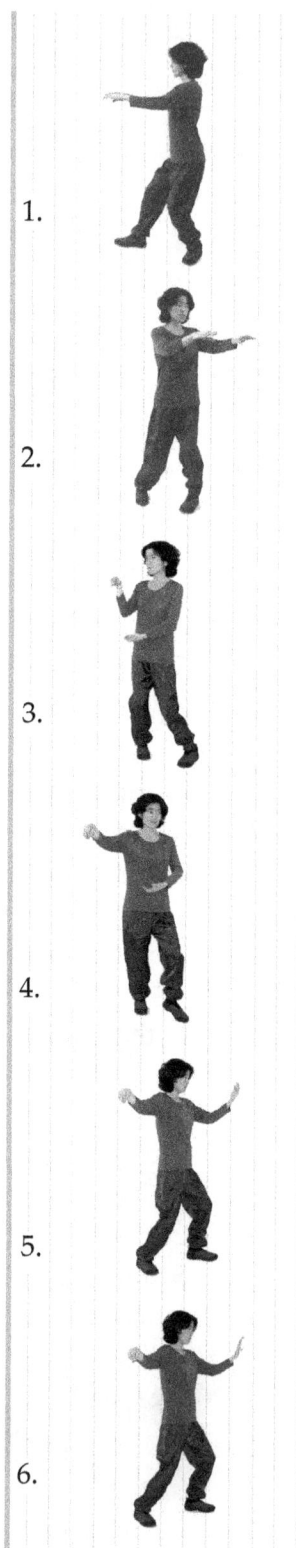

98. Wave Hands in Clouds (left)

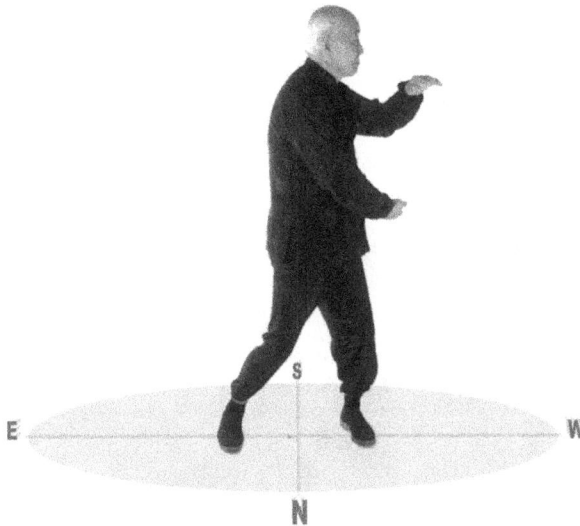

During the counts of:

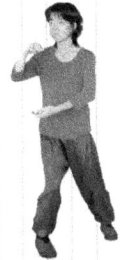

1. Shift your weight completely onto your right leg as you turn your torso to face northeast and your left foot, pivoting on the heel, to face north. At the same time open your right hand so that the palm is facing down and bring your left hand, palm facing up, in front of your waist so as to simulate holding a ball in front of your chest.

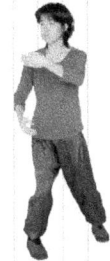

2. Turn both palms in to face your body and simultaneously bring your right hand down to your waist level and bring your left hand up to the level of your neck. The right hand passes on the inside of the left.

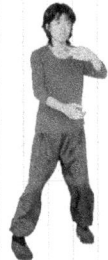

3. Turn your torso and hands as one unit to the left as you begin shifting your weight onto your left leg. On this beat your waist is now facing north.

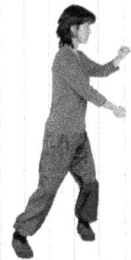

4. Shift 80% of your weight onto your left foot as you turn your torso to face west. Then turn both palms to face each other so that they are in a position of holding a ball in front of your chest.

99. Wave Hands in Clouds (right)

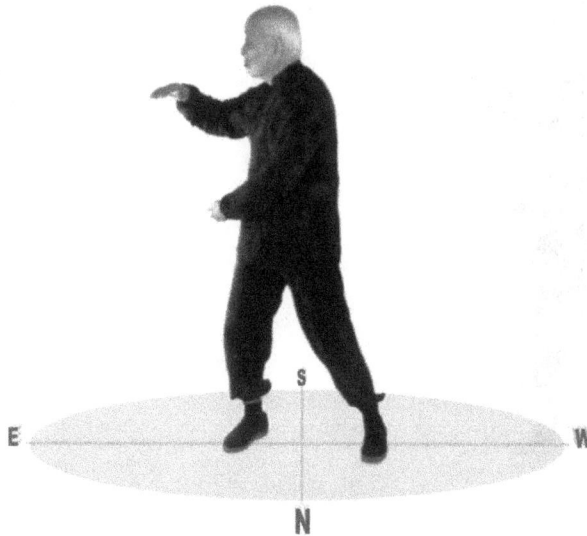

During the counts of:

1. Bring your left hand down to your waist level and simultaneously bring your right hand up to your neck level as you turn both palms to face inward. Your left hand passes on the outside of your right hand as they exchange positions.

2. Turn your torso clockwise to your right as you step backwards and to the east with your right foot, placing it parrallel to your left foot so that there is about 10" between them (less than a shoulders' width).

3. Continue to shift your weght onto right foot as you turn your torso and hands as one unit to the right. On the count of three you are facing directly north (not in picture).

4. Continue to turn your torso and hands to the right until you're facing east with 80% of your weight on your right leg. Your right hand now turns palm down and your left hand turns palm up. Again you are simulating holding a ball in front of your chest.

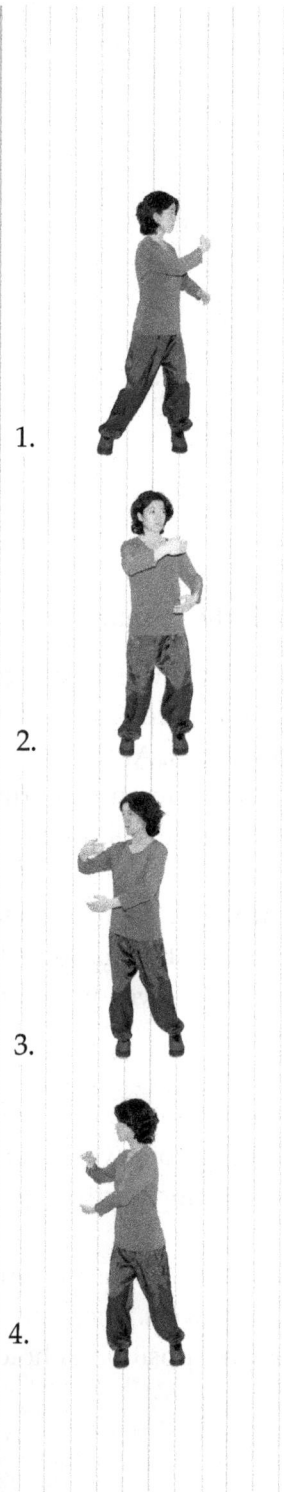

164

100. Wave Hands in Clouds (left)

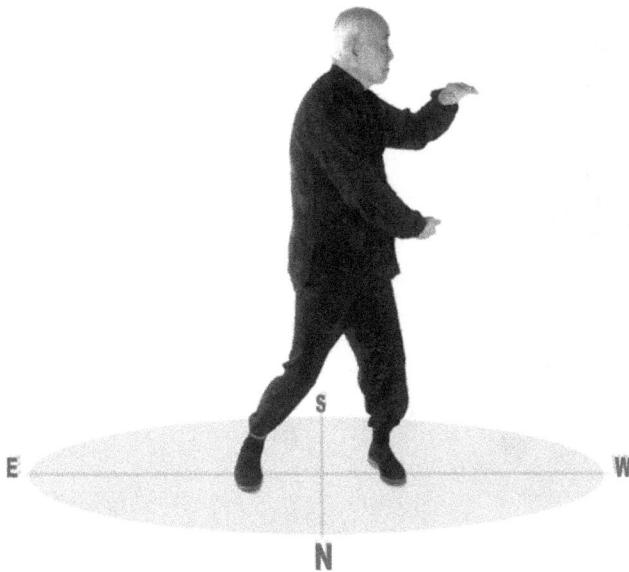

During the counts of:

1. Passing on the outside, bring your right hand down to your waist level and simultaneously bring your left hand, on the inside, up to your neck level as you turn both palms to face inwards.

2. As you turn your torso to your left, step and to the west with your right foot, placing it parralel to your left foot so that there is about 18" between them (more than a shoulders' width).

3. Continue to shift your weight onto left foot as you turn your torso and hands as one unit to the left.

4. Continue to turn your torso and hands to the left until you're facing west with 80% of your weight on your left leg. Your left hand now turns palm down and your right hand turns palm up. Again you are simulating holding a ball in front of your chest.

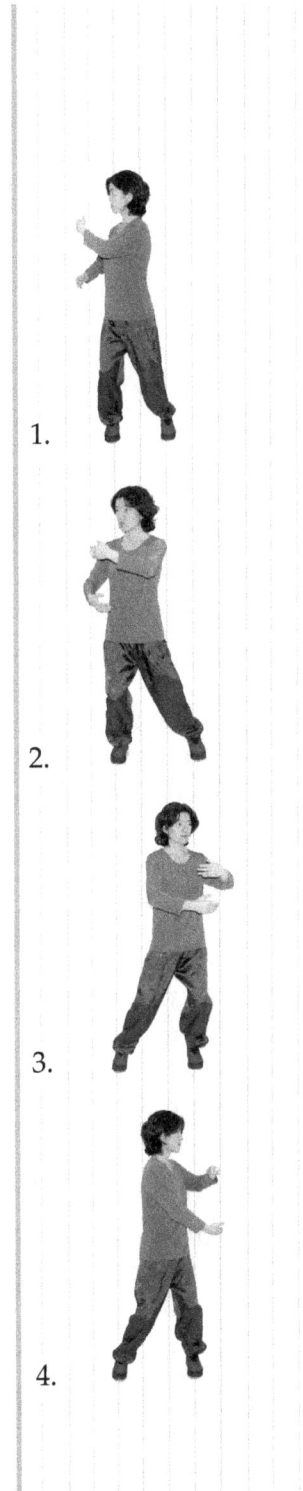

101. Wave Hands in Clouds (right)

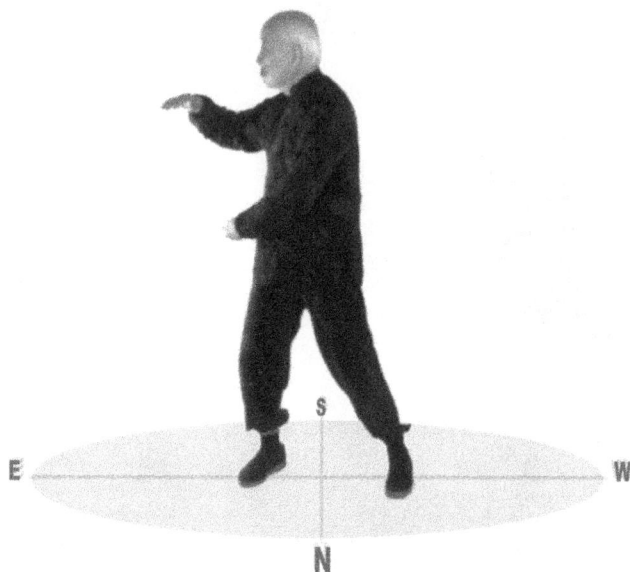

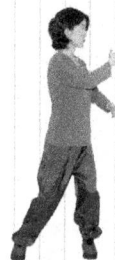

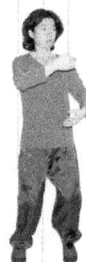

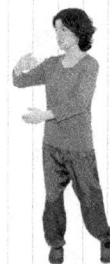

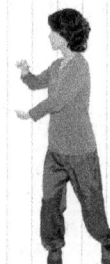

During the counts of:

1. Bring your left hand down to your waist level and simultaneously bring your right hand up to your neck level as you turn both palms to face inwards. Your left hand passes on the outside of your right hand as they exchange positions.

2. As you turn your torso to your right, step to the east with your right foot, placing it parrallel to your left foot so that there is about 8 to 10" between them (less than a shoulders' width).

3. Continue to shift your weght onto your right foot as you turn your torso and hands as one unit to the right. On the count of three you are facing directly north (not in picture).

4. Continue to turn your torso and hands to the right until you're facing east with 80% of your weight on your right leg. Your right hand now turns palm down and your left hand turns palm up. Again you are simulating holding a ball in front of your chest.

102. Wave Hands in Clouds (left)

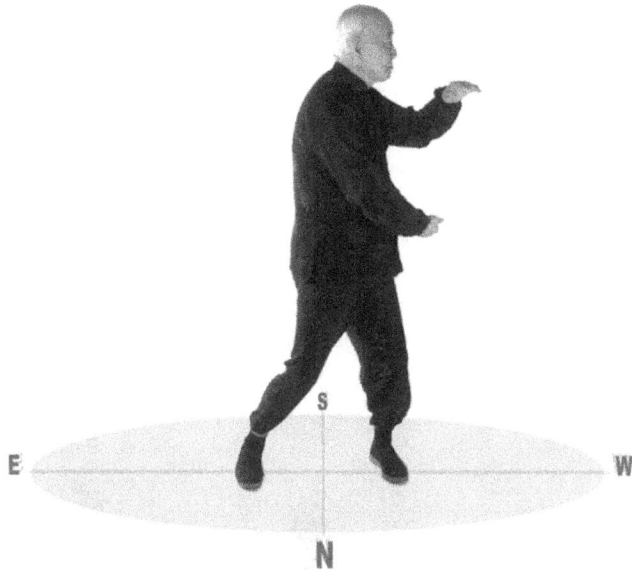

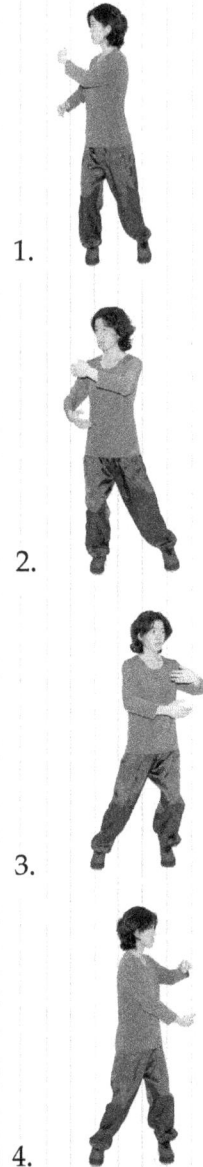

During the counts of:

1. Passing on the outside, bring your right hand down to your waist level and simultaneously bring your left hand, on the inside, up to your neck level as you turn both palms to face inwards.

2. As you turn your torso to your left, step and to the west with your right foot, placing it parralel to your left foot so that there is about 18" between them (more than a shoulders' width).

3. Continue to shift your weight onto left foot as you turn your torso and hands as one unit to the left.

4. Continue to turn your torso and hands to the left until you're facing west with 80% of your weight on your left leg. Your left hand now turns palm down and your right hand turns palm up. Again you are simulating holding a ball in front of your chest.

103. Single Whip

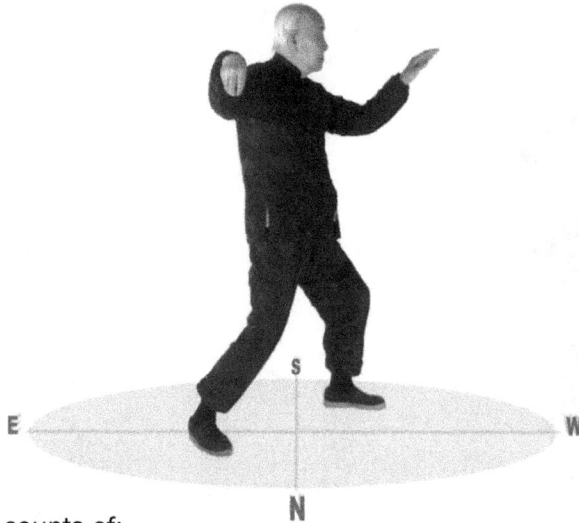

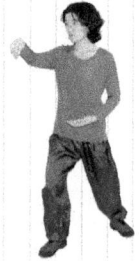

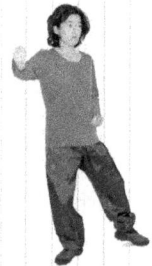

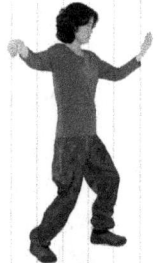

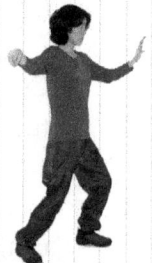

During the counts of:

1. Form a "hook" with your right hand, fingers pointing down, and strike out with it in a diagonal direction upwards to the northeast corner, as you take a step with your right foot in this same direction. At the same time lower your open left hand, palm up, in front of your stomach.

2. Shift your weight completely onto your right foot and turn your torso to the left facing northwest. Let this turning motion turn your left foot, pivoting on the toes to face west.

3. Continue to turn your torso to face west and step with your left foot, heel first, so as to form a shoulders' width stance facing west. The movement of your torso brings your left hand, palm facing in, up in front of your body at face level. At the same time let this movement turn your right foot, pivoting on the heel, to point northwest. The right hand "hook" does not move.

4. Complete the bow and arrow stance facing west by shifting your weight 70% into your left foot. At the same time turn your left hand palm outward being careful to leave your arm slightly bent. Your eyes gaze just over and past the fingertips.

104. Single Whip Squatting Down

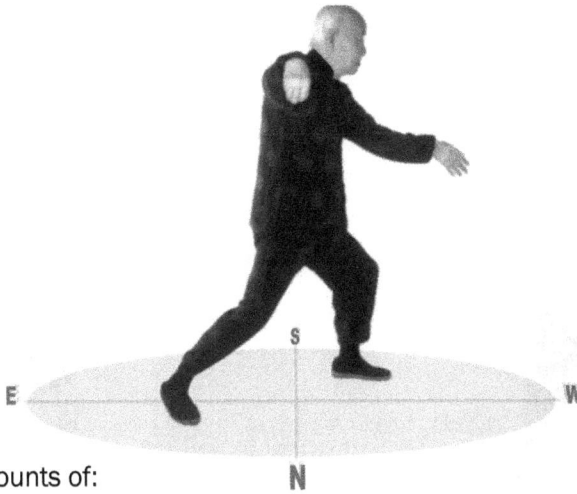

During the counts of:

1. Momentarily shift all of your weight onto your left leg and then turn your right foot, pivoting on the heel, to face northeast. Shift your weight onto the right foot as you turn your torso to face north/northeast and turn your left foot, pivoting on the heel, to point north. Let your left hand and arm, moving in conjunction with the waist, circle upwards in a clockwise motionto the northeast. The right hand "hook" remains where it is.

2. Turn the torso to face northwest/west and turn your left foot, pivoting on the heel, so the toes point west. Keeping your back straight and upright as much as possible, use the turning of your waist, continue to circle your left hand down inside of your left thigh to your left knee with the palm facing north and the fingers pointing west.

3. Shift your weight 60% onto your left leg and turn in your right foot, pivoting on the heel, 90 degrees to face northwest.

4. Completing your bow and arrow stance, shift 10% more of your weight into the left foot and let the forward motion of your body initiate a forward motion with the left hand (striking to the imaginary opponent's groin).

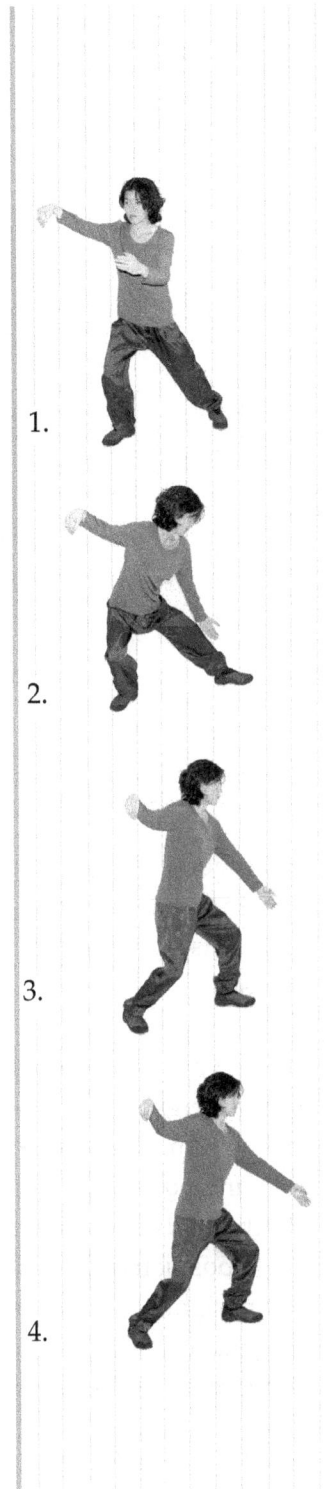

105. Golden Rooster Standing on One Leg (right)

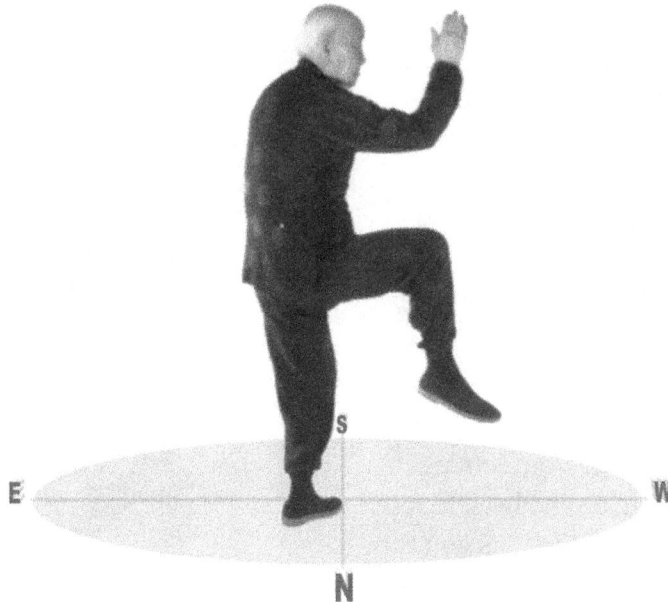

During the counts of:

1. Shift your weight back onto your right leg and turn your left foot out, pivoting on the heel, 45 degrees left so that it points southwest. Your hands open up in front of your chest.

2. Keep your waist facing west and don't rise up as you shift your weight entirely onto your left leg. With this shifting forward motion, raise your right knee up to groin level, leaving your right foot with the toes pointing down. Both hands circle down with your left hand coming into the "position of attention" next to your left hip and your open right hand, in conjunction with the upward motion of your right knee, comes up in front of your face. The fingers are pointing up and the palm is facing south.

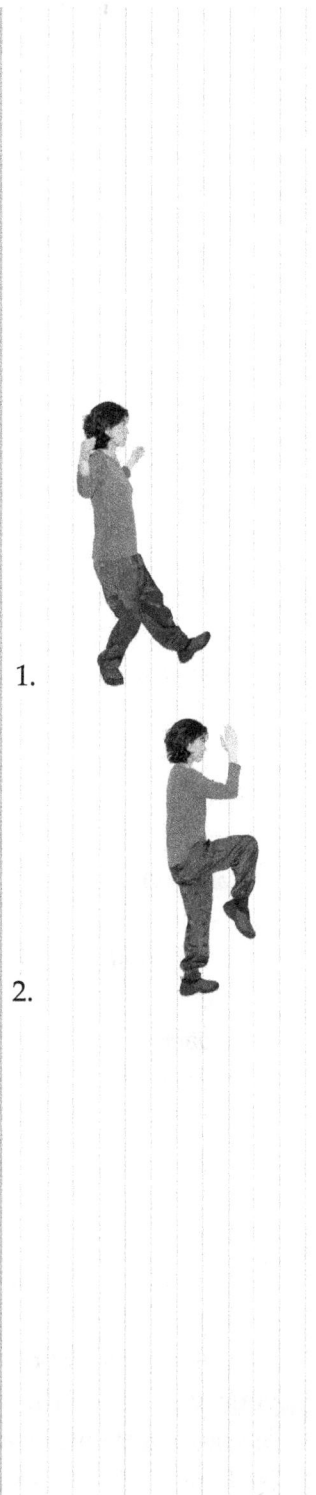

106. Golden Rooster Standing on One Leg (left)

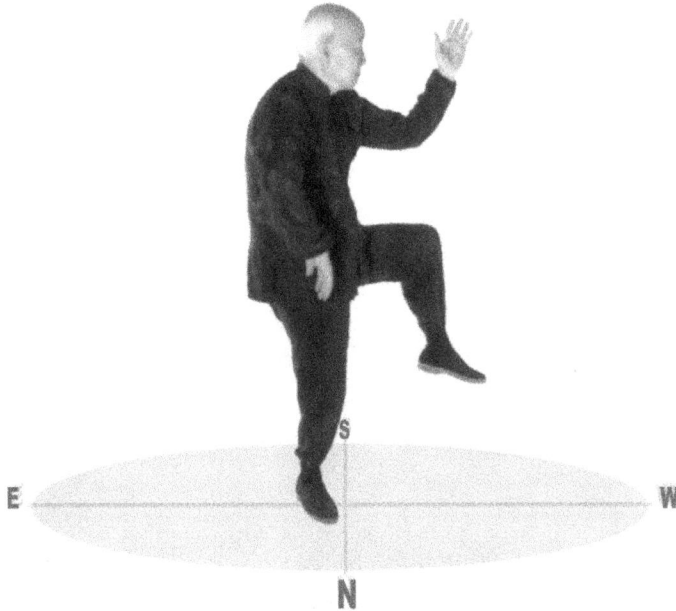

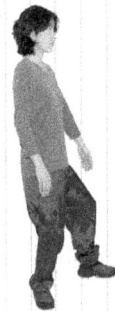

1.

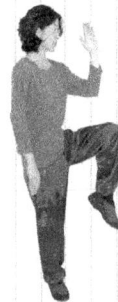

2.

During the counts of:

1. Take a relaxed step backward to the northeast with your right foot, setting it down at an angle so that the toes point northwest.

2. Keeping your waist facing west , shift your weight entirely to your right leg. Lower your right hand down to your right thigh into the "position of attention." Raise your left knee up to groin level, leaving your left foot with the toes pointing down. Your open left hand, in conjunction with the upward motion of your left knee, comes up in front of your face. The fingers are pointing up and the palm is facing north.

107. Step Back and Repulse Monkey (right style)

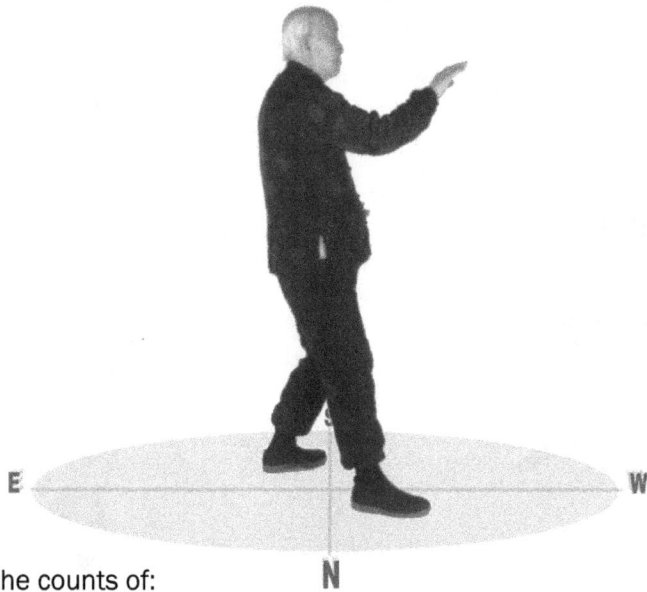

During the counts of:

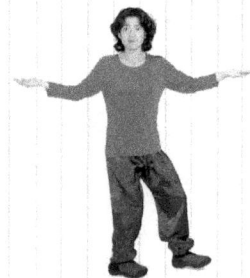

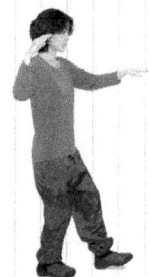

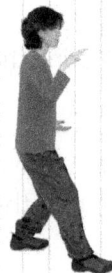

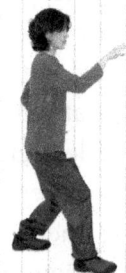

1. Keep your weight on your right leg and turn your torso to the right to face north. With this movement, extend both hands at shoulder level to the east and west. Your right hand circling to the east, palm open and facing up. Your left hand to the west with its palm open and facing down. Your left leg straightens out with the toes extended to the west but the foot does not touch the ground..

2. Turn your torso back to the left to face west and bring your right hand forward beside your right ear with palm and fingers pointing slightly forward. Your left foot remains slightly raised, toes pointing west.

3. Turn your left hand palm up and draw it back and down to your left thigh. At the same time step back with your left foot with the toes pointing straight ahead to the west and shift your weight back onto it. Your right foot, pivoting on the heel, turns inward so that both feet are parallel and pointing west.

4. Sink your weight into your left foot and push forward (issue*) with your right hand.

108. Step Back and Repulse Monkey (left style)

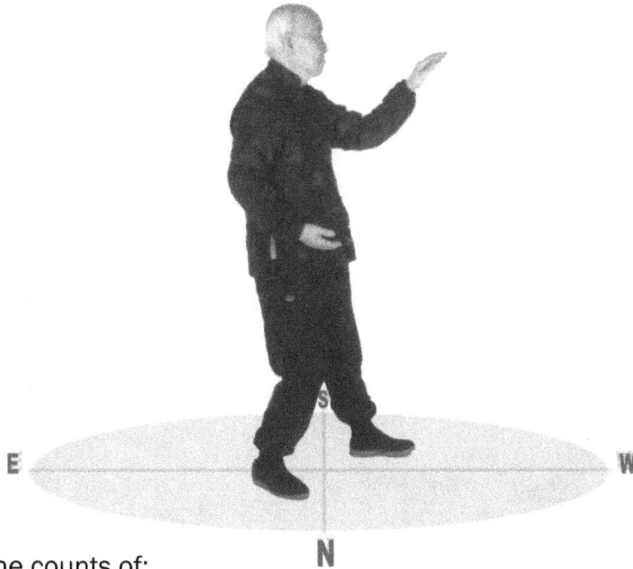

During the counts of:

1. Keep your weight on your left leg and turn your torso to your left to face south. With this movement, extend both hands at shoulder level to the east and west. Your left hand circling to the east, palm open and facing up. Your right hand to the west with its palm open and facing down.

2. Turn your torso back to your right to face west and bring your left hand forward beside your left ear with palm and fingers pointing slightly forward to the west.

3. Turn your right hand palm up as you draw it back and down to your right thigh. At the same time step back with your right foot with the toes pointing straight ahead to the west and shift your weight back onto it.

4. Sink your weight into your right foot and push forward (issue) with your left hand.

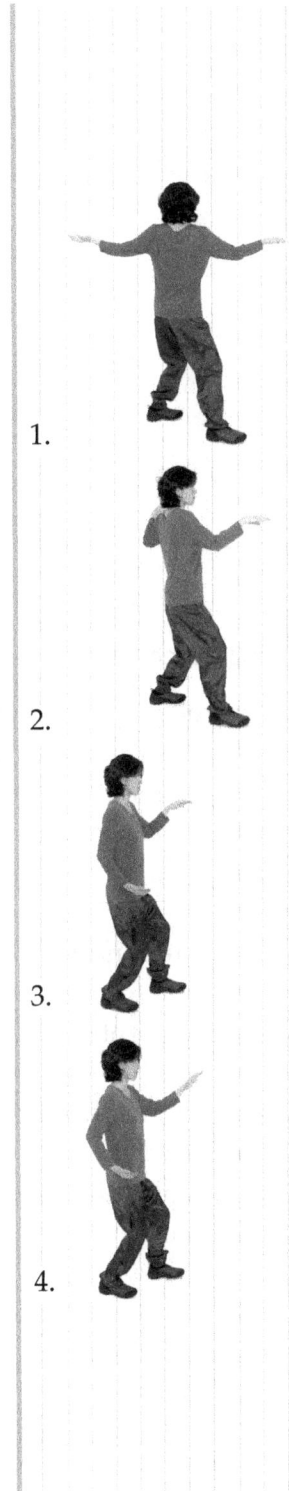

109. Step Back and Repulse Monkey (right)

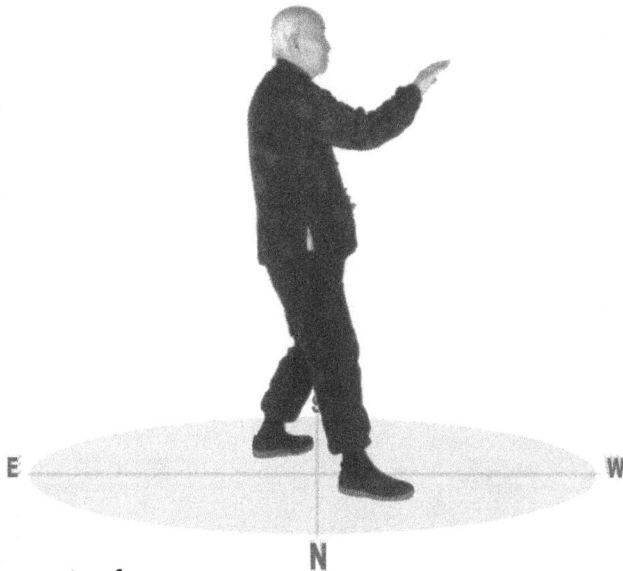

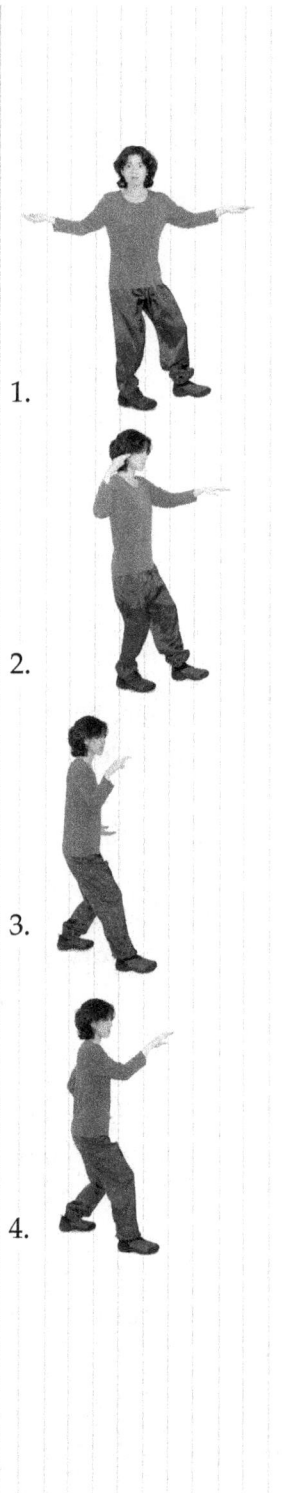

During the counts of:

1. Keep your weight on your right leg and turn your torso to the right to face north. With this movement, extend both hands at shoulder level to the east and west. Your right hand circling to the east, palm open and facing up. Your left hand to the west with its palm open and facing down.

2. Turn your torso back to the left to face west and bring your right hand forward beside your right ear with palm and fingers pointing slightly forward.

3. Turn your left hand palm up as you draw it back and down to your left thigh. At the same time step back with your left foot with the toes pointing straight ahead to the west and shift your weight back onto it.

4. Sink your weight into your left foot and push forward (issue) with your right hand.

110. Step Back and Repulse Monkey (left)

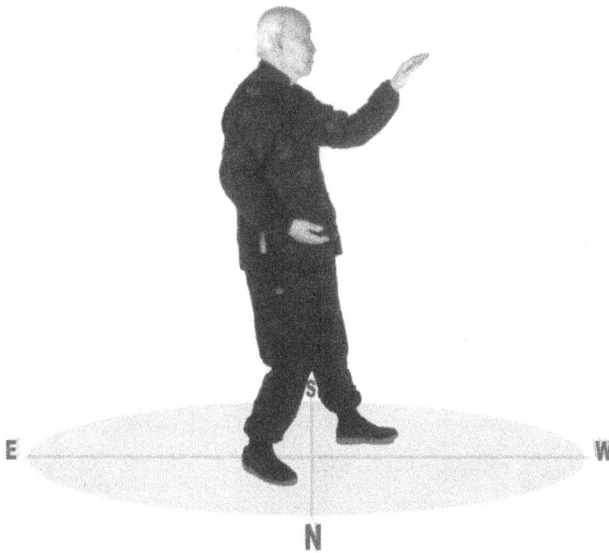

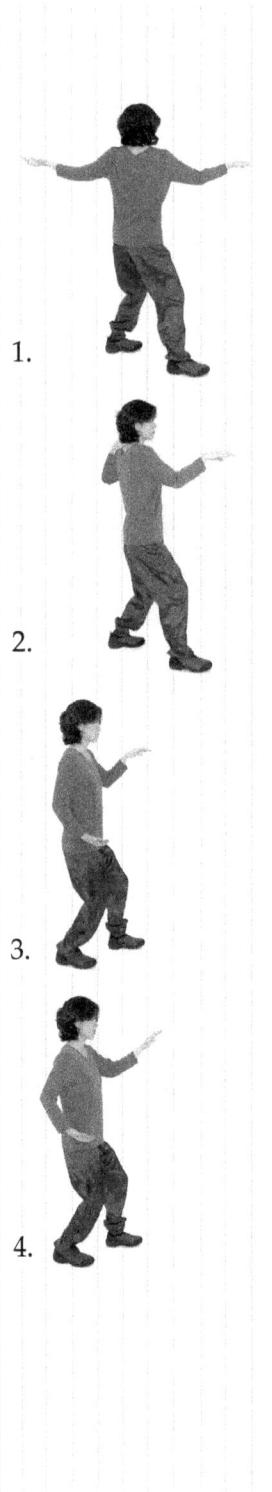

During the counts of:

1.   Keep your weight on your left leg and turn your torso to your left to face south. With this movement, extend both hands at shoulder level to the east and west. Your left hand circling to the east, palm open and facing up. Your right hand to the west with its palm open and facing down.

2.   Turn your torso back to your right to face west and bring your left hand forward beside your left ear with palm and fingers pointing slightly forward to the west.

3.   Turn your right hand palm up as you draw it back and down to your right thigh. At the same time step back with your right foot with the toes pointing straight ahead to the west and shift your weight back onto it.

4.   Sink your weight into your right foot and push forward (issue) with your left hand.

111. Step Back and Repulse Monkey (right)

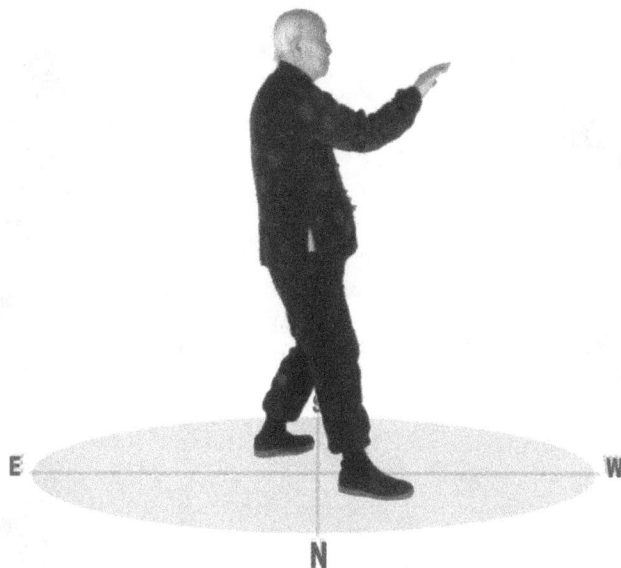

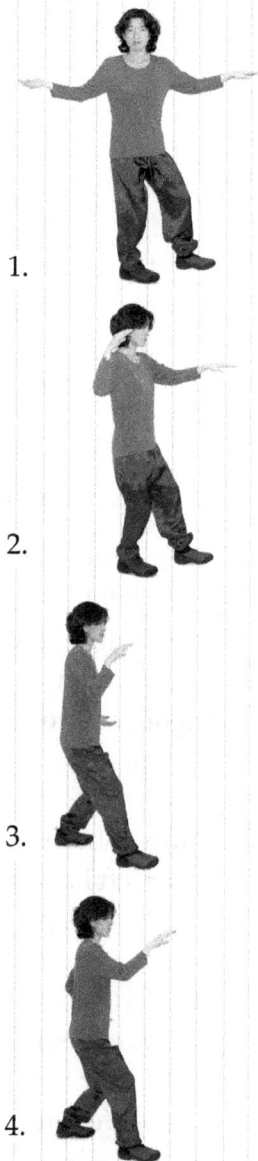

1.

2.

3.

4.

During the counts of:

1. Keep your weight on your right leg and turn your torso to the right to face north. With this movement, extend both hands at shoulder level to the east and west. Your right hand circling to the east, palm open and facing up. Your left hand to the west with its palm open and facing down.

2. Turn your torso back to the left to face west and bring your right hand forward beside your right ear with palm and fingers pointing slightly forward.

3. Turn your left hand palm up aas you draw it back and down to your left thigh. At the same time step back with your left foot with the toes pointing straight ahead to the west and shift your weight back onto it.

4. Sink your weight into your left foot and push forward (issue) with your right hand.

112. Diagonal Flying Posture

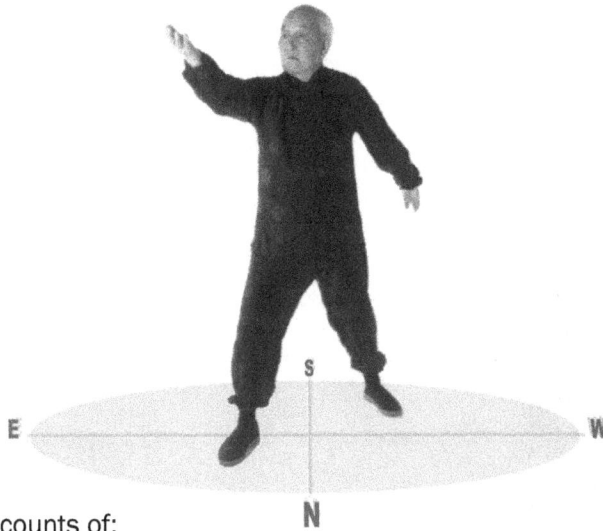

During the counts of:

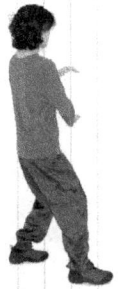

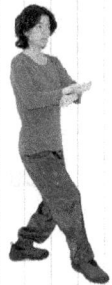

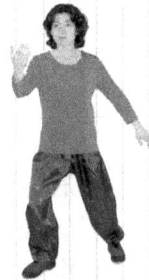

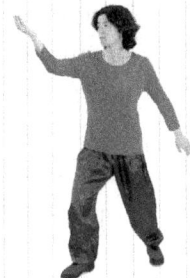

1. | Turn your torso 45 degrees to your left to face southwest. At the same time bring your hands in front of your chest with the palms facing each other as if holding a ball. Your left hand is ontop with the palm facing down and your right hand is on the bottom with the palm facing up.

2. | Turn your torso clockwise to your right to face northwest and at the same time bring your right hand inside of your left and place it ontop, crossed at the wrists. Your right palm remains facing up and the left palm facing down.

3. | Continue to turn your torso to your right and step with your right foot (almost a backward step) to the northeast with the heel landing first. Keep your right palm facing up and sweep, in a horizontal arching upward motion, your right arm across to the right in conjuncton with the turning of your torso. Shift your weight 60% to your right leg and turn your left foot in 90 degrees, pivoting on the heel, to point north.

4. | Shifting your weight another 10% onto your right leg, continue to move your right arm in a diagonally upward motion in conjuction with the torso as it turns to the northeast. At the same time extend your left hand, thumb down, diagonally downward behind your left thigh.

113. Lifting Hands

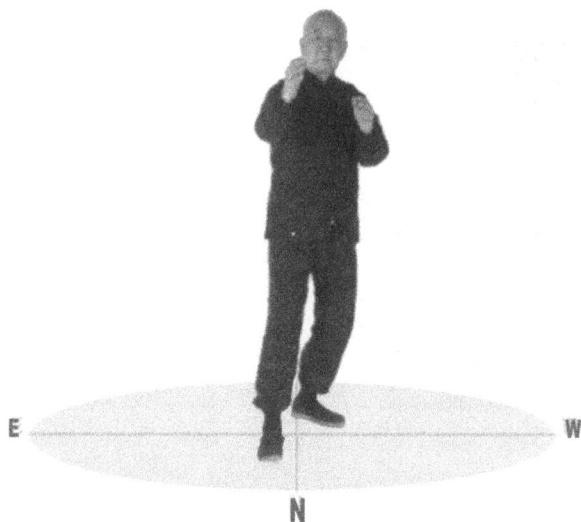

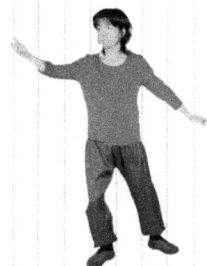

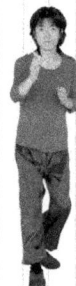

1.

2.

During the counts of:

1.   Shift your weight all the way onto your right leg and lift up your left foot and place it back down, adjusting the toes to face northwest.

2.   Turn your palms slightly inwards so that they face each other and shift your weight onto your left foot and then bring your right foot to the north in front of your body and place it heel down, with the toes slightly off the ground, about 12 inches in front (to the north of) your left heel. Your right leg remains slightly bent. At the same time bring your arms together horizontally, without dropping them down, so that your right arm, with the elbow slightly bent, is aligned over your right leg. Your left hand comes over opposite the inside of your right elbow - about 8-10″ away.

114. Shoulder Stroke

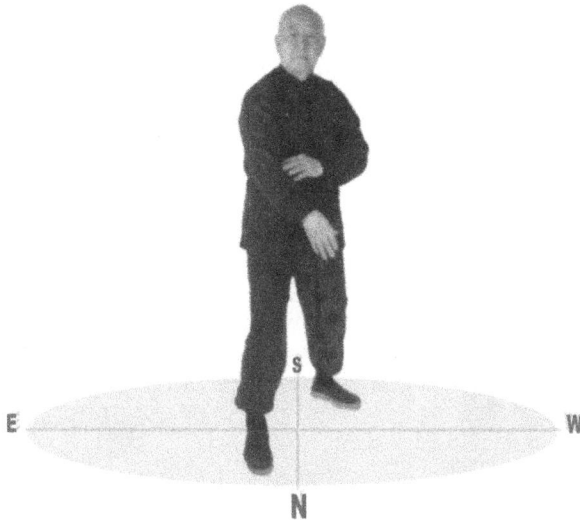

During the counts of:

1. Withdraw your right foot and place it down, heel up, toes touching the ground and pointing north, directly in front of your left heel. At the same time bring your arms down. Your right hand drops to the side of your right thigh with its palm facing backward toward the groin. Your left hand comes down with its palm facing the right palm.

2. Step forward to the north with your right foot (heel touching first and toes pointing very slightly to the northwest). Lightly adhere with your left fingers to the inside of your right forearm and simultaneously shift your weight about 70% forward onto your right foot, striking forward with your right shoulder and side.

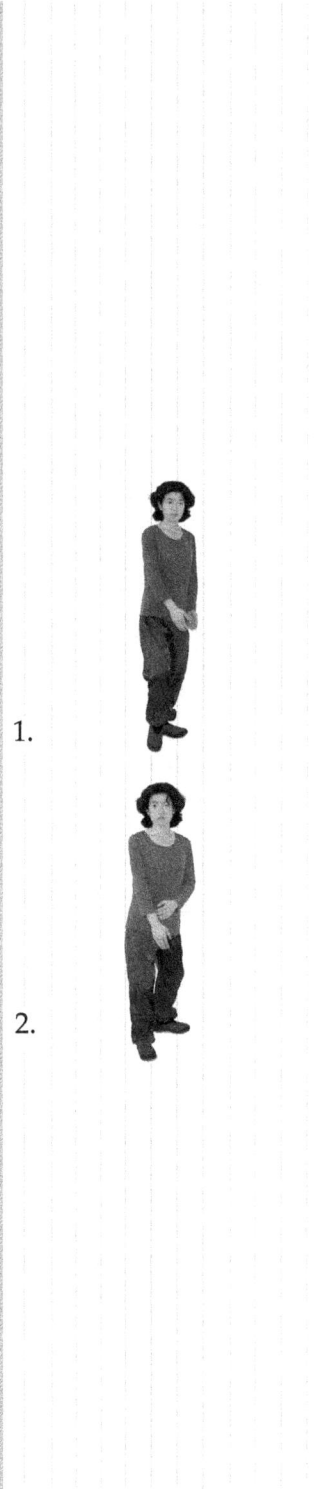

1.

2.

115. White Crane Spreading Its Wings

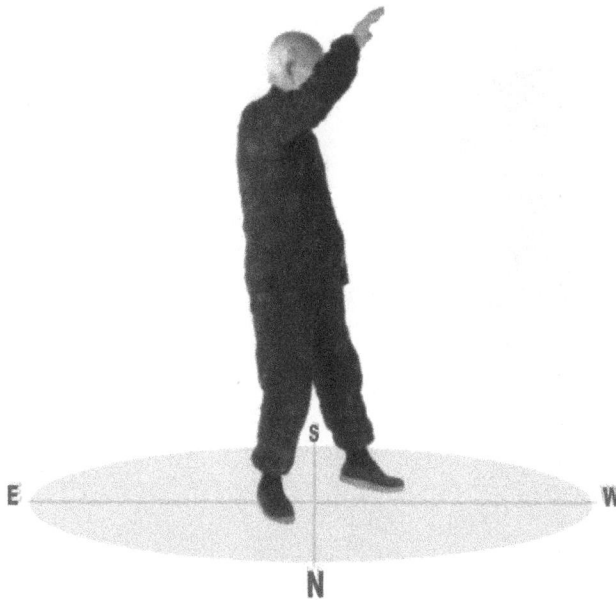

During the counts of:

1. Shift your weight to your right foot as you turn your torso to face west, letting your left foot pivot on the toes to point southwest.

2. Raise your body by straightening out your right leg. At the same time bring your left foot forward and place it toes down, heel up, in front of your right heel. Using this upward momentum, let your right arm come underneath your left and raise it up above your forehead, in a screw motion, to face diagonally outwards, elbow down. Your left hand simultaneously comes to the "position of attention" beside your left hip, palm facing backward.

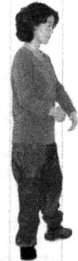

1.

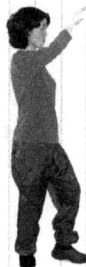

2.

116. Step forward and Brush Knee (left)

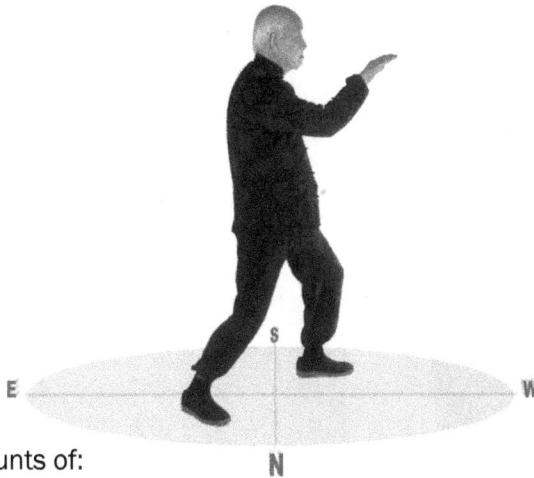

During the counts of:

1. Lower your body by bending your right knee and turn your torso slightly to the right. At the same time turn your right hand palm up to face you and let it begin to drop down in a counterclockwise motion.

2. Continue to turn your torso to the right until it is facing northwest (45 degrees) with your right hand continuing its counter-clockwise motion until it comes full circle to your right ear with the fingers pointing towards the west and the elbow bent and hanging downwards. During this turning motion of your torso your left hand rises up into a "ward off" position opposite your chest with the fingers pointing north.

3. Step with your left foot, heel first to the southwest, so as to form a shoulders' width stance facing west. Turn your torso to face west. In conjunction with this turn brush your left knee with your left hand and let it come to rest in the "position of attention" by your left hip pocket. Your right foot, pivoting on the heel, turns in 45 degrees to point northwest and your weight is now 60% forward on your left foot.

4. Complete the bow and arrow stance facing west by shifting 10% more of your weight into your left foot. At the same time using your whole body, push forward with your right hand, elbow slightly bent.

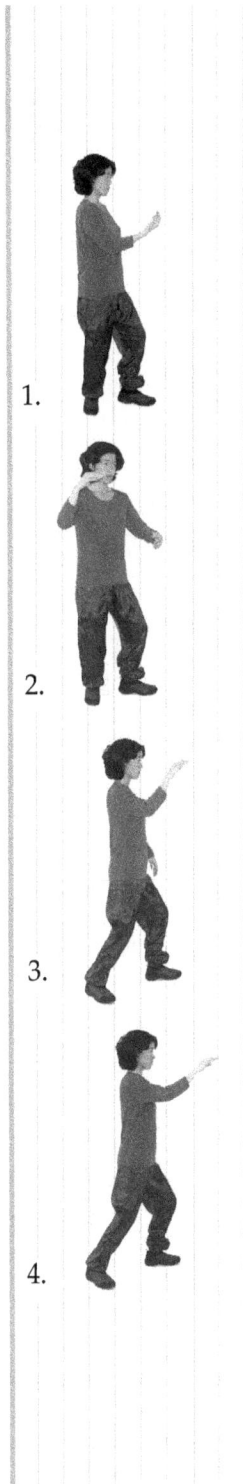

117. Needle at Sea Bottom

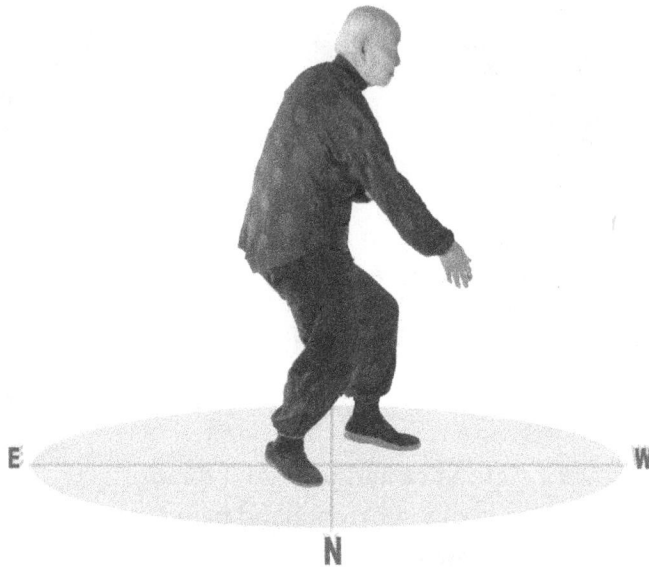

During the counts of:

1. Shift all of your weight onto your left foot and pick up your right foot and set it down again in the same position - with the toes pointing to the northwest.

2. Shift your weight onto your right foot and allow your right arm to straighten out slightly. Bring your left hand forward and lightly attach your left hand fingers to the inside of your right forearm. At the same time bring your left foot over and place it about 12" in front of your right heel with only the toes touching the ground.

3. Keeping your back straight and your weight on your back leg, sink down by bending your right knee.

4. Without leaning forward too much and keeping your waist facing west, continue to lower your right hand and your body so that your right fingers point directly to the ground in front of your right knee.

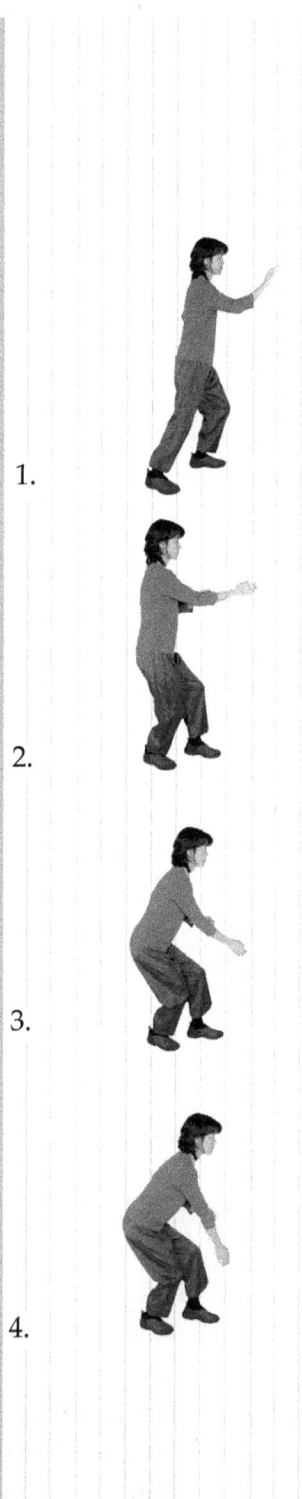

118. Fan Penetrates the Back

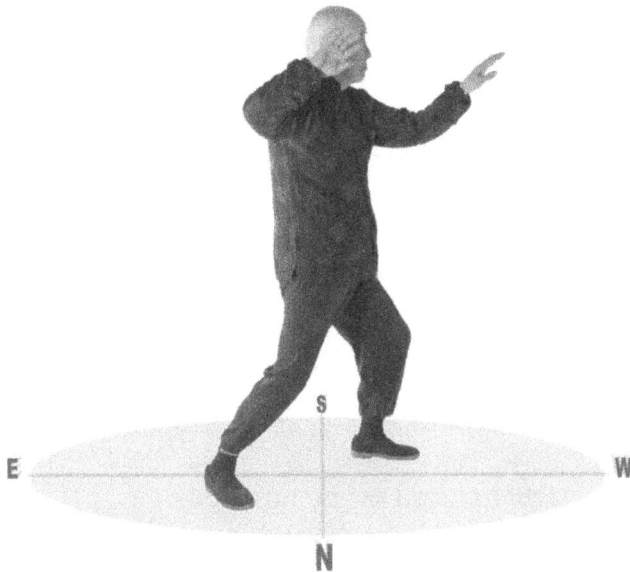

During the counts of:

1. Raise your body up and raise your right hand to your chest level with the palm facing south and with your left hand still attached to your right forearm.

2. Withdraw your right hand back near your right ear with the palm outward to the north. At the same time move your left hand forward with palm outward. Let both of your elbows remain bent downwards.

3. Take a half step forward with your left foot into a bow and arrow stance and shift 60% of your weight onto it.

4. Push through your left hand by shifting 10% more of your weight onto your left foot.

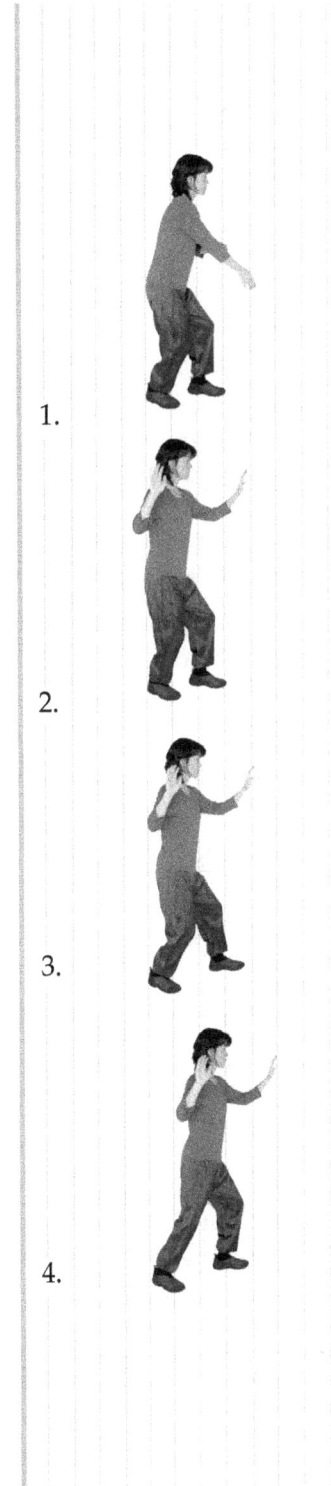

119. Turn Around and White Snake Puts Out Tongue

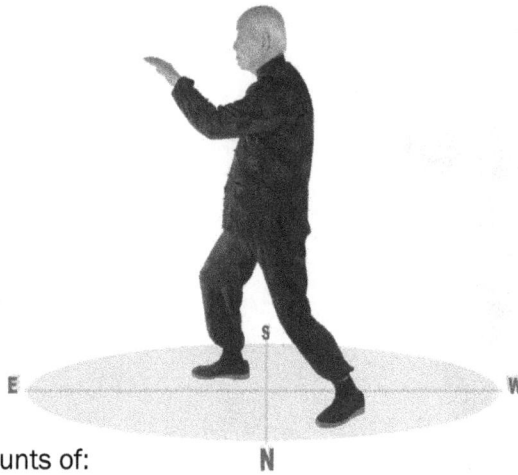

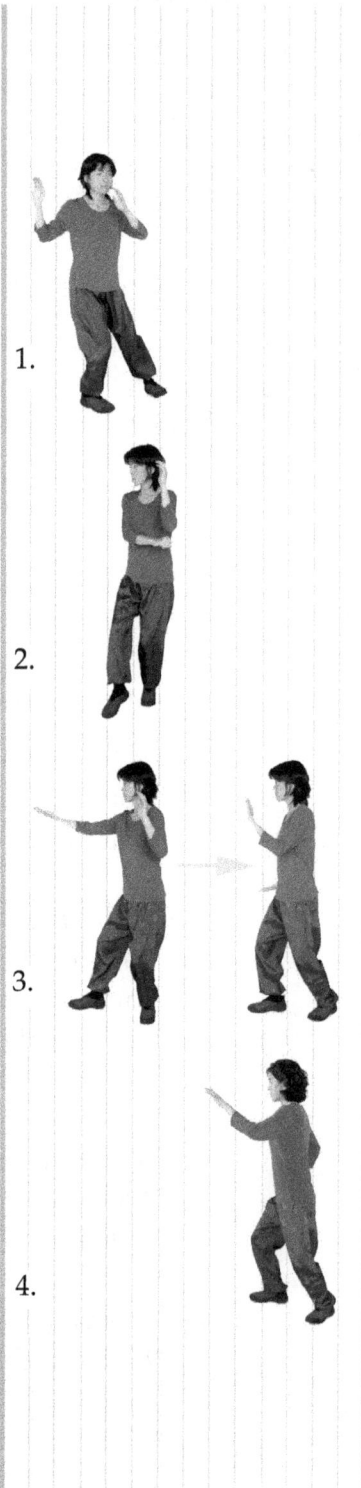

During the counts of:

1. Shift your weight back onto your right foot and as you turn your torso to face north, turn your left foot, pivoting on the heel, so the toes point north. Simultaneously circle your hands, without raising your elbows, in a clockwise motion.

2. Shift your weight back onto your left leg and continue to circle your hands clockwise until your left hand is near your left ear, with palm outward and elbow bent, and your right hand, clenched into a fist with the "tiger's mouth" facing your chest, comes under your right elbow. At the same time pivot your right foot on the toes to point north/northeast.

3. Step to the east with your right foot and chop to the east with your right fist. As your fist is just about to strike, open your fist to instead strike with your outstretched fingers (the snake puts out its tongue). When your strike is complete and pulling back, then shift your weight 60% onto your right foot and bring your open right hand, palm up, to your right hip. With the turning forward to the east of your torso simultaneously turn in your left foot, pivoting on the heel, to point northeast.

4. Complete the bow and arrow stance by shifting your weight about 70% onto your right foot and push forward (strike) with your left hand/palm.

120. Sep Forward, Deflect Downward, Intercept and Punch

During the counts of:

1. Shift your weight completely onto your right foot and pick up your left foot and place it back down, adjusting the toes to point north/northwest.

2. Shift your weight to your left foot and reach out with both hands at waist level to the northeast. Your palms are facing each other as though holding a ball with your right hand positioned slightly higher than your left.

3. Raise your right foot and place it diagonally forward to the right (without shifting any weight onto it) with the toes pointing south/southeast. At the same time make a fist with your right hand and circle it clockwise, in a deflecting motion, around to the right side of your waist and attach it to your hip, palm side facing up and "tigers mouth" facing south. In unison with this motion your left hand circles clockwise upward and forward in front of your face without raising your elbow to high. This motion is often described as emtying a bucket.

4. Facing east, shift your weight to your right foot (toes pointing to the south/southeast) and simultaneously deflect downward with your left hand to the level of your stomach with the palm facing the floor.

5. Step directly forward, to maintain a shoulders' width stance, with your left foot and shift 60% of your weight onto it. At the same time extend or intercept with your left hand forward and to the left. The left hand is open with the fingers pointing east and the palm is facing south. With this motion your right foot turns inwards, pivoting on the heel, toes pointing southeast.

6. Complete the bow and arrow stance facing west by shifting 10% more of your weight into your left foot. At the same time, using your whole body behind it, punch forward with your right fist ("tiger's mouth" facing up). As your right hand is punching forward let your left hand come over and cover the inner wrist of your right hand.

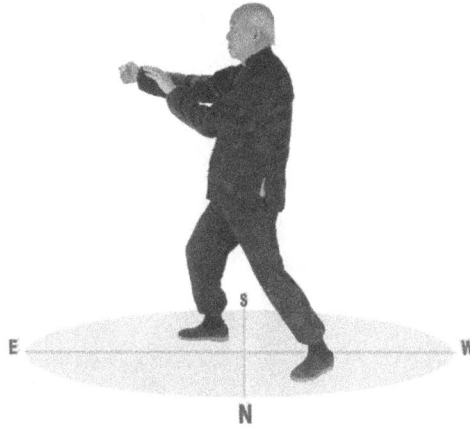

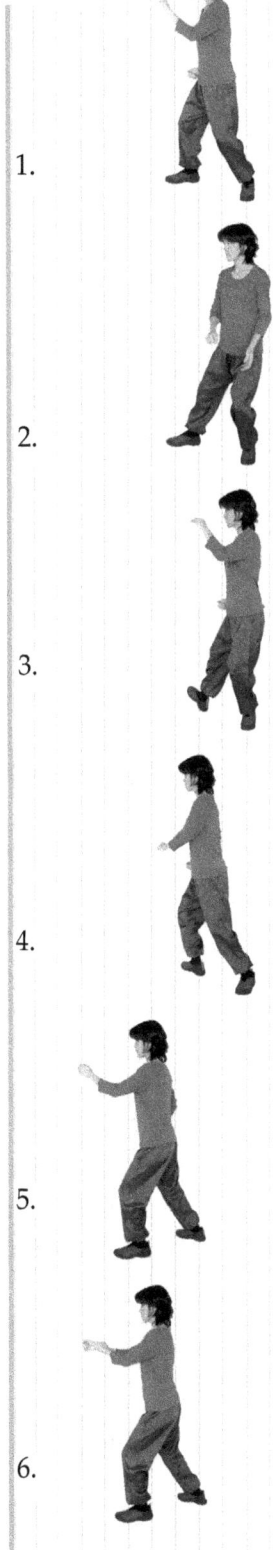

121. Ward Off Right

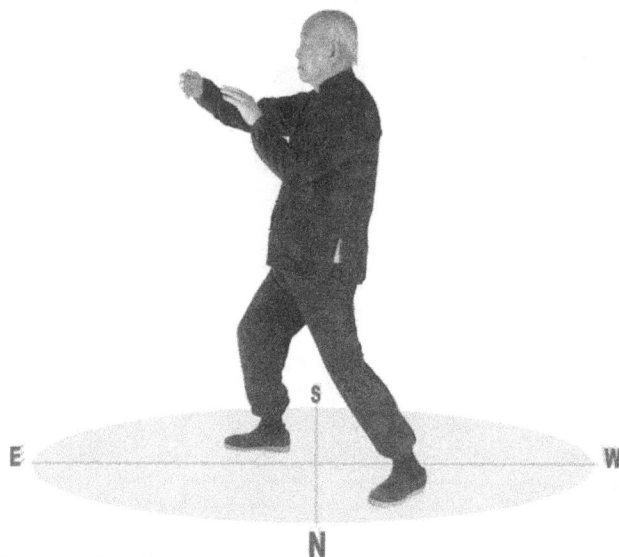

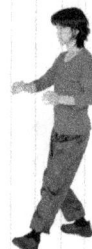

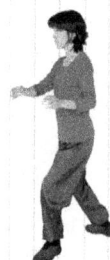

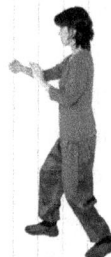

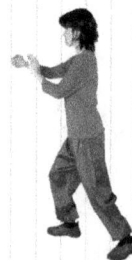

During the counts of:

1. Shift your weight back onto your right leg while turning your torso to face northeast and turning your palms to face each other. At the same time turn your left foot, pivoting on the heel, to point north/northeast.

2. Shift your weight onto your left foot ...

3. ... and step forward to the east into a bow and arrow stance with your right foot. Shift your weight 60% onto your right leg as you turn your torso to face east. Simultaneously pivot on your left heel, turning your left foot inward so the toes are pointing to the northeast. During this count, bring your right hand up in front of your chest/neck with the palm facing in. Your left hand faces your right palm, as if holding a small ball. Your right arm remains rounded out and your left elbow is lowered.

4. Complete the bow and arrow stance facing east by shifting an additional 10% of your weight onto your right foot. At the same time, using your whole body, push forward with the back of your right hand, both elbows remaining slightly bent.

186

122. Roll Back

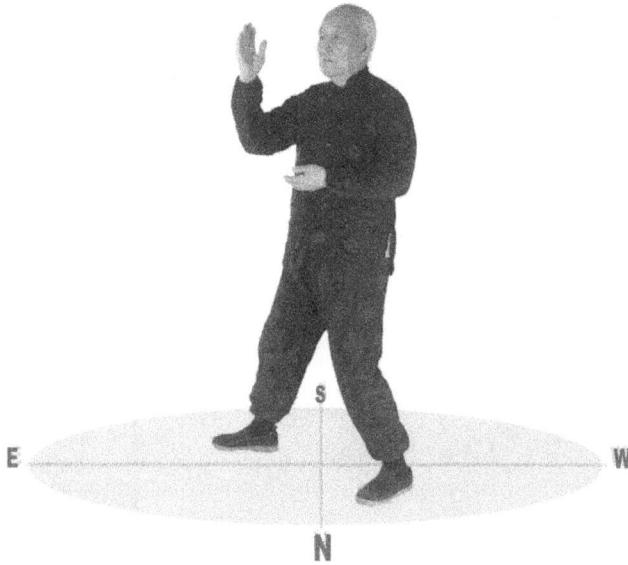

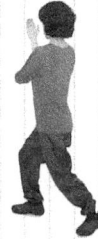

1.

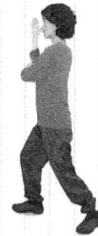

2.

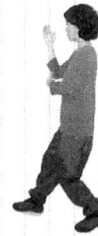

3.

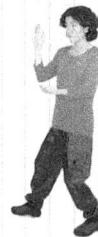

4.

During the counts of:

1. Turn your torso to the right 45 degrees and bring your right forearm up vertically and perpendicular to your chest. At the same time bring your left forearm across in front of the chest with your left palm facing in and the fingers almost touching your right elbow.

2. Keeping your weight on the right foot, turn your upper torso back to the left 45 degrees to face east again. Your waist, upper body, arms and hands move together as one unit.

3. With your torso facing straight ahead to the east, withdraw your weight back onto your left foot.

4. Turn your torso to the left 45 degrees to face northeast. At the same time turn your left palm upwards.

123. Press

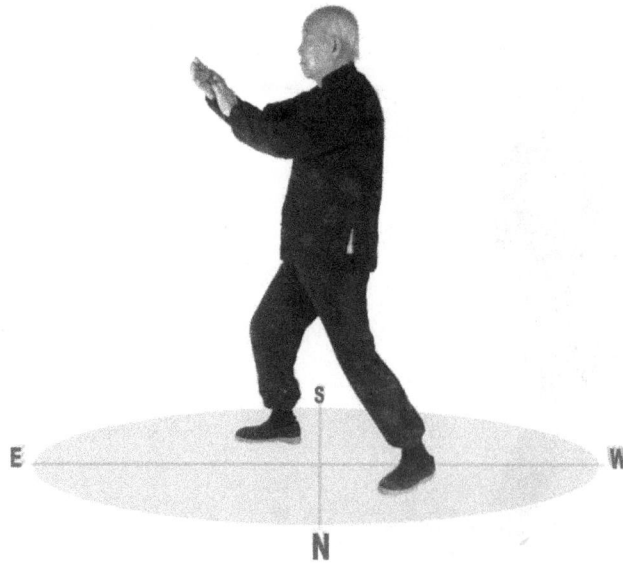

During the counts of:

1. Turn your torso 45 degrees to your left to face north. With the momentum of this turn let your left hand drop down and circle around (without lifting the elbow), heading up toward your left ear.

2. As your left hand is passing by your ear, turn your torso back 90 degrees to your right to face east and lightly attach your left fingers to the inside of your right wrist (as though you're feeling your pulse). Your right forearm drops slightly down into a diagonal position in front of your upper chest with the left elbow lowered.

3. Without letting your hands and arms move separately from your body, shift your weight onto the right leg and press forward with your right forearm. It's important here to move your whole body as one unit and not let your hands and arms move independently or initiate any movement.

4. Continue to press forward and slightly upwards until your right leg bears about 70% of your weight.

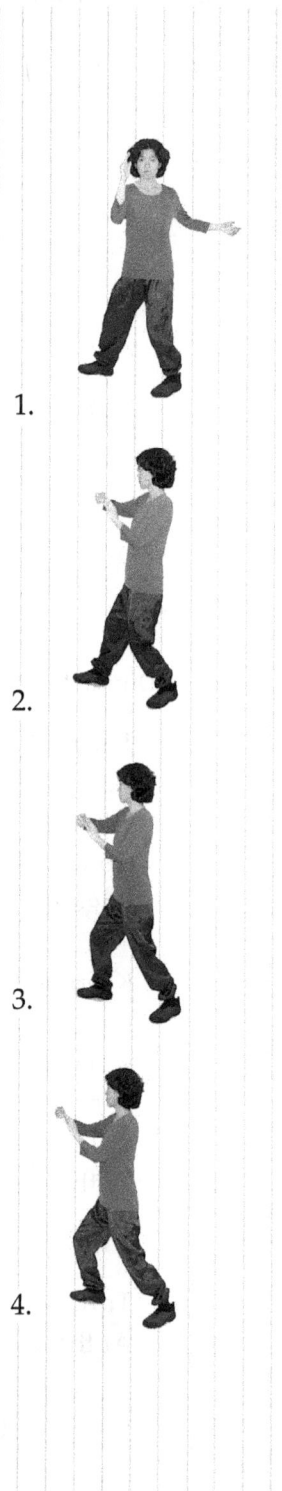

124. Push

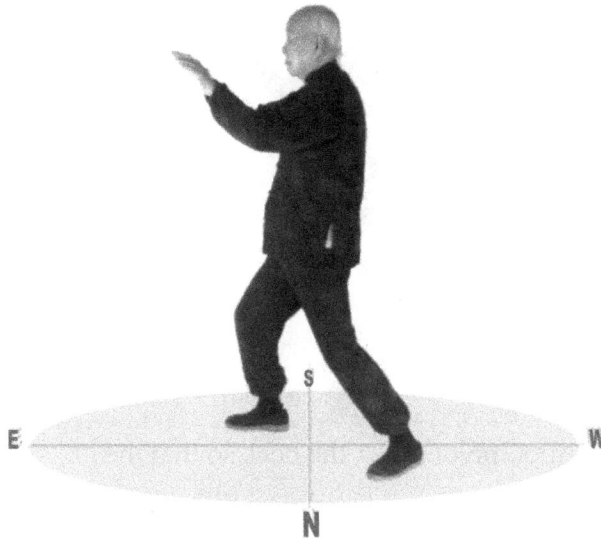

During the counts of:

1. | Separate your hands, palms down, at the level of your shoulders.

2. | Keeping your back straight, shift your weight back onto your left leg and simultaneously withdraw your hands slightly towards your upper chest. The fingers of both hands point forward and the elbows remain relaxed and bent downwards.

3. | Without moving your hands and arms separately from your body, shift 60% of your weight onto your right leg again. The push is coming from the forward movement of your whole body - not your arms.

4. | Complete the bow and arrow stance by shifting about 10% more of your weight into your right foot. At the same time slightly raise your fingertips so that the intention of the push is coming through your palms and directed to the east.

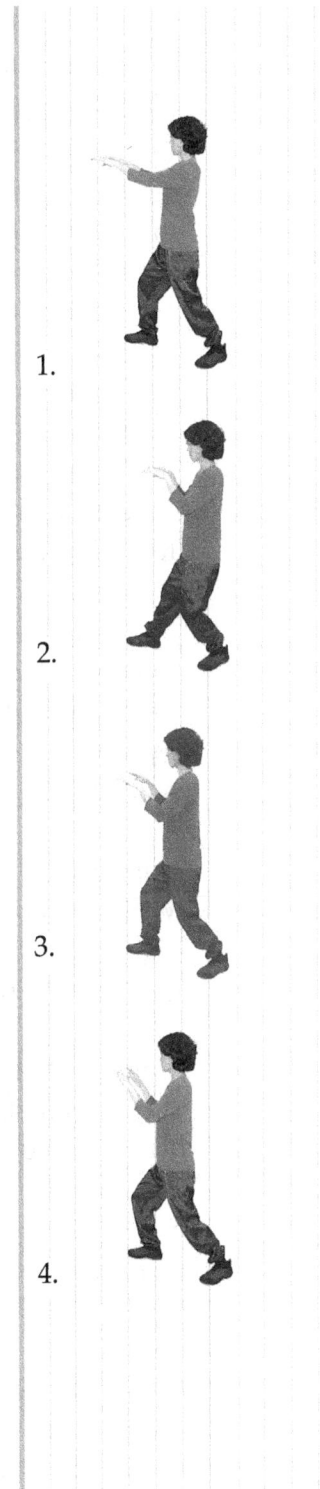

1.

2.

3.

4.

125. Single Whip

During the counts of:

1. Shift your weight back onto your left foot and let your arms stretch out slightly with the palms of the hands facing downward.

2. Turn your torso to the left until it faces northwest and at the same time turn your right foot, pivoting on the heel, so that the toes point north as well.

3. Shift your weight back to your right leg as you turn your torso to face northeast. Simultaneously withdraw both hands. The left hand comes down opposite the navel with its palm up and the right hand forms a "hook" (all 5 digits are touching at the tips and pointing downward) near your right armpit.

4. Turn your torso counterclockwise back to the northwest corner. With this movement strike to the northeast corner with your right hand "hook" and simultaneously pivot the left foot on the toes to point northwest.

5. Continue to turn your torso to face west and step with your left foot, heel first, so as to form a shoulders' width stance facing west with 60% of your weight on your left foot. The movement of your torso brings your left hand, palm facing in, up in front of your body at face level. At the same time let this movement turn your right foot, pivoting on the heel, to point northwest. The right hand "hook" does not move.

6. Complete the bow and arrow stance facing west by shifting your weight about 70% onto your left foot. At the same time turn your left hand palm outward being careful to leave your arm slightly bent. Your eyes gaze just over and past the fingertips.

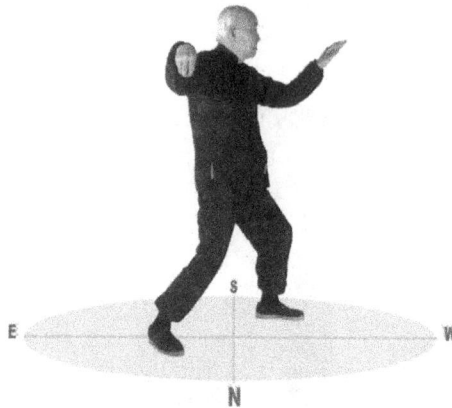

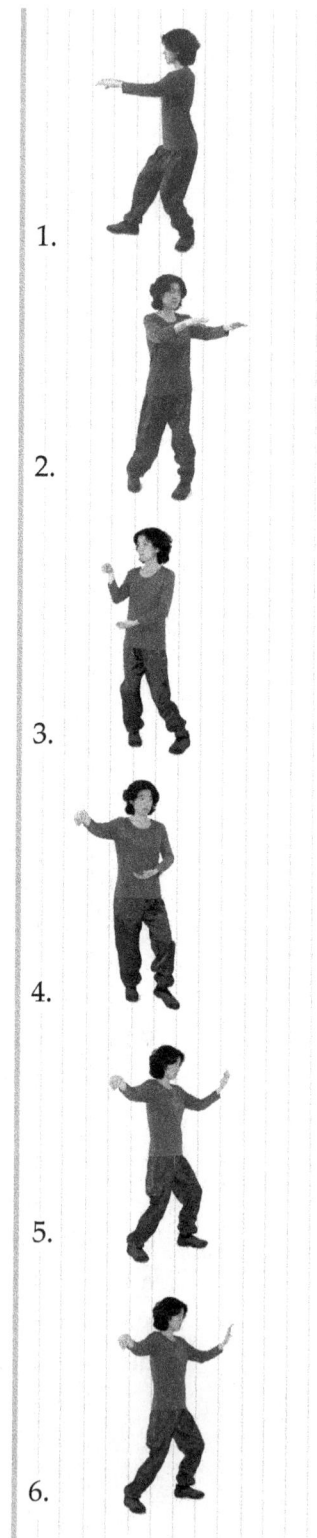

126. Wave Hands in Clouds (left)

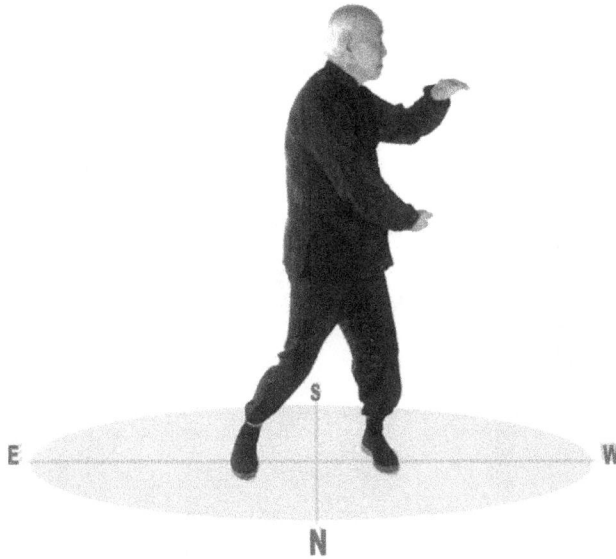

During the counts of:

1.   Shift your weight completely onto your right leg as you turn your torso to face northeast and your left foot, pivoting on the heel, to face north. At the same time open your right hand so that the palm is facing down and bring your left hand, palm facing up, in front of your waist so as to simulate holding a ball in front of your chest.

2.   Turn both palms in to face your body and simultaneously bring your right hand down to your waist level and bring your left hand up to the level of your neck. The right hand passes on the inside of the left.

3.   Turn your torso and hands as one unit to the left as you begin shifting your weight onto your left leg. On this beat your waist is now facing north.

4.   Shift 80% of your weight onto your left foot as you turn your torso to face west. Then turn both palms to face each other so that they are in a position of holding a ball in front of your chest.

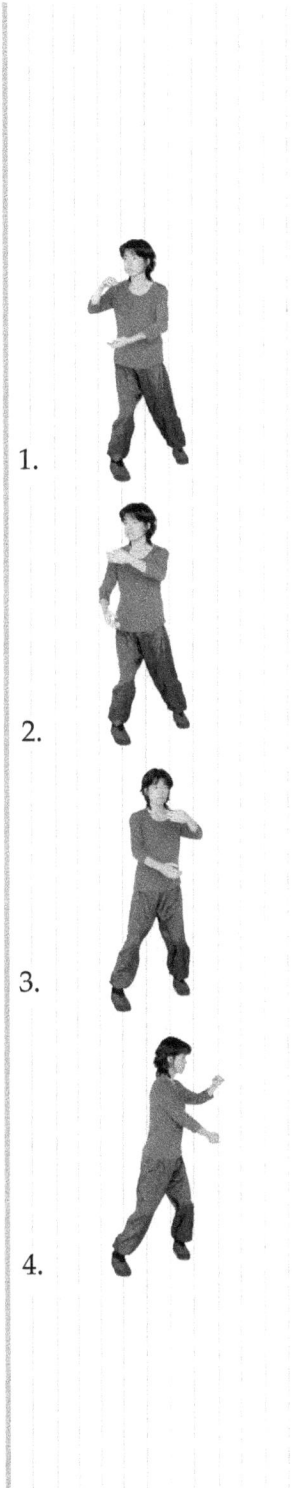

127. Wave Hands in Clouds (right)

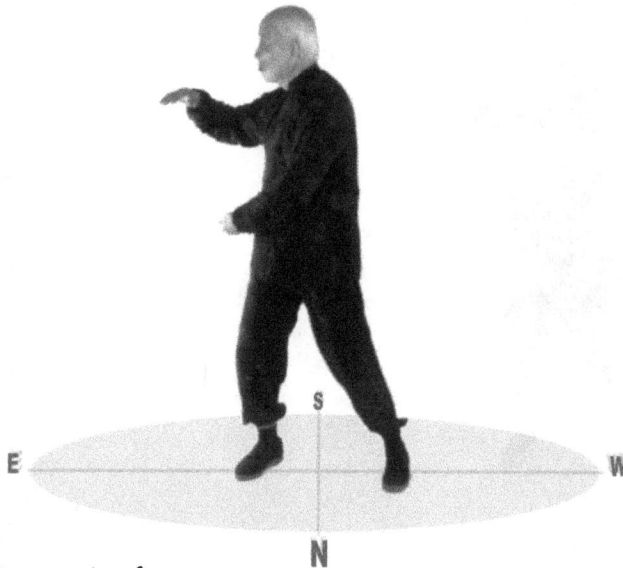

During the counts of:

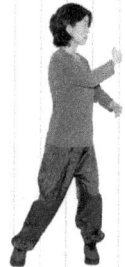

1. | Bring your left hand down to your waist level and simultaneously bring your right hand up to your neck level as you turn both palms to face inwards. Your left hand passes on the outside of your right hand as they exchange positions.

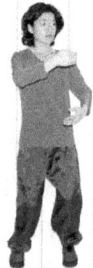

2. | As you turn your torso to your right, step backwards and to the east with your right foot, placing it parrallel to your left foot so that there is about 10" between them (less than a shoulders' width).

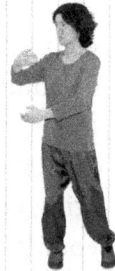

3. | Continue to shift your weght onto right foot as you turn your torso and hands as one unit to the right. On the count of three you are facing directly north (not in picture).

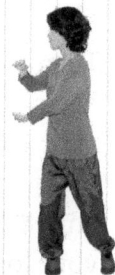

4. | Continue to turn your torso and hands to the right until you're facing east with 80% of your weight on your right leg. Your right hand now turns palm down and your left hand turns palm up. Again you are simulating holding a ball in front of your chest.

1.

2.

3.

4.

128. Wave Hands in Clouds (left)

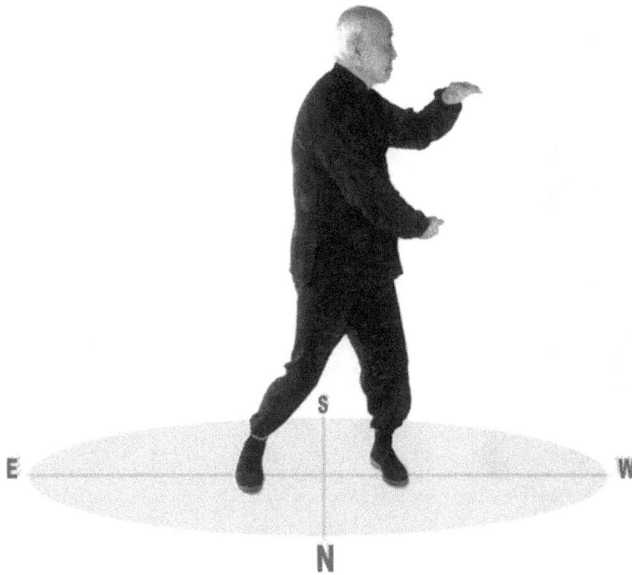

During the counts of:

1. Passing on the outside, bring your right hand down to your waist level and simultaneously bring your left hand, on the inside, up to your neck level as you turn both palms to face inwards.

2. As you turn your torso to your left, step and to the west with your right foot, placing it parralel to your left foot so that there is about 18" between them (more than a shoulders' width).

3. Continue to shift your weight onto your left foot as you turn your torso and hands as one unit to the left.

4. Continue to turn your torso and hands to the left until you're facing west with 80% of your weight on your left leg. Your left hand now turns palm down and your right hand turns palm up. Again you are simulating holding a ball in front of your chest.

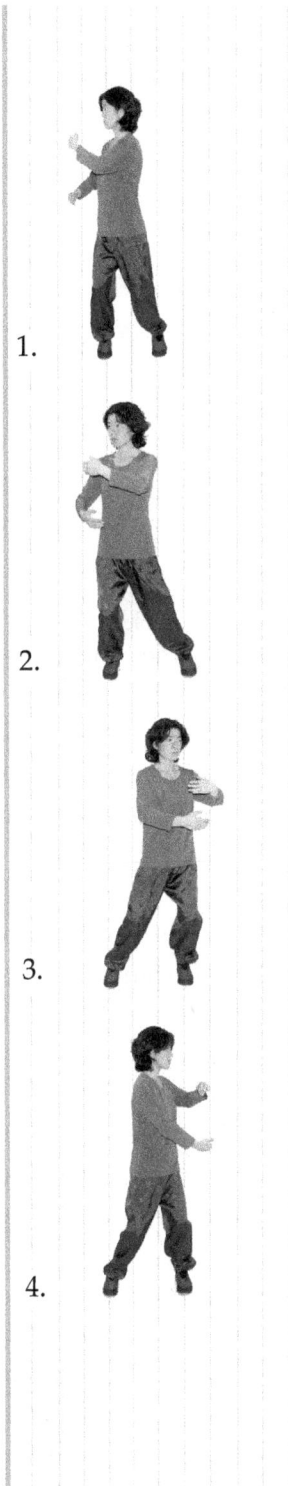

129. Wave Hands in Clouds (right)

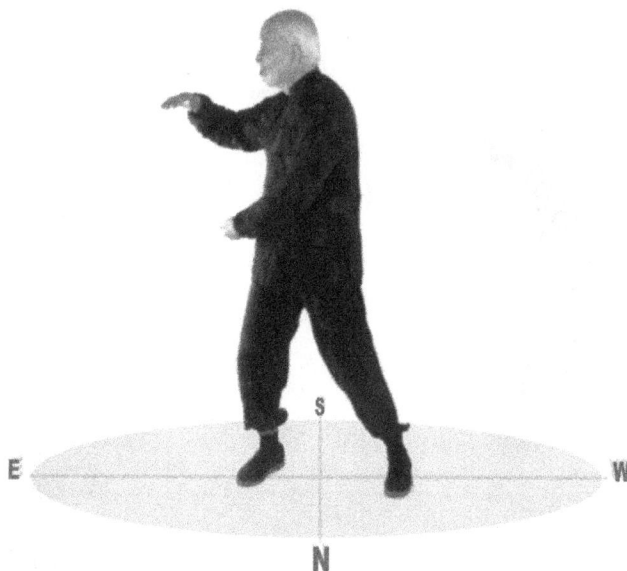

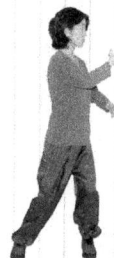

1.

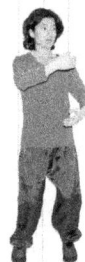

2.

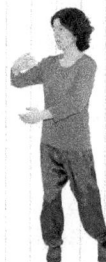

3.

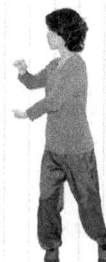

4.

During the counts of:

1. | Bring your left hand down to your waist level and simultaneously bring your right hand up to your neck level as you turn both palms to face inwards.Your left hand passes on the outside of your right hand as they exchange positions.

2. | As you turn your torso to your right, step to the east with your right foot, placing it parrallel to your left foot so that there is about 8 to 10" between them (less than a shoulders' width).

3. | Continue to shift your weght onto your right foot as you turn your torso and hands as one unit to the right. On the count of three you are facing directly north (not in picture).

4. | Continue to turn your torso and hands to the right until you're facing east with 80% of your weight on your right leg. Your right hand now turns palm down and your left hand turns palm up. Again you are simulating holding a ball in front of your chest.

130. Wave Hands in Clouds (left)

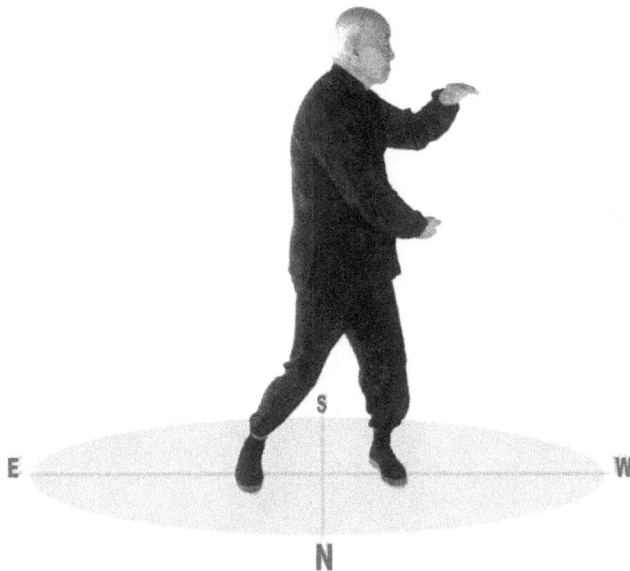

During the counts of:

1. Passing on the outside, bring your right hand down to your waist level and simultaneously bring your left hand, on the inside, up to your neck level as you turn both palms to face inwards.

2. As you turn your torso to your left, step and to the west with your right foot, placing it parralel to your left foot so that there is about 18" between them (more than a shoulders' width).

3. Continue to shift your weight onto left foot as you turn your torso and hands as one unit to the left.

4. Continue to turn your torso and hands to the left until you're facing west with 80% of your weight on your left leg. Your left hand now turns palm down and your right hand turns palm up. Again you are simulating holding a ball in front of your chest.

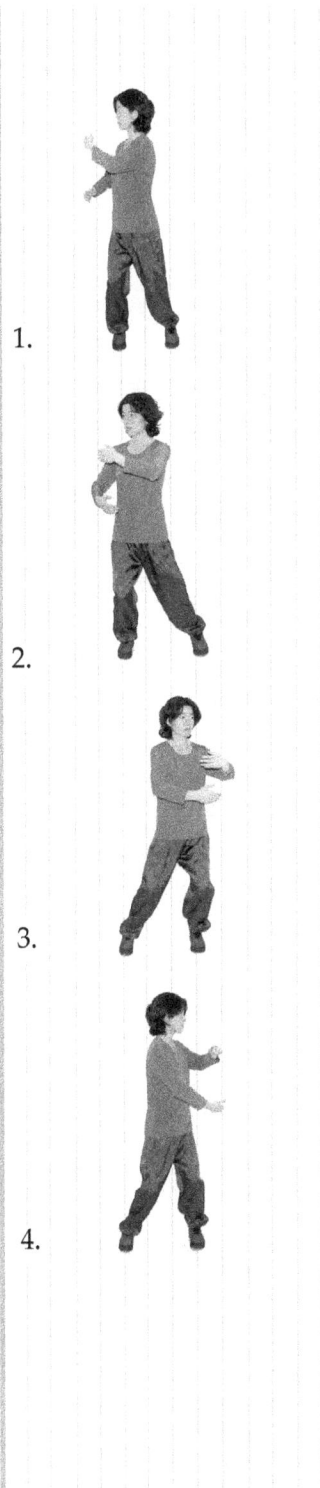

131. Single Whip

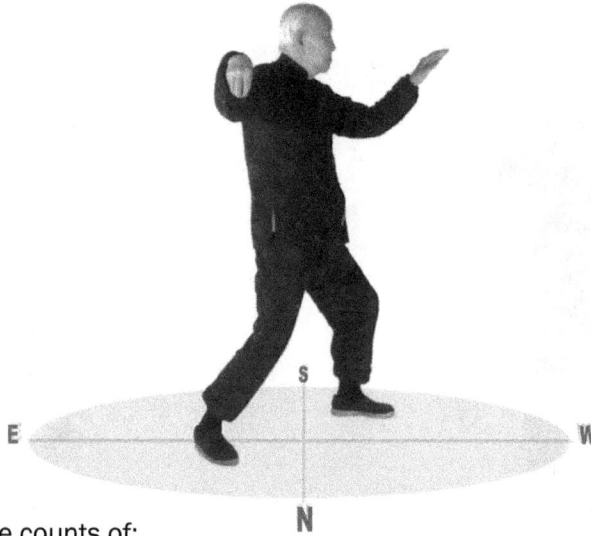

During the counts of:

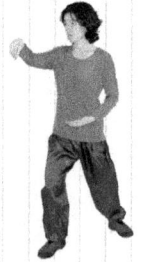

1. Form a "hook" with your right hand,[1] fingers pointing down, and strike out with it in a diagonal direction upwards to the northeast corner, as you take a step with your right foot in this same direction. At the same time lower your open left hand, palm up, in front of your stomach.

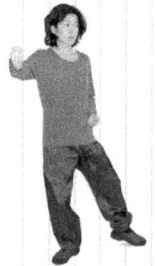

2. Shift your weight completely onto your right foot and turn your torso to the left facing northwest. Let this turning motion turn your left foot, pivoting on the toes to face west.

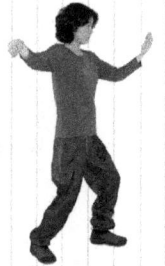

3. Continue to turn your torso to face west and step with your left foot, heel first, so as to form a shoulders' width stance facing west. The movement of your torso brings your left hand, palm facing in, up in front of your body at face level. At the same time let this movement turn your right foot, pivoting on the heel, to point northwest. The right hand "hook" does not move.

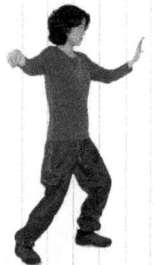

4. Complete the bow and arrow stance facing west by shifting your weight about 70% into your left foot. At the same time turn your left hand palm outward being careful to leave your arm slightly bent. Your eyes gaze just over and past the fingertips.

132. High Pat on Horse

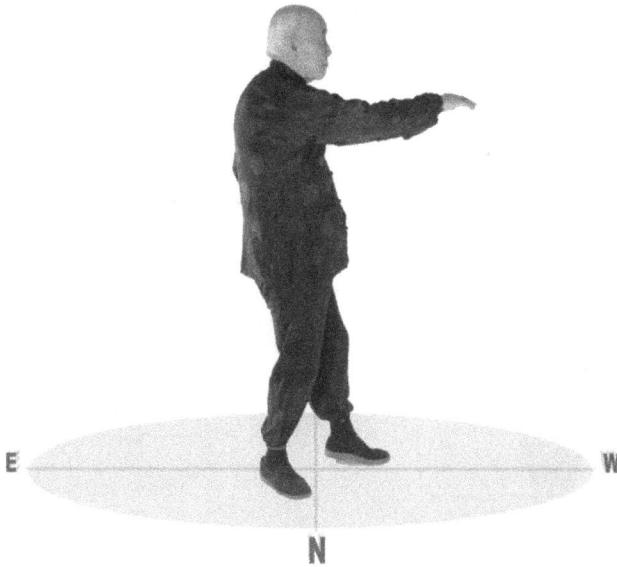

During the counts of:

1. Pick up your right foot, readjust it, and then place it back down with the toes once again pointing northwest.

2. Shift your weight back onto your right foot and place the toes of your left foot down about 12" in front of your right heel facing west. As soon as the toes touch the ground open your right hand so that the palm is facing the floor.

3. Bring your right hand over, palm still facing down, and cover your left inner elbow. At the same time turn your left hand so that the palm is facing up.

4. Withdraw your left hand, palm up, down to your left pocket and simultaneously strike forward with your right hand at neck level, palm facing down.

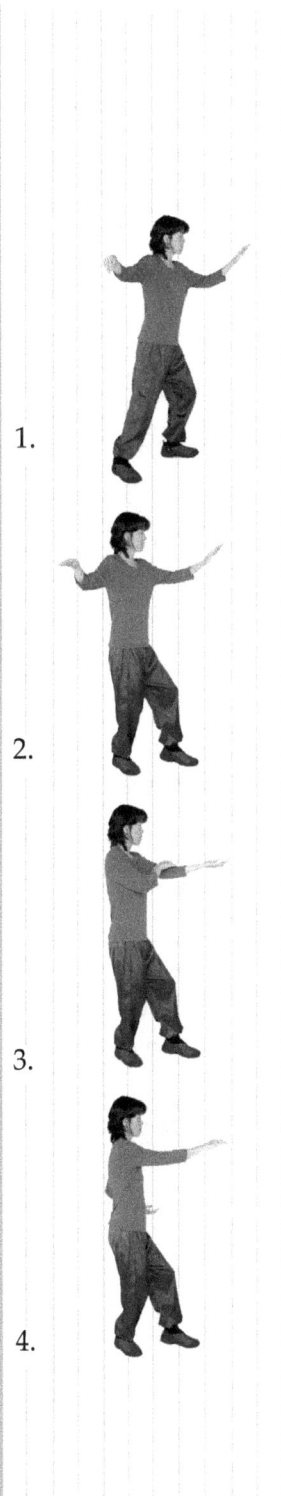

1.

2.

3.

4.

133. Thrusting Hand

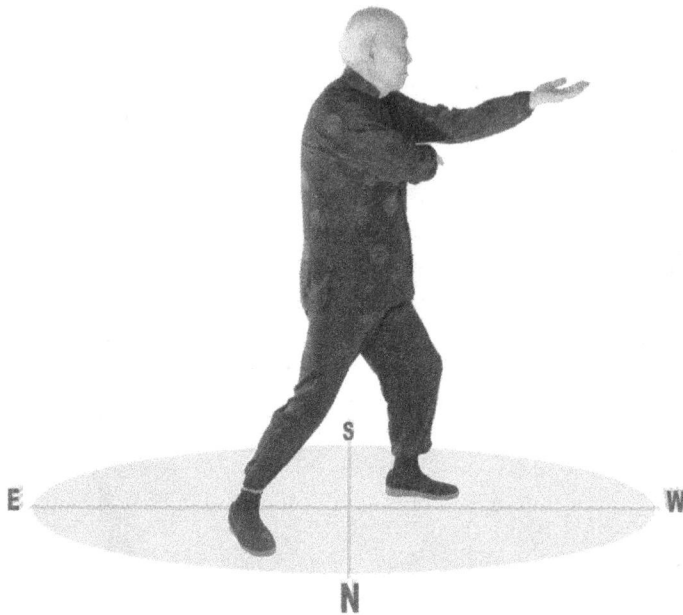

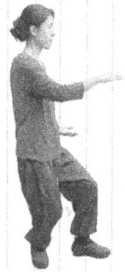

1.

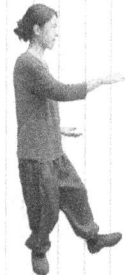

2.

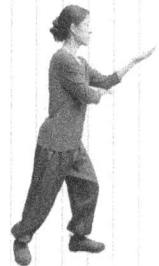

3.

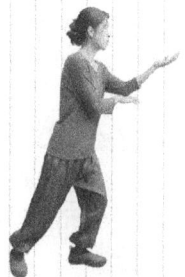

4.

During the counts of:

1. Bending at the knee, sink your weight down into your right leg and then ...

2. ... step forward and over to the left with your left foot (without shifting your weight onto it), toes pointing west, into a shoulders' width stance facing west.

3. Shift your weight onto your left leg as you ...

4. ... strike forward with your left hand with the palm turned up and the fingers thrusting forward. As your left hand strikes forward, bring your right hand, palm facing down, back under your left armpit. Your weight is now about 70% on your left leg.

134. Turn Round and Kick With Sole

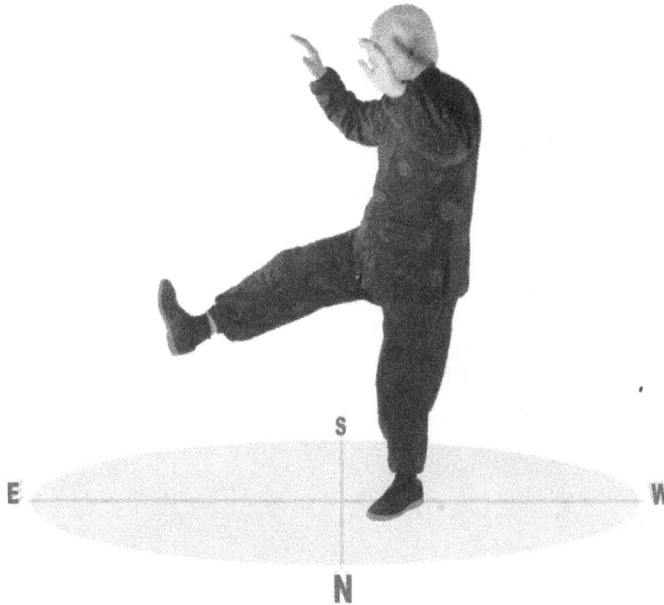

During the counts of:

1. | Shift your weight back onto your right leg and ...

2. | ... then turn your torso to face northeast. At the same time turn your left foot, pivoting on your heel, to point north/northeast and withdraw your left wrist back to cross your right wrist.

3. | Shift your weight onto your left foot and turn your torso to fully face east. At the same time raise your right knee and toes so that the sole of your right foot is facing east. Slip your left hand under your right hand and cross them at the wrists, with the palms facing out to the east, in front of your chest. Your left hand is now on the outside.

4. | Kick out with the sole of your right foot to the east and separate your hands to the north and south while leaving your forearms positioned vertically.

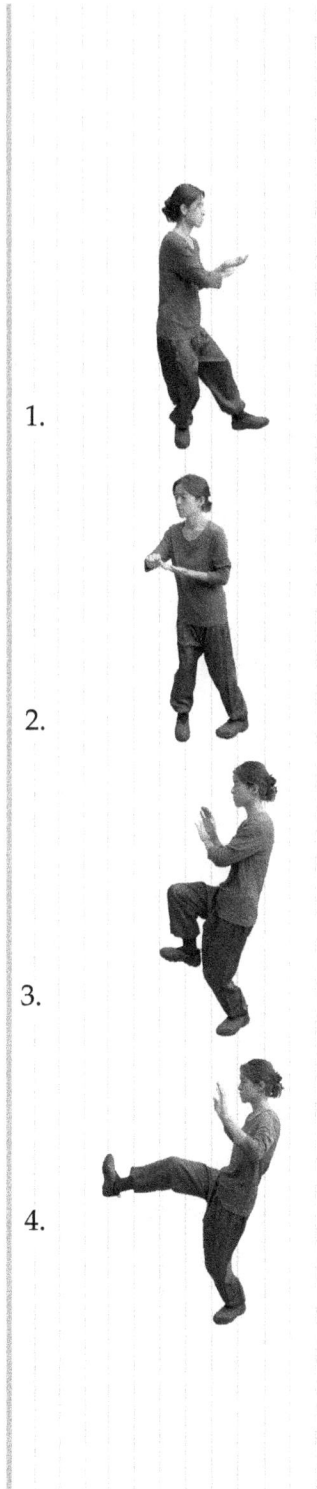

135. Step Forward, Brush Knee and Punch to Groin

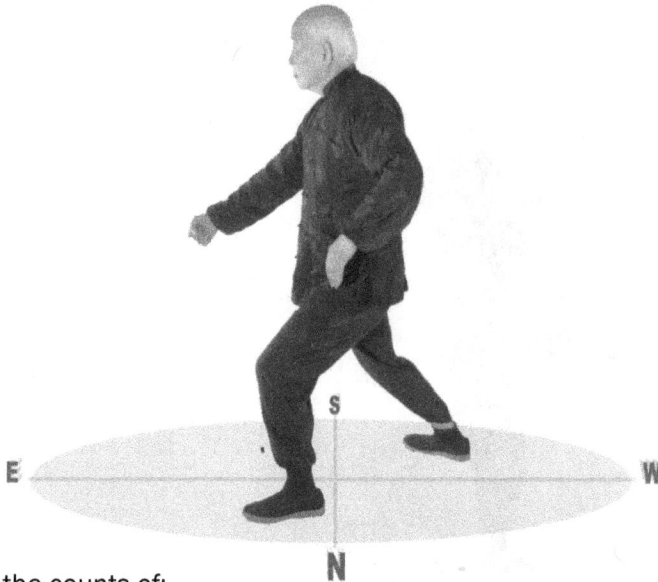

During the counts of:

1. Set your right foot down with the toes pointing south/
   southeast and, at the same time, form a fist with your right
   hand and attach it to your right thigh with the "tiger's
   mouth" pointing south. Your left hand comes up into a ward
   off position with fingers pointing south.

2. Turn your torso to the southeast and shift your weight onto
   your right foot.

3. Take a step directly forward into a shoulders' width bow
   and arrow stance with your left foot, heel touching first.
   Turn your torso to face east and shift 60% of your weight
   onto it. With the turning motion of your torso, brush your
   left knee with your left hand and bring it into the "position
   of attention" beside your left thigh while at the same time
   turning your right foot inward, pivoting on the heel, to point
   southeast.

4. Shift an additional 10% of your weight into your left foot and
   punch forward and slightly downward with your right hand
   to groin level, turning your fist "tigers mouth up."

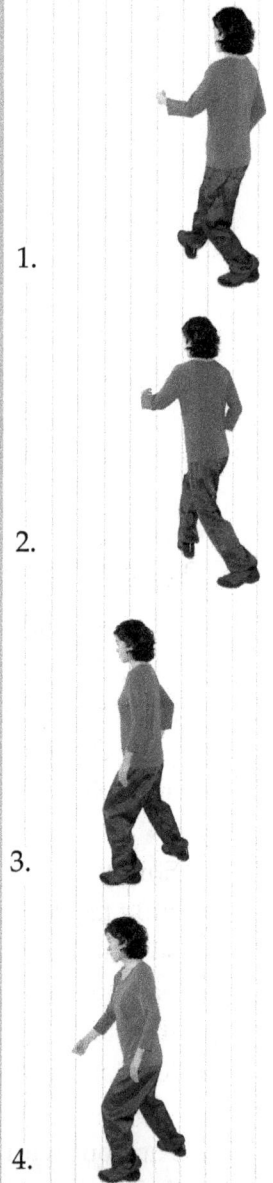

136. Step Forward and Ward Off Right

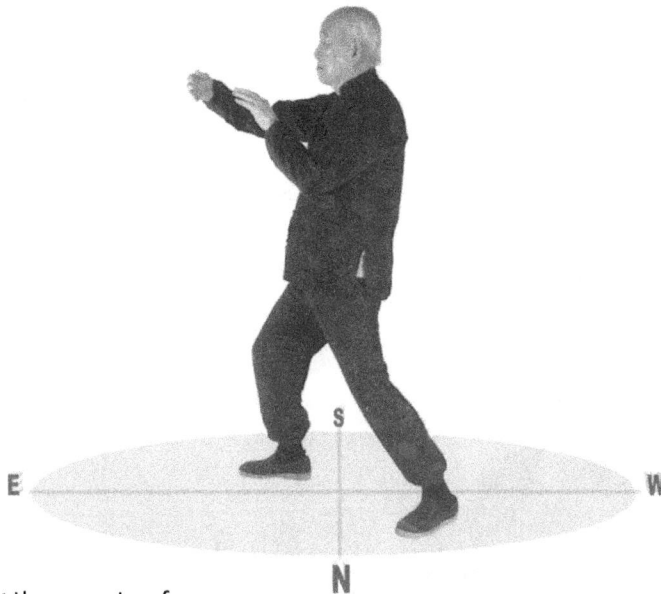

During the counts of:

1. Shift your weight back onto your right leg while turning your torso to face northeast and turning your palms to face each other. At the same time turn your left foot, pivoting on the heel, to point north/northeast.

2. Shift your weight onto your left foot ...

3. ... and step forward to the east into a bow and arrow stance with your right foot. Shift your weight 60% onto your right leg as you turn your torso to face east. Simultaneously pivot on your left heel, turning your left foot inward so the toes are pointing to the northeast. During this count, bring your right hand up in front of your chest/neck with the palm facing in. Your left hand faces your right palm, as if holding a small ball. Your right arm remains rounded out and your left elbow is lowered.

4. Complete the bow and arrow stance facing east by shifting an 10% more of your weight onto your right foot. At the same time, using your whole body, push forward with the back of your right hand, both elbows remaining slightly bent.

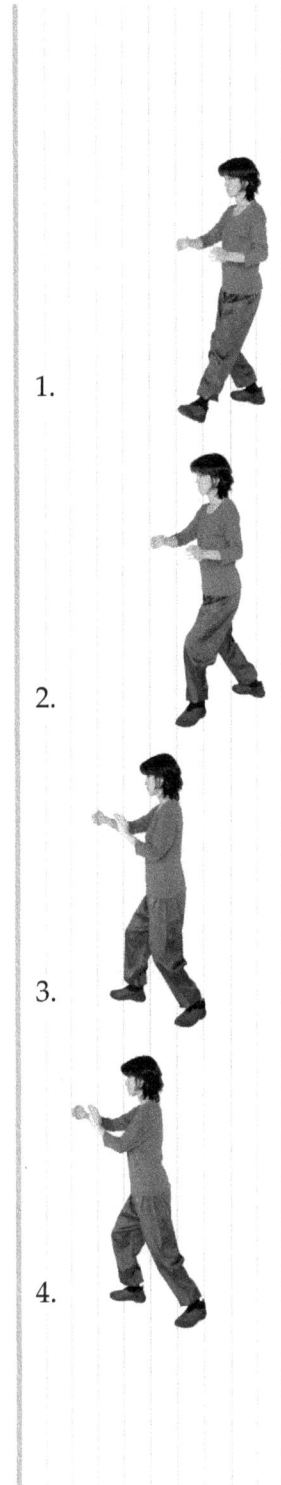

137. Roll Back

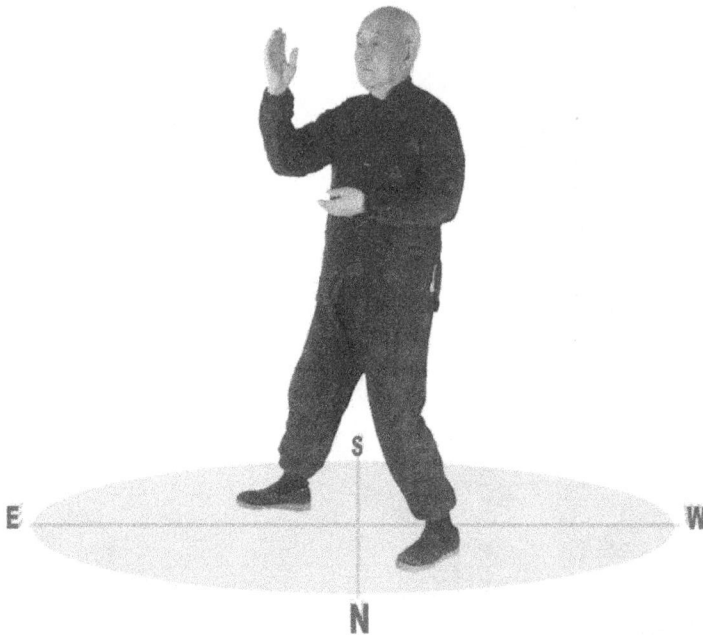

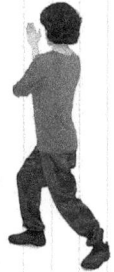

1.

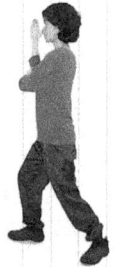

2.

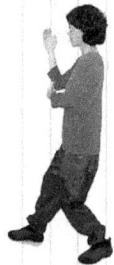

3.

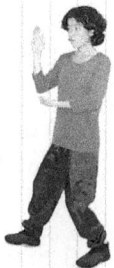

4.

During the counts of:

1. Turn your torso to the right 45 degrees and bring your right forearm up into a 90 degree angle, perpendicular to your body. At the same time bring your left forearm across in front of the chest with your left palm facing in and the fingers almost touching your right elbow.

2. Keeping your weight on the right foot, turn your upper torso back to the left 45 degrees to face east. Your waist, upper body, arms and hands move together as one unit.

3 With your torso facing straight ahead to the east, withdraw your weight back onto your left foot.

4. Turn your torso to the left 45 degrees to face northeast. At the same time turn your left palm upwards.

138. Press

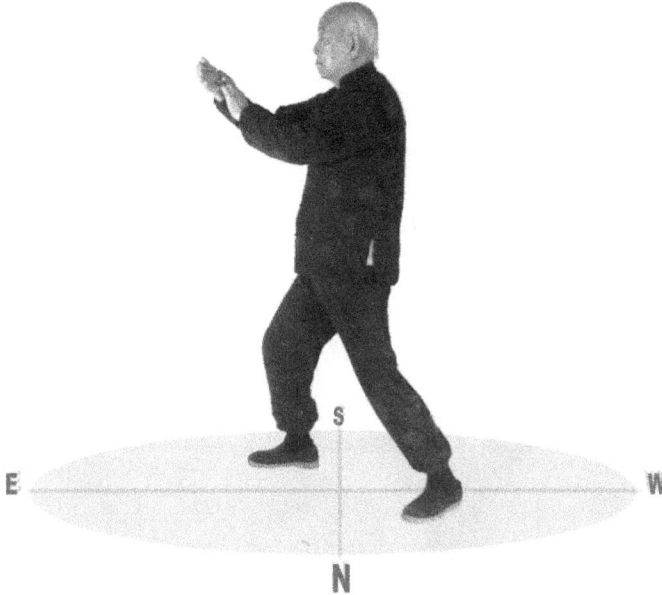

During the counts of:

1. Turn your torso 45 degrees to your left to face north. With the momentum of this turn let your left hand drop down and circle around (without lifting the elbow), heading up toward your left ear.

2. As your left hand is passing by your ear, turn your torso back 90 degrees to your right to face east and lightly attach your left fingers to the inside of your right wrist (as though you're feeling your pulse). Your right forearm drops slightly down into a diagonal position in front of your upper chest with the left elbow lowered.

3. Without letting your hands and arms move separately from your body, shift your weight onto the right leg and press forward with your right forearm. It's important here to move your whole body as one unit and not let your hands and arms move independently or initiate any movement.

4. Continue to press forward and slightly upwards until your right leg bears about 70% of your weight.

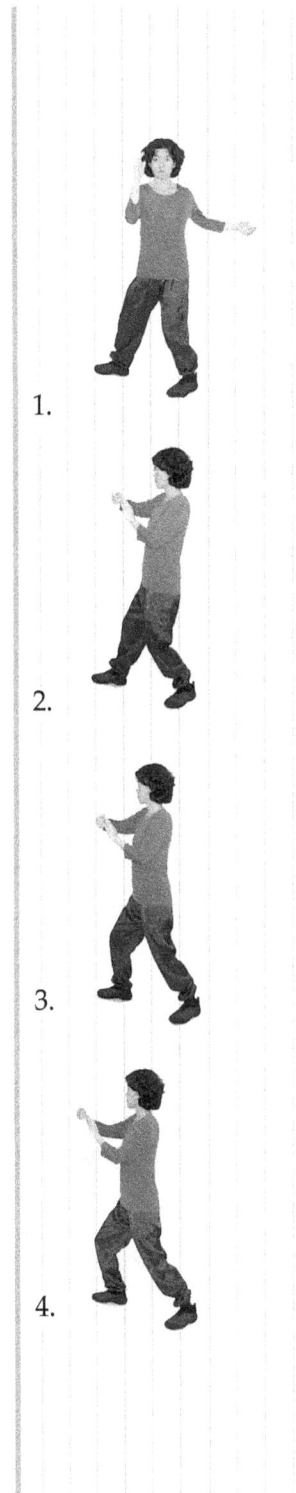

139. Push

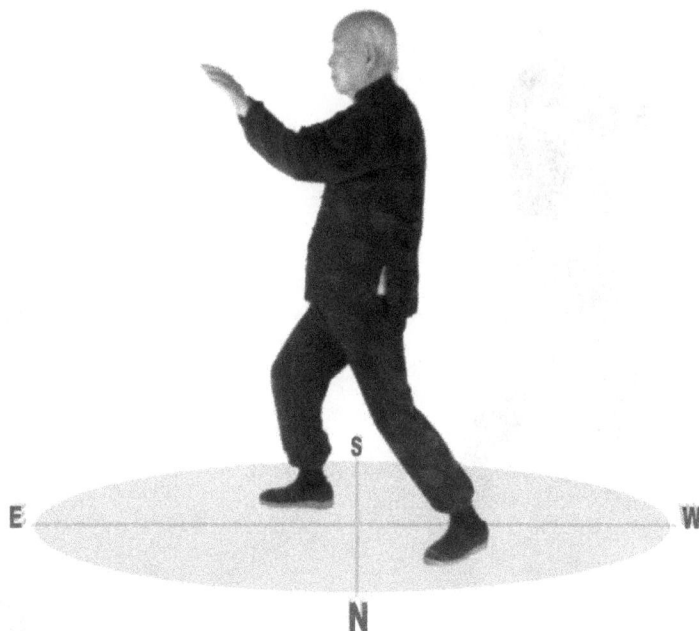

During the counts of:

1. | Separate your hands, palms down, at the level of your shoulders.

2. | Keeping your back straight, shift your weight back onto your left leg and simultaneously withdraw your hands slightly towards your upper chest. The fingers of both hands point forward and the elbows remain relaxed and bent downwards.

3. | Without moving your hands and arms separately from your body, shift 60% of your weight back onto your right leg. The push is coming from the forward movement of your whole body - not your arms.

4. | Complete the bow and arrow stance by shifting an additional 10% more of your weight into your right foot. At the same time slightly raise your fingertips so that the intention of the push is coming through your palms and directed to the east.

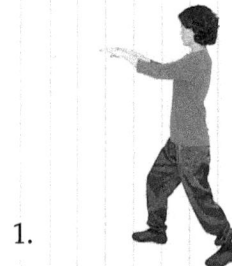

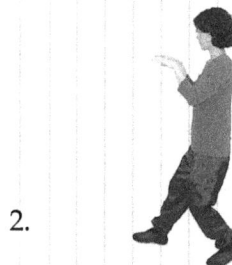

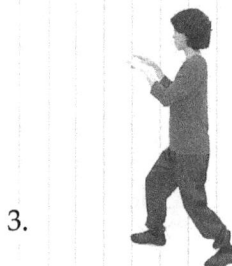

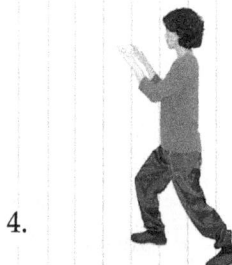

140. Single Whip

During the counts of:

1. Shift your weight back onto your left foot and let your arms stretch out slightly with the palms of the hands facing downward.

2. Turn your torso to the left until it faces northwest and at the same time turn your right foot, pivoting on the heel, so that the toes point north.

3. Shift your weight back to your right leg as you turn your torso to face northeast. Simultaneously withdraw both hands. The left hand comes down opposite the navel with its palm up and the right hand forms a "hook" (all 5 digits are touching at the tips and pointing downward) near your right armpit.

4. Turn your torso counterclockwise back to the northwest corner. With this movement strike to the northeast corner with your right hand "hook" and simultaneously pivot the left foot on the toes to point northwest.

5. Continue to turn your torso to face west and step with your left foot, heel first, so as to form a shoulders' width stance facing west with 60% of your weight on your left foot. The movement of your torso brings your left hand, palm facing in, up in front of your body at face level. At the same time let this movement turn your right foot, pivoting on the heel, to point northwest. The right hand "hook" does not move.

6. Complete the bow and arrow stance facing west by shifting 10% more of your weight onto your left foot. At the same time turn your left hand palm outward being careful to leave your arm slightly bent. Your eyes gaze over and past the fingertips.

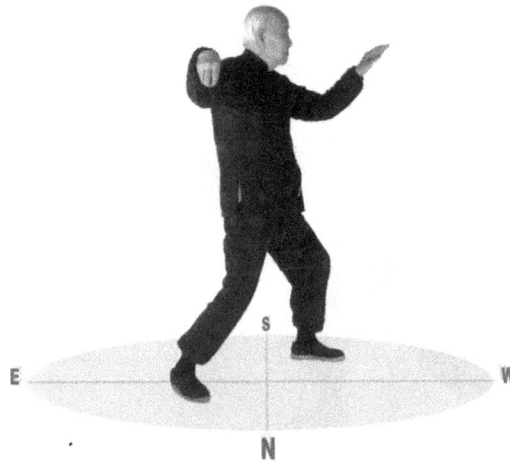

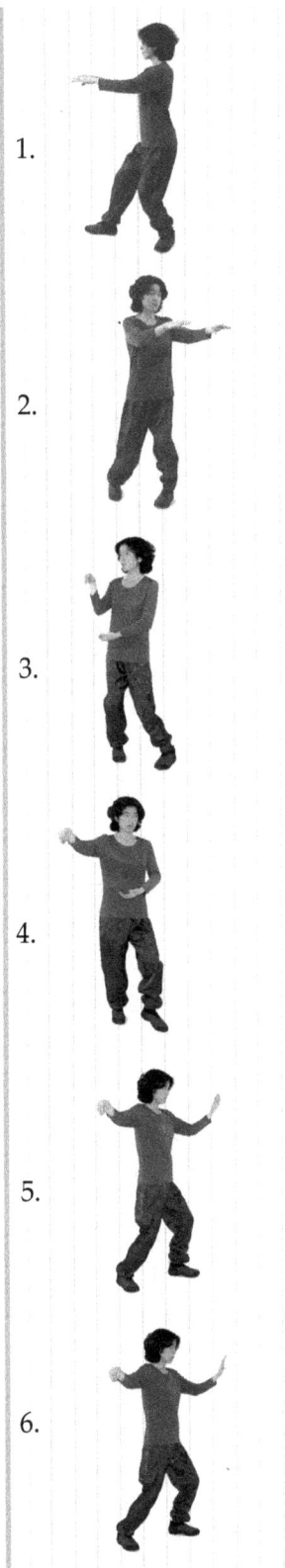

205

141. Single Whip Squatting Down

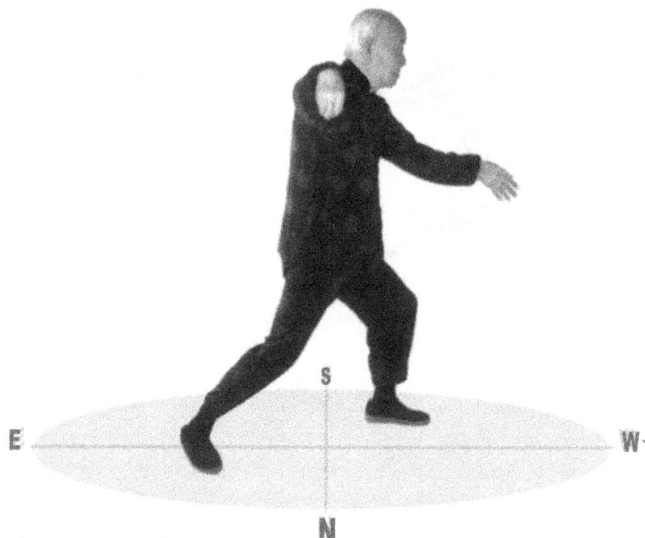

During the counts of:

1. Momentarily shift all of your weight onto your left leg and then turn your right foot, pivoting on the heel, to face northeast. Shift your weight onto the right foot as you turn your torso to face northwest and turn your left foot, pivoting on the heel, to point north. Let your left hand and arm, moving in conjunction with the waist, circle upwards in a clockwise motionto the northeast. The right hand "hook" remains where it is.

2. Turn the torso to face nothwest/west and turn your left foot, pivoting on the heel, so the toes point west. Keeping your back straight and upright as much as possible, continue to circle your left hand down inside of your left thigh to your left knee with the palm facing north and the fingers pointing west.

3. Shift your weight 60% onto your left leg and turn in your right foot, pivoting on the heel, 90 degrees to face northwest.

4. Completing your bow and arrow stance, shift 10% more of your weight into the left foot and let the forward motion of your body initiate a forward motion with the left hand (striking to the imaginary opponent's groin).

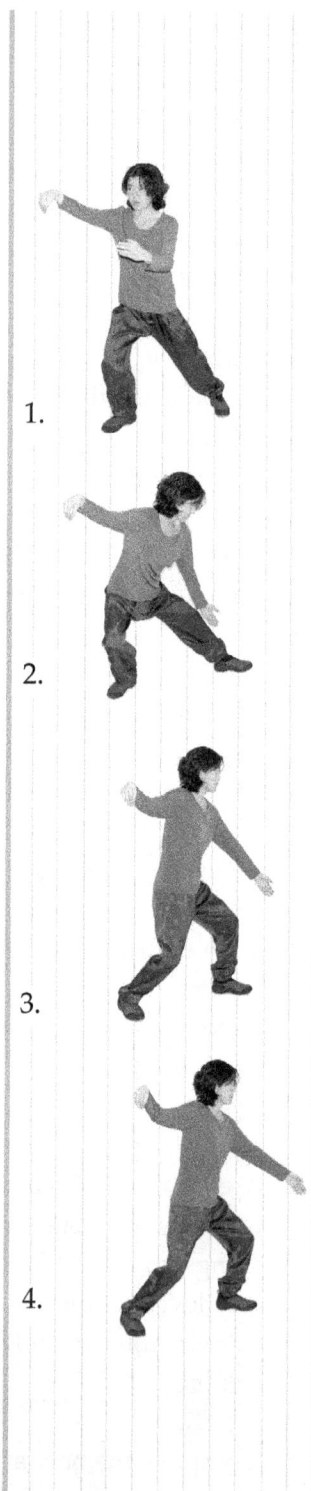

206

142. Step Forward to the Seven Stars

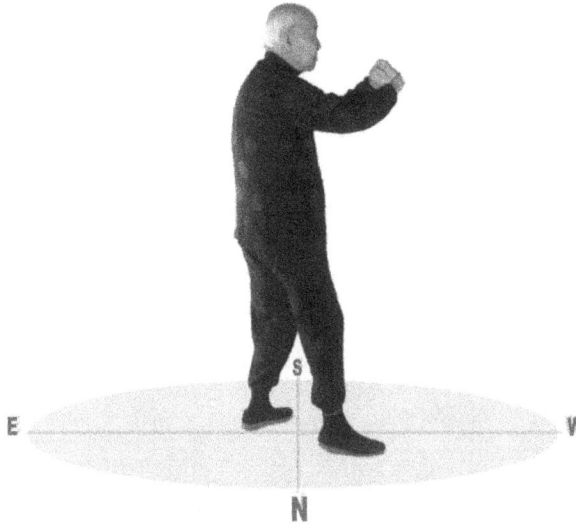

During the counts of:

1. Shift your weight back onto your right foot and turn the left foot, pivoting on the heel, 45 degrees to the left so the toes point southwest. Both hands circle up and out with the palms facing down.

2. Shift all of your weight forward onto your left foot and step forward with your right foot, placing it in front of the left foot (without shifting your weight forward) with the heel up and the toes touching the ground. Simultaneously both hands continue to circle around (out, down and up) until they form two fists joined at the wrists. The left fist is on the inside of the right fist and both "tiger mouths" are facing back to your face. The wrists cross at the same time the right toes touch the ground.

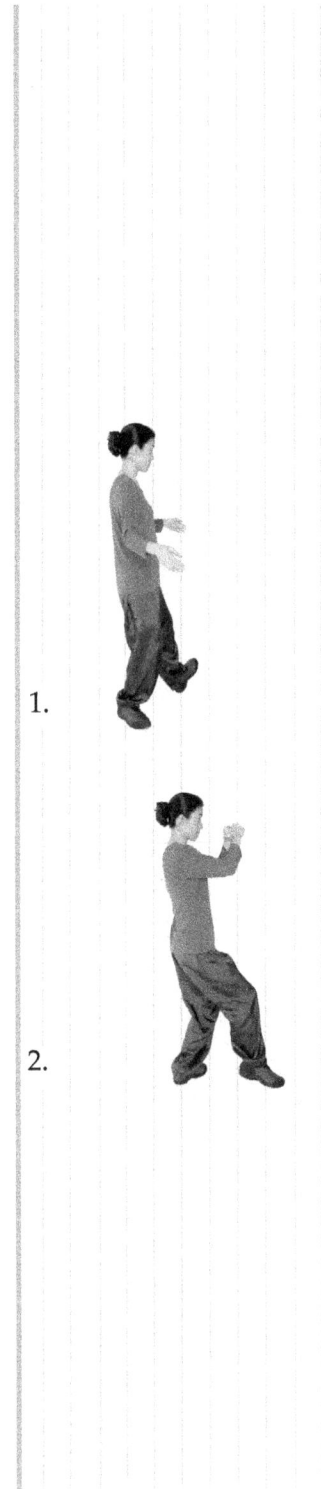

143. Step Back to Ride the Tiger

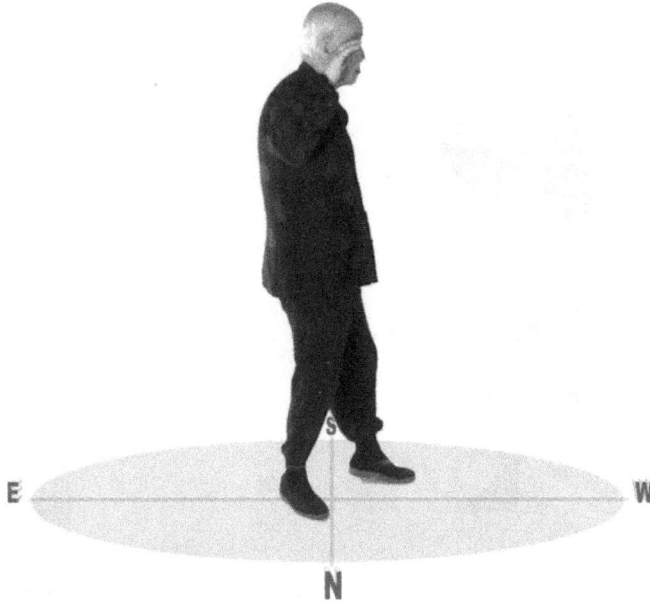

During the counts of:

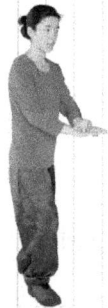

1. Turn your waist to the northwest and simultaneously step back with your right foot to the northeast, placing it down with the toes pointing northwest and then shift your weight onto it. Keep your wrists attached and open your fists as you bring them down to your waist level while turning them so that the right palm faces down and the left palm faces up.

1.

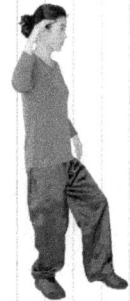

2. Turn your torso to face west. With this motion, simultaneously circle your right hand around to your right ear keeping the fingers up with the palm facing forward (leaving your elbow relaxed and down) and dropping the left hand down into the "position of attention" at the left hip. The left foot steps over to the right in a slight curve and lands in line in front of the right heel with the toes touching the ground, heel up. Your weight remains on your right foot.

2.

144. Turn Round and Sweet with Leg (right foot)

During the counts of:

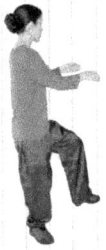

1. Turn your torso to the left facing southwest and raise your left foot slightly off the ground so that it turns with the torso and the toes end up pointing to the southwest as well. At the same time extend both hands at chest level to the southwest with the palms facing each other and the fingers pointing out.

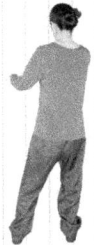

2. Using the windup motion of the first count to the left, spin on the ball of your right foot about 225 degrees to your right (clockwise) to face east/south east. Place your left foot down pointing southwest (do not shift your weight) in front of your right foot. During this spinning motion your palms turn face down with fingers pointing out.

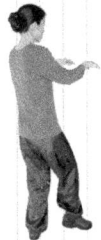

3. Shift your weight onto your left foot and continue to turn your body, with hands still outstretched in front of your chest, clockwise to your right until ...

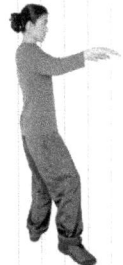

4. ... you are facing west. With your weight entirely on the left foot, pick up your right foot and place it a shoulder's width to your right (to the northwest corner) with the toes on the ground pointing northwest.

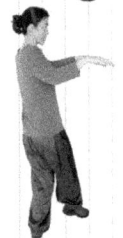

5. Slide your right foot with toes scraping the ground to the left ...

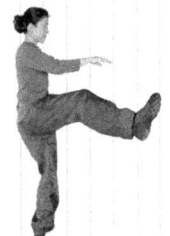

6. ... and then circle the right foot upward in a clockwise motion in front of your waist so that the toes brush the bottoms of your outstretched fingers at the top of the circle. Your right foot continues to circle down to your hip level where it stops with the sole of the foot facing northwest.

145. Bend the Bow and Shoot the Tiger

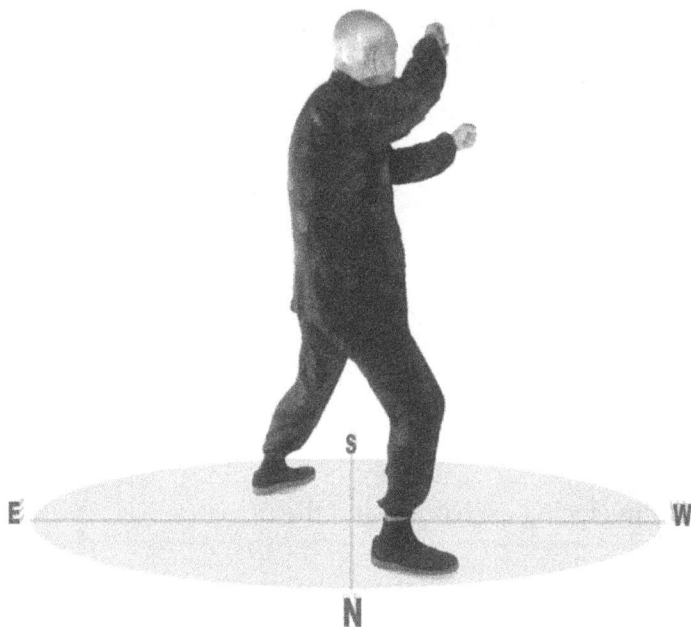

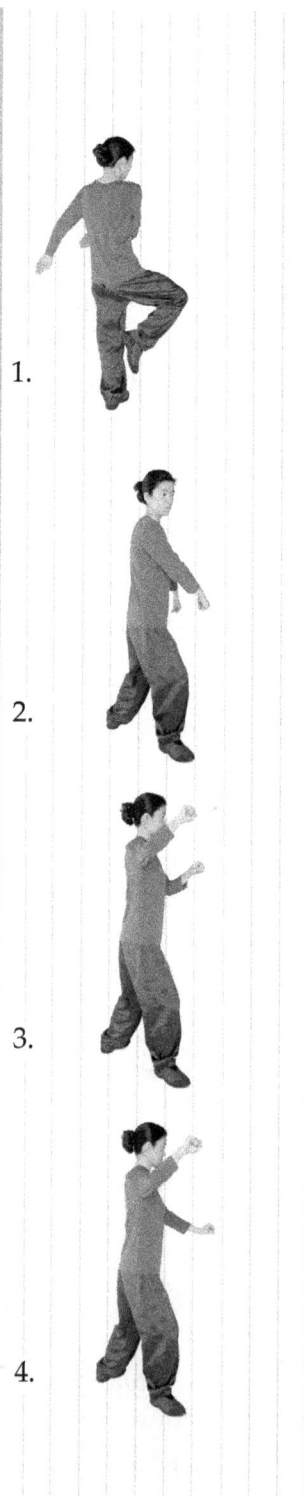

During the counts of:

1. Lower both hands diagonally backwards to the southeast with the palms facing in (northeast). Lower your right leg bending at the knee so that the toes point down.

2. Step diagonally to the northwest with your right foot. Form two fists with your hands.

3. Shift your weight onto your right foot and turn in the left foot, pivoting on the heel, so that the toes point west. Circle your fists around, keeping them aligned together, with the "tiger's mouths" facing each other (as though holding a stick with fists positioned about 18" apart) so that your right fist is near your right ear and your left fist is down in front of your chest.

4. Extend your left fist forward (sliding it down the imaginary stick) to the southwest. Your right hand remains by the ear with the elbow down and bent.

146. Turn Body and Chop

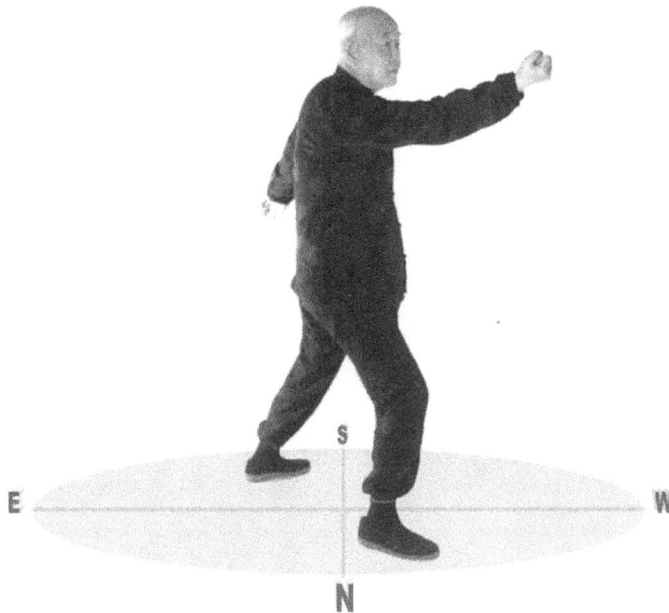

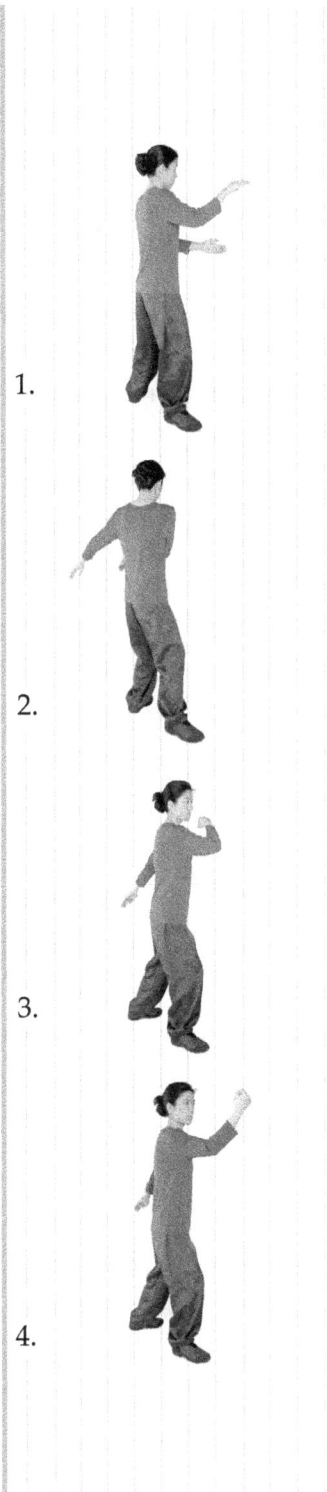

1.

2.

3.

4.

During the counts of:

1.   Pick your left foot up and set it down, heel first, with the toes pointing to the southwest.

2.   Shift your weight to the left foot and lower your hands, with palms facing down, diagonally backwards to the southeast.

3.   Step with your right foot to the northwest and, as you shift your weight to it, turn your torso to the right to face northwest. With the turning of your torso, turn your left foot, pivoting on the heel, so that the toes point west. Make a fist with your right hand
and ...

4.   ... circle it diagonally upward - chopping to the northwest corner. Leave your left hand extended down and backwards, palm down, to the southeast.

147. Step Forward, Deflect Downward, Intercept and Punch

During the counts of:

1. Pick up your left foot and set it down, heel first, with the toes pointing to the southwest.

2. Shift your weight back onto your left foot and turn your torso to the left to face southwest as you reach out in that direction with both hands. Your palms are facing each other as though holding a ball with your right hand positioned above.

3. Turning your waist to the west, raise your right foot and step forward diagonally to the right. At the same time make a fist with your right hand and circle it clockwise around to the right side of your waist and attach it to your right hip, palm side facing up. In unison with this motion your left hand circles clockwise upward and forward in front of your face. Your left elbow remains relaxed and down.

4. Facing west, shift your weight to your right foot (toes pointing to the north/ northwest) and simultaneously bring your left hand forward, deflecting downward to the level of your stomach, palm facing the floor.

5. Step directly forward, maintaining a shoulders' width stance, with your left foot and shift 60% of your weight onto it. At the same time extend or intercept with your left hand forward and to the left. The left hand is open with the fingers pointing west and the palm is facing north. With this motion your right foot turns inwards, pivoting on the heel, so that the toes are pointing northwest.

6. Complete the bow and arrow stance facing west by shifting 10% more of your weight into your left foot. At the same time, using your whole body (not just your arm), punch forward with your right fist ("tiger's mouth" facing up). As your right hand is punching forward let your left hand come over and cover the inner wrist of your right hand.

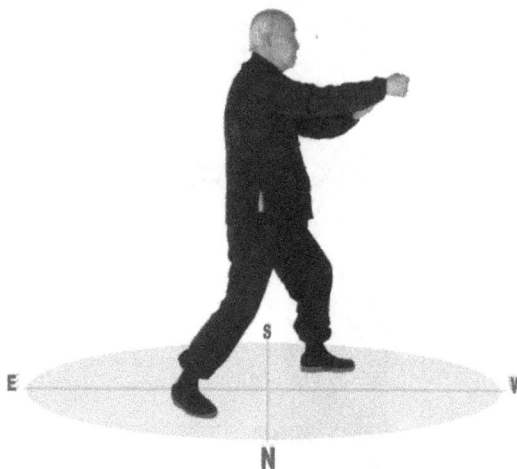

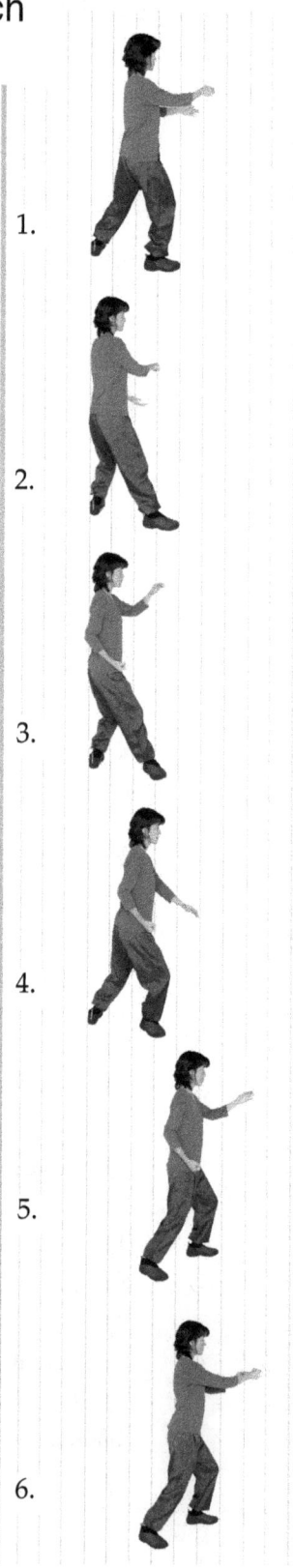

212

148. Withdraw and Push

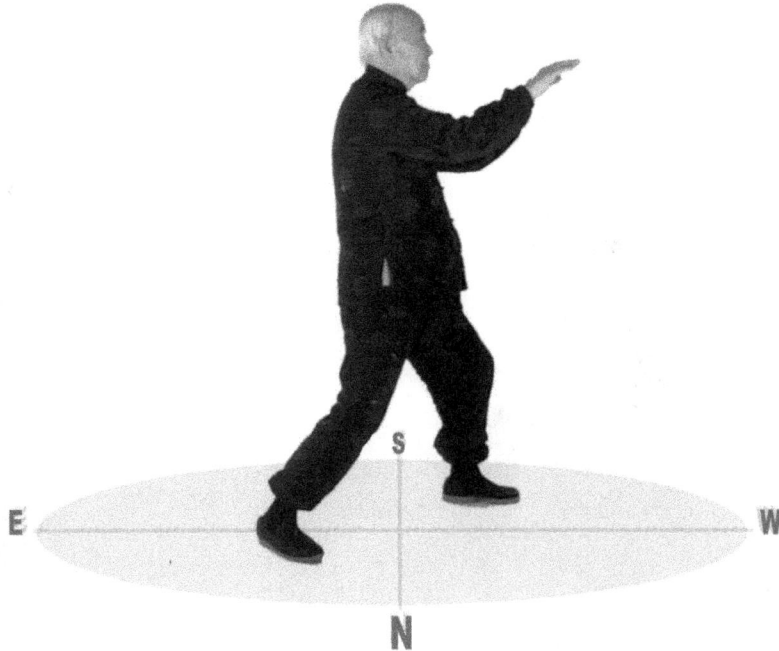

During the counts of:

1. Slide your left hand, palm up, under your right wrist and open the right fist so that both palms are now open and facing upwards with your hands crossed at the wrists.

2. Shift your weight back onto your right foot and draw both hands back with your palms facing your chest. Separate your hands ...

3. ... and then turn both palms outward to face west. Without moving your hands and arms separately from your body, push forward by shifting your weight forward onto your left leg. The push is coming from the forward movement of your body - not your arms.

4. Complete the bow and arrow stance by shifting an additional 10% of your weight into your left foot. At the same time slightly raise your fingertips so that the intention of the push is coming from your palms.

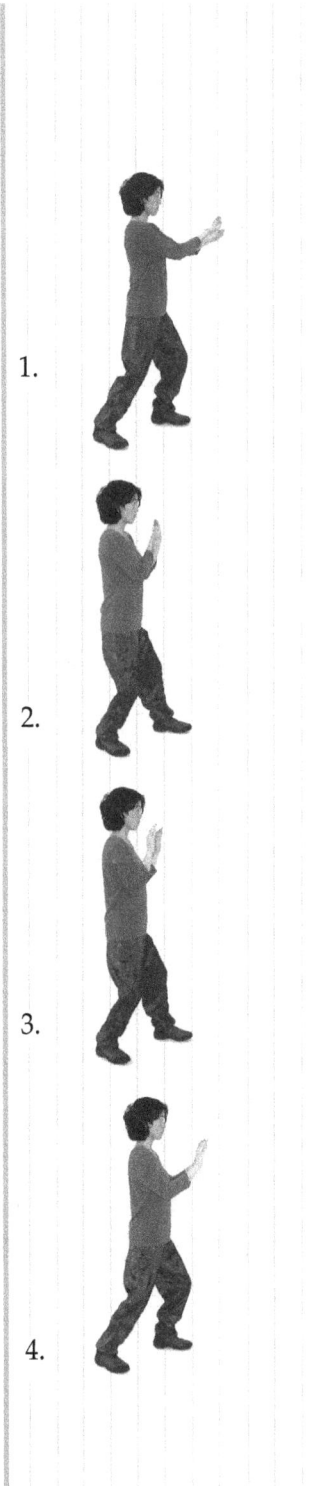

149. Crossing Hands

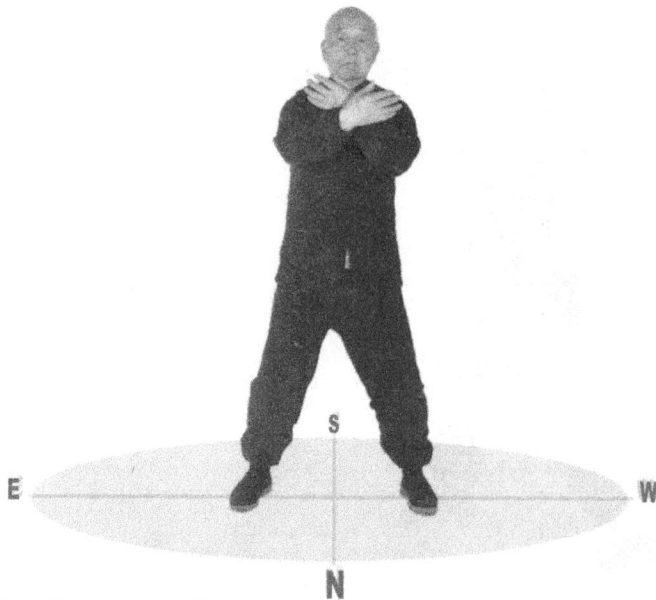

During the counts of:

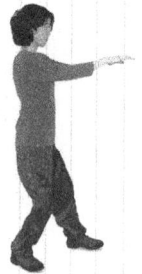

1. Keep your back straight and shift your weight back onto your right leg, and as you do this, let your arms straighten out.

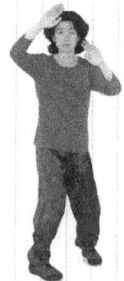

2. Turn your torso to face north and, bending at your elbows, circle your hands in front of your face with both palms facing out to the north. Your right hand is slightly higher than your left.

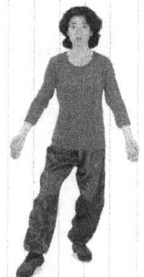

3. Shift your weight back onto your left foot and circle both hands out and down.

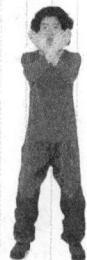

4. Step back with your right foot and place it down a shoulders' width distance from your left foot and parallel to it. At the same time bring your hands (your right hand outside the left) up in front of your face, crossing them at the wrists with both palms facing to the south. Your eyes gaze just over the fingertips. Your weight shifts slightly more than 50% onto your left leg.

150. Conclusion of Tai Chi

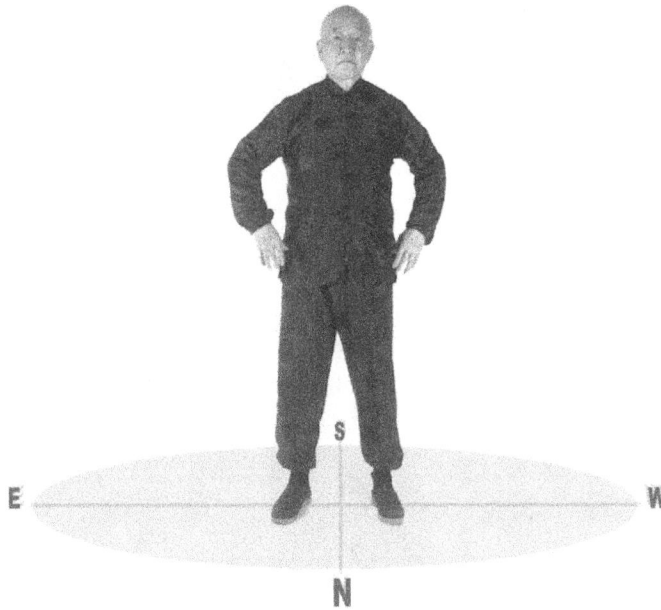

During the counts of:

1.   Shift your weight equally to both feet and ...

2.   ... begin to rise up by straightening your legs and lowering your hands in front of your body.

3.   Bring your hands, palms facing back and fingers pointing down, to beside your thighs.

4.   Bend your elbows and raise both of your hands into the "position of attention."

Hold this posture for extra beats....

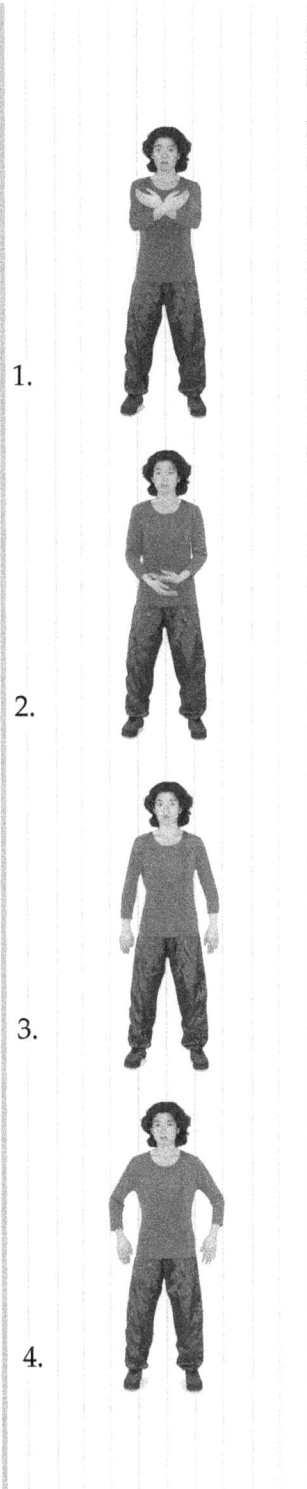

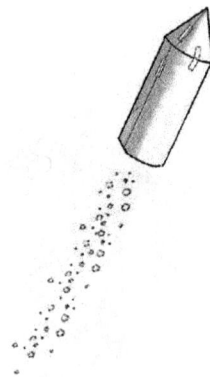

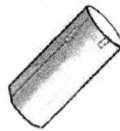

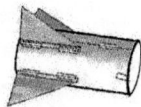

"Tai Chi Ch'uan is an ancient form of calisthenics created by a Taoist priest named Chan San Feng about 700 years ago. Tai Chi means "round form" as pictured in the Yin Yang symbol (Tai Chi Shu) so when you practice you must simulate that form, everything a round shape. You must practice it slowly, effortlessly and continuously, then it will be good for your health. Tai Chi is first for Health, second for Self-defense, third for mental accomplishment and last to become an Immortal."

T.T. Liang

10 Liang's Four Stages of Tai Chi

Liang saw the study of Tai Chi as progressing in four stages or levels. First, one practices it for health, learning how to relax the body and gain a sense of balance; secondly, as a mastery of the physical movements for self-defense; thirdly for what Liang called "mental accomplishment" where the cultivation of a focused attention is stressed. And, lastly, the final stage is what Liang fondly referred to as "becoming an Immortal." By this I understood him to mean that the practitioner was able to achieve a heightened state of awareness: a highly focused, detachment of mind. For each of the above stages Liang used rhythm or beats in correspondingly unique ways to help the student learn and progress.

So far I've mostly focused on how Liang used beats in the first two stages to carefully guide the student through the postures, while at the same time I've been able to introduce some of the more intricate concepts that are integral to understanding Tai Chi. In the more advanced stages of study, Liang describes the beats as being used in an entirely different way.

Stage One - Health: the student will master the use of rhythm and gain an understanding of how to move one's body correctly. The beats are used as a structure within which the student learns the correct timing and positioning of the body. Students will observe themselves in motion and correct any defects of alignment, using the beats as a guide. They will learn how to relax the muscles and move the body as a single unit – meaning they have found the center, or core, of their body (tan tien) and can initiate movements from within it so that there are no extraneous, unconnected gestures of their outer limbs. With a focus on balance, breathing and blood circulation the emphasis is on health.

Stage Two - Self-Defense: When the student has accomplished the first stage, the beats can then be used to learn the practical application of each posture. Practitioners learn to position their bodies correctly with each successive beat and to conclude each posture by issuing a directed force to a single point. Successful execution depends entirely on the student's degree of relaxation, correct movement and weight distribution. Particular attention is paid to matching and following the beat exactly. It is during this stage that two-person exercises are introduced. Performing the functional use of the postures with another student helps to reflect both practitioners' defects. They are advised, while working with a partner, not to try to win or "score a point" but instead to relax and observe their own responses during interactions. This is sometimes referred to as "Quiet minding while investing in loss." This is a "feedback tool" allowing the practitioners to see themselves in active use of the solo form postures. Weapons are introduced at this stage as well. The use of an object in the hand helps the student project force (in a wave-like motion) beyond their hands (through the weapon). Typical Tai Chi weapons are the double-edged sword, spear and saber.

Stage Three - Mental Accomplishment: After a period of study, the once difficult and hard to master postures now become automatic. You no longer have to think about every little complex motor movement and adjustment of the body. You have brought all the movements down to a single common denominator, the turning and positioning

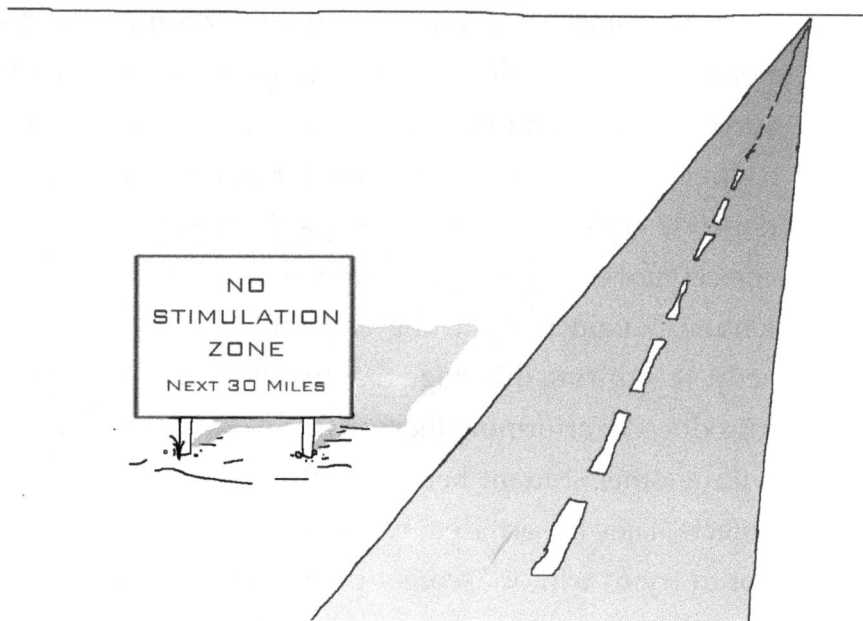

NO
STIMULATION
ZONE
NEXT 30 MILES

of the waist (tan tien). The body, in a sense, can now go on autopilot. Your skill has reached such a level that your mind is now free from having to think about the details of movements, and thus is able to focus on deeper aspects of the Tai Chi exercise. The beats and rhythm formerly used to guide the body, are now used to focus the mind: they become a tool you use to help you forget about the body. The emphasis of the Tai Chi form now becomes primarily an exercise of directing one's consciousness.

The practitioner now focuses his attention entirely on the beats and works to keep all other distractions away; to shut his mind off from everything and attend only to the process of counting the beats. Liang likened this to the Buddhist practice of counting one's breath in order to suspend one's random thoughts – what he liked to call your "monkey thoughts." He described it as follows:

> "More than 1000 years ago a Chinese monk named Chan Chung developed a method of concentration during meditation. He told people to repeat silently, 'What did I look like before I was born?' Later this method was handed down to Japan as Zen Dao, using the question 'what is Mu (nothing)?' for concentration. We often say that a human's heart is like a monkey, jumping in and around all the time, and the mind is like a horse galloping without pause. When one begins to practice meditation, the heart and mind are fully occupied with short-cut thoughts. When one thought is gone, it is immediately replaced by another, giving the heart and mind no chance to rest and concentrate. So, the monk Chan Chung used his way of concentrationto cut out the other short confused thoughts and not let distractions in. The question, 'what did I look like before I was born?' can never be solved, you have to repeat it over and over again for a long time. Gradually your heart and mind will become peaceful, quiet, and only one thing will be left to think of – 'What did I look like before I was born?'"

By focusing on the beats, the practitioner is able to let go of any kind of automatic, rational or sequential thinking; he gives up normal thinking patterns, verbal associations, conceptual ideas and thoughts and uses the beats to help him suspend this "normal" awareness.

Stage Four - By keeping your attention on the rhythm, or using the beats as a means to focus your mind to exclude other thoughts, you will eventually progress to the final stage of Liang's Tai Chi: what he called "becoming an immortal." This he described as an opening up of awareness or a clear state of attentiveness; a state where you will come to forget about the beats entirely. As Liang says: "The application or functioning of Tai Chi will now hinge entirely upon the player's (practitioner's) consciousness."

Liang describes this fourth stage as follows: "After sufficient practice, you will master the 150 postures so thoroughly that you will forget the rhythm, the movement, even yourself - although you are proceeding as usual. At this stage, you are in a trance; your five attributes (form, perception, consciousness, action, and knowledge) are all empty - this is meditation in action and action in meditation. When you finish and come to the end of the postures, suddenly you are back. Where have I been? What have I been doing? I don't know and I don't remember. This is complete relaxation of body and mind lasting 30 minutes. For 30 minutes I really was in another world. It was an ideal world, peaceful and quiet. After that total relaxation of body and mind for these 30 minutes in the ideal world, I return to this one."

"I should say that the principles and theories of Tai Chi are so profound and abstruse and the applications so subtle and ingenious that you must find out the absolutely accurate and correct way to learn and practice. If what you have learned is not quite correct and accurate, the minimal error will keep you handicapped and you will fall behind by ten thousand miles and you will also lose the functional use of Tai Chi and then there is no use talking about mental accomplishment and the way to immortality."

T. T. Liang

11   Conclusion

Tai Chi in the 21st century

I have attempted to explain the function and implementation of Liang's use of rhythm in the practice of Tai Chi Ch'uan, and in conclusion I would like to say something about its use in the West today.

This art was designed and developed for people living 700 years ago – an entirely different time, and in a very different cultural environment: a time when the philosophy behind it grew out of and was part of the culture. The study required dedication not only to the exercise, but to the philosophy behind it as well, which would already be imbued in the society. Thus, it is not applicable or available to 21st century Western students. In those days, as Liang indicated in the quotation at the end of the last chapter, implicit in the study is the enlightened teacher who had experienced "immortality." Such a teacher would, as he states, know how to "suit the teaching to the different dispositions of the students, [because] the slightest divergence will take one far from the path."

Liang liked to say that he developed the use of beats in Tai Chi as a way to make the exercise "more scientific and more aesthetic." He strove to make a then relatively obscure ancient exercise relevant to his contemporary students. Since he started teaching in the United States in the 1960's, Tai Chi has grown in popularity. Now there is keen interest from the sports and medical fields alike as to its health and mental benefits. Athletes are adopting it as a supplement to their workout routines and much research has been conducted looking at the uses of Tai Chi for rehabilitation and prevention regimens for the many health conditions that affect our modern Western lives.

Dr. Herbert Benson, author of The Relaxation Response*, has found that exercises like Tai Chi positively alter the physical and emotional responses to stress. They can decrease one's heart rate, blood pressure, rate of breathing, as well as muscular tension.

The soft and yielding principles behind the martial aspects of Tai Chi establish flexibility and adaptation. They are employed for positive coping strategies in business and personal matters. One divorce lawyer I know uses these principles as a foundation for his clients to "listen" to each other in order to achieve conflict negotiation and resolution.

Rotem Shacham, a Doctoral Fellow from Bar-Ilan University in Israel, specializes in the psychological study of negotiation and personal negotiating skills. He uses the Tai Chi self-awareness techniques of responding to incoming stimuli to enhance training and consulting strategies.

Examples like these highlight the importance for those of us interested in this art to continue to bring Tai Chi into alignment with our own cultural understanding and necessities. As Liang experimented with adding beats to enhance the study of Tai Chi, it is appropriate in the same way for instructors to look for ways to make the benefits of this exercise more approachable to a wider audience. I hope that Tai Chi instructors will avail themselves of the current research being done today so they are better able to serve their students and collaborate more effectively with the conventional medical, business and educational communities.

To this end, I recommend a book titled The Harvard Medical School Guide to Tai Chi by Peter M. Wayne, Ph.D.*, which brings together much of the current research on Tai Chi being done today and offers a clear contemporary perspective on how it might be used and understood. As the author states, he "seeks to show, in a scientifically balanced and objective manner, the clinical promise for Tai Chi and to provide insights into the underlying physiological processes that explain how Tai Chi improves health."

*The Harvard Medical School Guide to Tai Chi, Peter M. Wayne, Ph.D., with Mark L. Fuerst. Harvard Health Publications, Harvard Medical School. Shambala Publications, Inc, 2013.

Personal Experience

For my part, the study of Tai Chi has been a framework for self-observation. Practicing the Tai Chi form has been my personal self-awareness laboratory. It is in the practice of the exercise that I can pay close attentionto and study what is happening in my body as I move. I observe where I am holding tension and how my balance shifts and falls. And most importantly, I feel how my center of gravity rises and sinks as I move and respond to incomeing stimuli (even a thought can throw me off balance!).

Tai Chi has taught me to look for refined aspects of movement. In the process of practicing the Tai Chi forms I have noticed that what I once perceived as simple gestures, in both myself and others, can instead contain complex nuances of movement that lay beneath the obvious. In this light, for me the Tai Chi symbol known to most people as the "Yin-Yang" symbol is not a representation of opposites, as it is commonly understood (hard & soft - black & white) but it instead describes the infinite degrees between them. In other words, if we think of Yin and Yang as black and white, then the study of Tai Chi could be analogous to the awareness of the infinite possible shades of grey between them (at least more than 50…).

Finding a teacher

Liang constantly admonished me to go back to school saying, "you must learn and study your whole life!" And to prove his point, at 78 years of age, he enrolled himself in a class at Harvard

University studying 19th century English literature (Dickens'
Bleak House, Austens' Emma, etc). I always felt that studying
with him was an invitationto join him in his enthusiastic quest
to deepen his knowledge about everything, not just Tai Chi. This
was perhaps, in his mind, because everything was in fact related
to Tai Chi.

Our classes together were always more about the latest things
he was studying, local current news, or even what his wife was
up to. Often we'd go grocery shopping instead. When he did
teach me something about Tai Chi, it was always with a twist.
For example, he asked me one morning to meet him at 6:00am
at a local park. He wanted to show me a weapons form, the Tai
Chi Saber. I showed up and for two hours we worked our way
through a set of 40 postures. At the end of our lesson a number of
other students started showing up and by 8:00 A.M. there were
about 15 people standing around. I asked Liang what was up,
and he explained that they were here to learn the saber form that
he had just showed me. He then picked up his things and said to
me, "you teach them, I'm going home."

There are many people now teaching Tai Chi that I'm sure are
a lot more qualified than I was with my poor fellow saber students. But one thing I learned is that the exercise of teaching is
often much more instructive for the teacher than it is for students.
If someone is putting himself or herself in the position of an instructor, he/she will hopefully be learning as much, if not more
from the experience.

The difficulty with finding a Tai Chi teacher is that there is no
standard training or licensing to be "certified." Interested per-

spective students will need to look for outside recommendations and find someone who will work with them while taking into account their health and physical fitness.

Anyone can "hang a shingle" and set himself or herself up as a Tai Chi teacher, claiming some kind of lineage or "spiritual" credentials. Some will go so far as to adopt an Eastern name, claiming a relationship of special distinction with a past teacher(s), knowledge of the inheritance of secret teachings, and so on. When Tai Chi is taught with this approach, it distorts what could be a valuable, specialized educational pursuit and turns it into a cult. This kind of approach has absolutely nothing to do with what T.T. Liang was interested in.

As Liang always said to me: "the best way to practice Tai Chi is to treat it as a hobby."

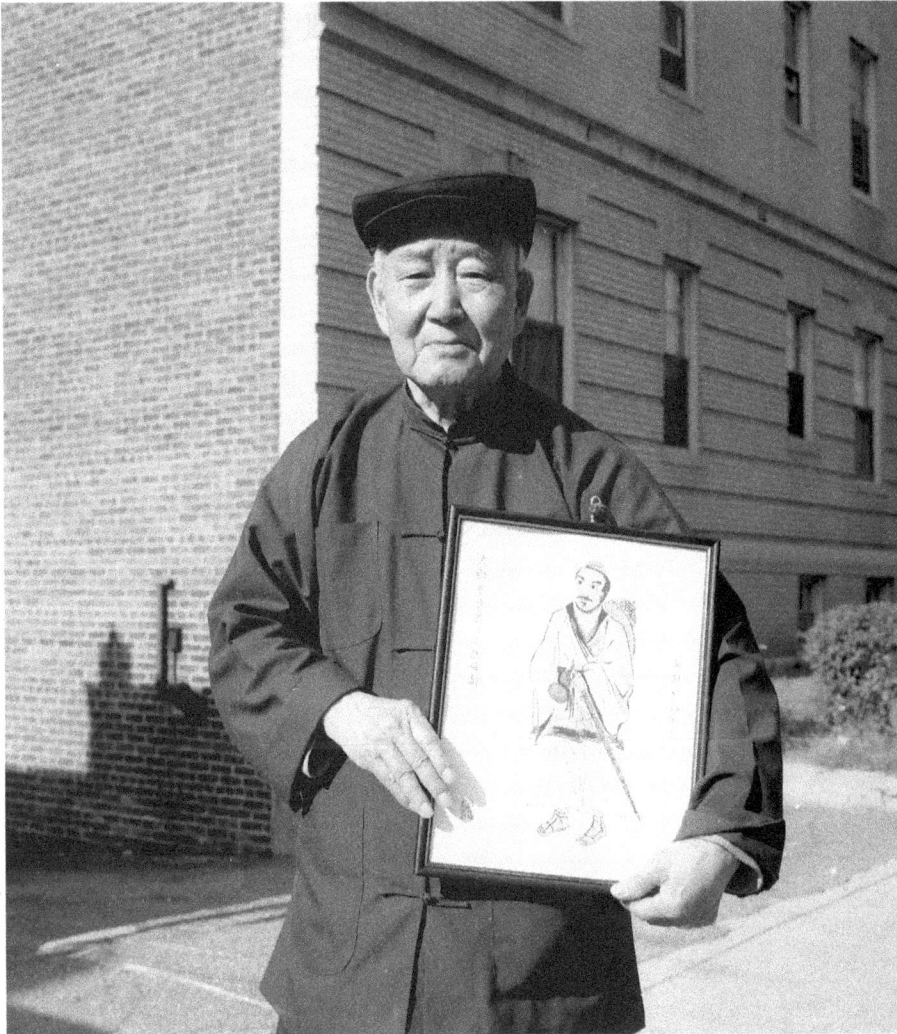

T.T. Liang with his painting of Chang San Feng, 1980

Appendix

Tai Chi Ch'uan
Posture Reference Guide

Name	Body Direction Upon Completion	Rhythm
1. Preparation	N.	2
2. Beginning	N.	6
3. Ward Off Left	N.	6
4. Ward Off Right	E	4
5. Roll Back	NE	4
6. Press	E	4
7. Push	E.	4
8. Single Whip	W	6
9. Lifting Hands	N	2
10. Shoulder Stroke	N	2
11. White Crane Spreading Wings	W	2
12. Step Forward and Brush Knee (left)	W	4
13. Playing the Guitar	W	2
14. Step Forward and Brush Knee (left)	W	4
15. Step Forward and Brush Knee (right)	W	4

16. Step Forward and Brush Knee (left)	W	4
17. Playing the Guitar	W	2
18. Step Forward and Brush Knee (left)	W	4
19. Chop With Fist	NW	2
20. Step Forward, Deflect Downward, Intercept and Punch	W	6
21. Withdraw and Push	W	4
22. Crossing Hands	N	4
23. Embrace the Tiger to Return to the Mountain	SE	4
24. Roll Back	E	4
25. Press	SE	4
26. Push	SE	4
27. Slanting Single Whip	NW	6
28. Punch Under the Elbow	W	6
29. Step Back to Repulse the Monkey (right)	W	4
30. Step Back to Repulse the Monkey (left)	W	4
31. Step Back to Repulse the Monkey (right)	W	4
32. Step Back to Repulse the Monkey (left)	W	4
33. Step Back to Repulse the Monkey (right)	W	4
34. Diagonal Flying Posture	NE	4
35. Lifting Hands	N	2
36. Shoulder Stroke	N	2
37. White Crane Spreading Wings	W	2
38. Step Forward and Brush Knee (left)	W	4
39. Needle at Sea Bottom	W	4
40. Fan Penetrates the Back	W	4
41. Turn Round and Chop	E	4
42. Step Forward, Deflect Downward, Intercept and Punch	E	6
43. Step Forward and Ward Off (right)	E	4
44. Roll Back	NE	4
45. Press	E	4

46. Push	E	4
47. Single Whip	W	6
48. Waving Hands in the Clouds (left)	W	4
49. Waving Hands in the Clouds (right)	E	4
50. Waving Hands in the Clouds (left)	W	4
51. Waving Hands in the Clouds (right)	E	4
52. Waving Hands in the Clouds (left)	W	4
53. Single Whip	W	4
54. High Pat on Horse	W	4
55. Separating Right Foot	NW	6
56. Separating Left Foot	SW	6
57. Turn Round and Kick with Sole (left foot)	E	4
58. Step Forward and Brush Knee (left)	E	4
59. Step Forward and Brush Knee (right)	E	4
60. Step Forward and Punch Downward	E	4
61. Turn Back and Chop With Fist	W	4
62. Step Forward, Deflect Downward, Intercept and Punch	W	6
63. Kick Upward with Right Foot	NW	4
64. Strike Tiger (left style)	SW	4
65. Strike Tiger (right style)	NW	4
66. Kick Upward with Right Foot	NW	4
67. Strike with Both Fists	NW	4
68. Kick Upward with Left Foot	SW	4
69. Turn Round and Kick with Sole (right foot)	W	6
70. Chop with Fist	NW	2
71. Step Forward, Deflect Downward, Intercept and Punch	W	6
72. Withdraw and Push	W	4
73. Crossing Hands	N	4
74. Embrace the Tiger to Return to the Mountain	SE	4
75. Roll Back	E	4

76. Press	SE	4
77. Push	SE	4
78. Horizontal Single Whip	N	6
79. Parting Wild Horse's Mane, Right	SE	4
80. Parting Wild Horse's Mane, Left	NE	4
81. Parting Wild Horse's Mane, Right	SE	4
82. Ward Off Left	N	4
83. Ward Off Right	E	4
84. Roll Back	NE	4
85. Press	E	4
86. Push	E	4
87. Single Whip	W	6
88. Fair Lady Weaving at Shuttle (1)	NE	6
89. Fair Lady Weaving at Shuttle (2)	NW	6
90. Fair Lady Weaving at Shuttle (3)	SW	6
91. Fair Lady Weaving at Shuttle (4)	SE	6
92. Ward Off Left	N	4
93. Ward Off Right	E	4
94. Roll Back	NE	4
95. Press	E	4
96. Push	E	4
97. Single Whip	W	6
98. Waving Hands in the Clouds (left)	W	4
99. Waving Hands in the Clouds (right)	E	4
100. Waving Hands in the Clouds (left)	W	4
101. Waving Hands in the Clouds (right)	E	4
102. Waving Hands in the Clouds (left)	W	4
103. Single Whip	W	4
104. Single Whip Squatting Down	W	4

105. Golden Rooster Standing on One Leg (right)	W	4
106. Golden Rooster Standing on One Leg (left)	W	4
107. Step Back to Repulse the Monkey (right)	W	4
108. Step Back to Repulse the Monkey (left)	W	4
109. Step Back to Repulse the Monkey (right)	W	4
110. Step Back to Repulse the Monkey (left)	W	4
111.Step Back to Repulse the Monkey (right)	W	4
112. Diagonal Flying Posture	NE	4
113. Lifting Hands	N	2
114. Shoulder-Stroke	N	2
115. White Crane Spreading Wings	W	2
116. Brush Left Knee	W	4
117. Needle at Sea Bottom	W	4
118. Fan Penetrates Back	W	4
119. Turn Round and White Snake Puts Out Tongue	E	4
120. Step Forward, Deflect Downward, Intercept and Punch	E	6
121. Step Forward and Ward Off Right	E	4
122. Roll Back	NE	4
123. Press	E	4
124. Push	E.	4
125. Single Whip	W.	6
126. Waving Hands in the Clouds (left)	W	4
127. Waving Hands in the Clouds (right)	E	4
128. Waving Hands in the Clouds (left)	W	4
129. Waving Hands in the Clouds (right)	E	4
130. Waving Hands in the Clouds (left)	W	4
131. Single Whip	W	4
132. High Pat on Horse	W	4
133. Thrusting Hand	W	4

The Tai Chi Dance Association
PO Box 2762
Berkeley, CA 94702
Phone (415) 902-4350
www.TaiChiSF.com   Email: jr@taichisf.com

www.ingramcontent.com/pod-product-compliance
Lightning Source LLC
Chambersburg PA
CBHW080327270326
41927CB00014B/3128